NCA Review for the
Clinical Laboratory Sciences

NCA Review for the Clinical Laboratory Sciences

Third Edition

Edited by
Susan J. Beck, PhD, CLS (NCA)
Associate Professor
Division of Laboratory Sciences
University of North Carolina at Chapel Hill School of Medicine
Chapel Hill, North Carolina

Associate Editors
Kathryn Doig, PhD, CLS (NCA)
Year One Curriculum Director
Michigan State University College of Human Medicine
East Lansing, Michigan

Susan J. Leclair, MC, CLS (NCA)
Professor
Department of Medical Laboratory Science
University of Massachusetts Dartmouth
North Dartmouth, Massachusetts

Sharon M. Miller, PhC, CLS (NCA)
Professor and Associate Dean
School of Allied Health Professions
Northern Illinois University College of Health and
Human Sciences
DeKalb, Illinois

Bernadette F. Rodak, MS, CLSpH (NCA)
Assistant Professor
Indiana University School of Allied Health Sciences
Education Coordinator—Hematology
Department of Pathology and Laboratory Medicine
Indiana University Medical Center
Indianapolis

Linda L. Seefried, MA, CLS, CLSup (NCA)
Education Coordinator
Clinical Laboratory Science Program
Duke University Medical Center
Durham, North Carolina

Michelle S. Wright, PhD, CLS (NCA)
Associate Professor
Department of Clinical Laboratory Science
University of Louisville School of Medicine
Louisville, Kentucky

Joyce A. Zook, CLS (M) (NCA)
Laboratory Manager
Oregon State Hospital
Salem, Oregon

Little, Brown and Company
Boston   New York   Toronto   London

Library of Congress Cataloging-in-Publication Data

NCA review for the clinical laboratory sciences.—3rd. ed. / edited
   by Susan J. Beck ; associate editors, Kathryn Doig ... [et al.]
        p.   cm.
     Includes bibliographical references.
     ISBN 0-316-59942-5
     1. Diagnosis, Laboratory—Examinations, questions, etc.   I. Beck,
Susan.   II. Doig, Kathryn.   III. National Certification Agency for
Medical Laboratory Personnel (U.S.)
     [DNLM: 1. Technology, Medical—examination questions.
2. Diagnosis, Laboratory—examination questions.   3. Certification—
examination questions.   QY 18.2 N337 1996]
   RB38.25.N34   1996
   616.07′5′076—dc20
   DNLM/DLC
   for Library of Congress   96-16315
                                                             CIP

Printed in the United States of America
SEM

Editorial: Suzanne Jeans
Production Services: Colophon
Production Supervisor/Designer: Mike Burggren
Cover Designer: Mike Burggren

Contents

Preface

The *NCA Review for the Clinical Laboratory Sciences* was developed to assist candidates preparing for the Clinical Laboratory Scientist (CLS) and Clinical Laboratory Technician (CLT) certification and recertification examinations. This, the third edition of the book, reflects changes in the NCA examinations resulting from a national job analysis. This job analysis prompted the development of new *content outlines* for both the CLS and CLT examinations. Because all the items on the NCA examinations are directly related to a specific task on a content outline, these content outlines provide the best guide for determining the range of materials that could be included on an NCA certification examination. The introduction to this book includes the CLT- and CLS-content outlines and an explanation of the taxonomic levels of items used in the examinations.

As in the previous editions of this book, the review sections consist of sample items, the correct answers, and explanations of each item. The sample tests at the end of the book have been expanded to represent the length and composition of the CLT and CLS examinations. We recommend that candidates complete the review sections before taking the sample tests. Mastery of the items provided in the review sections or in the sample tests in this book does not ensure that a candidate will pass a certification examination. Careful review of performance on the items presented in this book should, however, help a candidate identify areas of weakness that may be strengthened through additional study and review. The references at the end of each review section may serve as a guide for further study.

The NCA provides high-quality, clinically relevant peer-review certification examinations for laboratory personnel. This book and the NCA certification examinations are the result of the efforts of clinical laboratory practitioners who are committed to certification *by the profession and for the profession.* The authors hope that this book will help candidates prepare for NCA examinations and attain the distinguished credentials of Clinical Laboratory Technician or Clinical Laboratory Scientist.

S.J.B.

Acknowledgments

The National Certification Agency for Medical Laboratory Personnel gratefully acknowledges the efforts of all the people who have contributed to each edition of *NCA Review for the Clinical Laboratory Sciences*. We are particularly indebted to James L. Bender, editor of the first edition, and Sharon L. Zablotney, editor of the second edition of this book. The current edition is the result of the hard work of the associate editors and the many clinical laboratory scientists who contributed questions and explanations for each section. The dedication and expertise of these outstanding clinical laboratory professionals exemplifies the best in the profession and serves as the foundation for the NCA peer-review certification process.

Contributing Authors

Shauna C. Anderson, PhD, CLS (NCA)
Professor, Department of Microbiology, Brigham Young University, Provo, Utah

Susan J. Beck, PhD, CLS (NCA)
Associate Professor, Division of Clinical Laboratory Sciences, University of North Carolina at Chapel Hill School of Medicine, Chapel Hill, North Carolina

Nancy A. Brunzel, BA, CLS (NCA)
Laboratory Manager, Division of Medical Technology, Department of Laboratory Medicine and Pathology, University of Minnesota Medical School—Minneapolis, Minneapolis

Suzanne H. Butch, MA, CLDir (NCA)
Chief Technologist, Blood Bank and Transfusion Service, Department of Pathology, The University of Michigan Hospitals, Ann Arbor, Michigan

Susan Cockayne, PhD, CLS (NCA)
Assistant Professor, Department of Microbiology, Brigham Young University, Provo, Utah

Suzanne W. Conner, MA, CLS, CLDir (NCA)
Program Director and Safety Manager, Medical Technology Program, Children's Hospital Medical Center, Akron, Ohio

Kathryn Doig, PhD, CLS (NCA)
Year One Curriculum Director, Michigan State University College of Human Medicine, East Lansing, Michigan

Rebecca Janine Fithen, CLS (NCA)
Mingo Junction, Ohio

Margaret J. H. Fuller, MS, MPA, CLS (NCA)
Outpatient Laboratory Supervisor, Methodist Hospital Plainview, Plainview, Texas

Jean D. Holter, EdD, CLS (NCA)
Professor and Program Director, Medical Technology Program, West Virginia University School of Medicine, Morgantown, West Virginia

M. Kathleen Huck, MS, CLS (NCA)
Assistant Director, Laboratory Department, St. Francis Hospital and Health Centers, Beech Grove, Indiana

William B. Hunt, CLS (NCA), CLS p(H)
William Pepper Laboratory, University of Pennsylvania Medical Center, Philadelphia

Judy C. Jones, BS, CLDir (NCA)
Supervisor, SmithKline Beecham Clinical Lab, New Port Richey, Florida

Marcia A. Kilsby, MS, CLS (NCA)
Chair, Allied Health Department, Andrews University, Berrien Springs, Michigan

Rosemary Kuhn, CLSup (NCA)
Administrative Supervisor, Endocrine Testing, Ltd., Melrose Park, Pennsylvania

Hal S. Larsen, PhD, CLS (NCA)
Professor and Chair, Department of Clinical Laboratory Science, Texas Tech University Health Sciences Center, School of Medicine, Lubbock, Texas

Susan J. Leclair, MS, CLS (NCA)
Professor, Department of Medical Laboratory Science, University of Massachusetts Dartmouth, North Dartmouth, Massachusetts

Mary Ann McLane, PhD, CLS (NCA)
Postdoctoral Fellow, Department of Basic Sciences, Thrombosis Research Center, Temple University School of Medicine, Philadelphia, Pennsylvania

Sharon M. Miller, PhC, CLS (NCA)
Professor and Associate Dean, School of Allied Health Professions, Northern Illinois University College of Health and Human Sciences, DeKalb, Illinois

Frances A. Morgenstern, MS, SM, CLS (NCA)
Associate Professor Emeritus, Department of Medical Technology, State University of New York Health Science Center at Syracuse, College of Health Related Professions, Syracuse, New York

Donna L. Oblack, PhD, CLDir (NCA)
Technical Director, Laboratory Corporation of America, Herndon, Virginia

Joan E. Polancic, MS, EdD, CLS (NCA)
Associate Professor, Department of Clinical Laboratory Science, University of Illinois at Springfield, Springfield, Illinois

Joan A. Radtke, MS, MT (ASCP) SC, CLS (NCA)
Assistant Research Professor, Division of Medical Laboratory Sciences, University of Illinois at Chicago, School of Biomedical and Health Information Sciences, Chicago, Illinois

Bernadette F. Rodak, MS, CLSpH (NCA)
Assistant Professor, Indiana University School of Allied Health Sciences; Education Coordinator—Hematology, Department of Pathology and Laboratory Medicine, Indiana University Medical Center, Indianapolis

John P. Seabolt, EdS, CLS (NCA)
Senior Clinical Technologist, Clinical Microbiology Laboratories, University of Kentucky College of Medicine, A.B. Chandler Medical Center, Lexington, Kentucky

Linda L. Seefried, MA, CLS, CLSup (NCA)
Education Coordinator, Clinical Laboratory Science Program, Duke University Medical Center, Durham, North Carolina

Catherine Sheehan, MS, SI, CLS (NCA)
Professor, Department of Medical Laboratory Science, University of Massachusetts Dartmouth, North Dartmouth, Massachusetts

Barbara Snyderman, BS, CLSup (NCA)
Technical Consultant, Clinical Laboratory Services, Lindenwold, New Jersey

Betty Lynn Theriot, MHS, SBB, CLS (NCA)
President, Creative Educators, Pass Christian, Mississippi

Linda M. Ubelacker, BS, SC, CLSup (NCA)
Technical Supervisor, Laboratory Department, Endocrine Testing, Ltd., Melrose Park, Pennsylvania

Kathy V. Waller, PhD, CLS (NCA)
Assistant Professor, Department of Medical Technology, Ohio State University College of Medicine, Columbus, Ohio

Michelle S. Wright, PhD, CLS (NCA)
Associate Professor, Department of Clinical Laboratory Science, University of Louisville School of Medicine, Louisville, Kentucky

Patricia Etnyre-Zacher, EdD
Assistant Professor, School of Allied Health Professions, Northern Illinois University College of Health and Human Sciences, DeKalb, Illinois

Joyce A. Zook, CLS (M) (NCA)
Laboratory Manager, Oregon State Hospital, Salem, Oregon

Introduction

The NCA certification examinations for clinical laboratory technicians (CLTs) and clinical laboratory scientists (CLSs) are designed to assess candidates' ability to function with competence in a clinical laboratory as entry-level practitioners. The NCA offers generalist examinations for CLTs and CLSs and categorical examinations at the CLS level. This review book is designed to help candidates prepare for the CLT- or CLS-level examinations by (1) explaining the examination content, format, and scoring method; (2) reviewing some test-taking strategies; and (3) providing practice items and explanations. A careful review of the material in this book should help candidates identify areas of weakness that can be strengthened through additional study.

Examination Content

The NCA examinations are designed to be job-related. A national job analysis was conducted to ensure that the items on the NCA examinations are related to current practice. The CLT- and CLS-content outlines were derived from this national job analysis, and they specify the tasks that are expected of CLT and CLS practitioners at the entry level. All items on the NCA examinations are directly related to tasks in the content outlines.

The NCA-content outlines that follow list the number of examination items in each section of the exam and the cognitive level of those items. The CLT- and CLS-content outlines differ in some of the job tasks included and in the cognitive level of the items in each section of the examinations.

The three cognitive levels on the examination are recall, application, and analysis. *Recall* (R) refers to the ability to remember previously learned material. This may involve remembering a wide range of material from specific facts to complete theories. *Application* (AP) involves translating or applying information to new situations. This could involve transforming data, explaining information, or calculating results. *Analysis* (AN) involves breaking down material into its component parts so that its organizational structure may be understood. Items at this level involve evaluation and problem-solving skills and usually require judgments or choices regarding the appropriate course of action to resolve issues or problems.

Clinical Laboratory Technician Content Outline

	R	AP	AN
1. CHEMISTRY/URINALYSIS	**13**	**26**	**9**
A. Chemistry	11	19	8

1. CHEMISTRY/URINALYSIS

A. Chemistry

   1. Determine specimen suitability considering patient preparation; type of specimen; collection, handling, and storage of specimen; presence of interfering substances

   2. Preparation for a test run, including sample and reagent preparation; use of standards and controls; instrument calibration, performance, and maintenance checks; malfunction identification and trouble-shooting

   3. Perform analytical procedures recognizing method and instrument limitations; prepare and read manual or computer calculations; prepare and read data from a calibration curve

   4. Intepretation and reporting of results, including identification of analyte reference values; recognition of normal/abnormal results; identify values that are significantly different (e.g., risk values, panic values, analytical errors) and action required; correlate laboratory results with patient information

B. Urinalysis   2   7   1

   1. Preparation for testing, including instrument set-up, calibration, and maintenance; evaluation of reagent/dipstick acceptability; specimen collection, handling, and storage; quality control procedures

   2. Performance of macroscopic examination of urine including physical and chemical tests, identification of normal/abnormal values, corrections for abnormal constituents or temperature, definition of method limitation(s)

   3. Performance of microscopic examination of urine including selection of appropriate microscopy; preparation of reagents and controls; identification and enumeration of casts and other formed elements (e.g., cells, bacteria, crystals, artifacts)

   4. Performance of confirmatory test(s) and quantitative 24-hour test(s), including specimen collection and preparation of reagents and controls, determination of analyte concentration by calculation or reading of charts and graphs, identification of interfering substances or analytic interference, determination of method limitation(s)

   5. Interpretation and reporting of results including identification of questionable or contradictory results, correlation of laboratory data with normal/abnormal physiologic conditions or situations, identification of values that are significantly different (e.g., risk values, panic values) and action required

2. HEMATOLOGY   **15**   **23**   **0**

A. Hematology   10   14   0

   1. Determine specimen acceptability by evaluating type and age of specimen, additive, ratio of blood to additive, proper mixing, and proper labeling

   2. Prepare specimen for analysis by mixing specimen or checking for clots

   3. Prepare acceptable peripheral blood films (as described by NCCLS) considering size/width, thickness, feather edge (straight and free of streaks), homogeneity, and labeling

   4. Properly stain blood films with Romanowsky's stain

   5. Perform manual cell counts for leukocytes, platelets, and eosinophils

   6. Perform a microhematocrit

	R	**AP**	**AN**

7. Perform manual hemoglobin determinations

8. Calculate erythrocyte indices (MCV, MCH, MCHC)

9. Perform erythrocyte sedimentation rates (Wintrobe, Westergren, or their modifications) by making the appropriate blood dilution, if necessary, filling the ESR tube, and accurately reading the results

10. Perform reticulocyte counts

11. Perform manual peripheral blood differentials

12. Perform screening solubility tests

13. Perform physical and quantitative analysis of body fluids and process bone marrow aspirates or biopsies

14. Instrumentation

B. Hemostasis   5   9   0

1. Determine specimen acceptability by considering collection techniques, transport conditions, time, temperature, what, if any, additives are present, blood-to-anticoagulant ratio, as well as patient hematocrit

2. Prepare specimen for analysis by checking for clots or hemolysis; centrifuging, if necessary; and maintaining specimen acceptability relative to time, temperature, and pH

3. Perform routine procedures

4. Perform quality control on procedures; recognize out-of-range values

5. Correlate results of various hemostasis determinations and recognize discrepant results, interfering substances, or other sources of error

6. Take appropriate action when quality control specimens are out of range, results do not correlate, or a known source of error is recognized

7. Set up, calibrate, maintain, and shut down instruments used in hemostasis testing

8. Operate instruments used in hemostasis testing

3. IMMUNOHEMATOLOGY   15   23   0

A. Donors and donor blood   2   3   0

1. Select suitable donors

2. Collect single unit of blood from donor

3. Process donor blood

4. Harvest components from single donor units

5. Package and ship products

B. Basic techniques in blood-group serology   11   18   0

1. Prepare saline suspensions of red blood cells to specified concentrations (e.g., 2%, 4%)

2. Read and grade tube agglutination tests

3. Use a cell washer for antiglobulin testing

4. Wash cells manually for antiglobulin testing

5. Perform antiglobulin test procedure including use and interpretation of Coombs' control (check) cells

6. Balance and use a serologic centrifuge

7. Determine suitability of specimens for any given test including analysis of relevant factors

8. Perform elution techniques

9. Perform absorption/adsorption

10. Peform antibody titration and interpret results

11. Perform microtiter testing; read agglutination

	R	AP	AN

12. Perform antigen typings

13. Perform antibody screening and identification

14. Perform routine pretransfusion testing

15. Perform and interpret direct antiglobulin testing including use of polyspecific and monospecific reagents

16. Perform routine testing for administration of Rh immune globulin

17. Investigate suspected transfusion reactions

18. Investigate hemolytic disease of the newborn

C. Issue blood and blood products	2	2	0

1. Maintain adequate supply of blood and blood products

2. Issue blood and blood products

3. Receive unused or returned blood components

4. MICROBIOLOGY	**15**	**23**	**0**
A. Bacteriology	10	15	0

1. Basic principles of diagnostic bacteriology

2. Laboratory examinations of specimens for bacteriology

B. Mycology	2	2	0

1. General mycology

2. Laboratory examination of specimens for fungi

3. Clinically important fungal agents and infectious diseases

4. Quality control

C. Parasitology	2	3	0

1. Process, collect, handle, preserve specimens; examine macroscopically

2. Calibration of ocular micrometer

3. Direct microscopic examination

4. Concentration methods, permanent staining techniques

5. Preparation, staining, and examination of thick and thin smears, and concentration procedures for blood parasites

6. Detection and identification of parasites

D. Virology	1	2	0

1. Selection, collection, and transport of specimens

E. Infection control	0	1	0

1. Surveillance—confirmation of nosocomial cases and epidemics

2. Surveillance—handling and disposal of biohazardous wastes

5. IMMUNOLOGY	**4**	**16**	**0**
A. Serology	3	13	0

1. Perform radial immunodiffusion

2. Perform electrophoretic procedures

3. Perform flocculation tests (e.g., VDRL, RPR)

4. Perform agglutination assays (e.g., latex, red cell, bacterial)

5. Perform immunofluorescence assays [e.g., ANA, FTA-ABS]

6. Perform ligand assays

7. Perform neutralization assays (e.g., ASO, Anti-DNAse B)

B. Miscellaneous serologic assays	1	3	0

1. Perform differential absorption test for infectious mononucleosis (i.e., heterophil antibody)

2. Perform titrations (e.g., ASO, cold agglutinin, etc.)

	R	AP	AN
6. LABORATORY PRACTICE	5	10	3
A. Safety	1	2	1

6. LABORATORY PRACTICE
   A. Safety
      1. Establish and conform to guidelines for safety
      2. Enforce established guidelines for safety

   B. Management 1 2 0
      1. Comply with laws, regulations, and guidelines: federal, state, and local (e.g., HHS, CDC, OSHA, EEOC, CLIA, OPA)
      2. Voluntary accrediting and inspection agency requirements (e.g., CAP, JCAHO)
      3. Supervise laboratory personnel and operations
      4. Communicate/coordinate laboratory services to physician, institution, suppliers, and client
      5. Perform quality assessment activities

   C. Information management 0 1 0
      1. Record and retrieve laboratory data from work produced on site and from reference laboratories

   D. Reagent preparation 1 1 0
      1. Prepare and label reagents
      2. Store stock and working reagents properly

   E. Instrumentation and equipment 1 2 1
      1. Operate and perform preventive maintenance
      2. Calibrate and monitor instruments

   F. Specimen collection and handling 1 2 1
      1. Identify specimen collection procedures for venous blood, arterial blood, capillary blood, blood cultures, throat cultures, and other cultures
      2. Instruct patients and healthcare providers on the proper procedure for collection of semen, urine, feces, and other body fluids
      3. Evaluate acceptability of specimens
      4. Processing and preanalytic preparation of specimens (e.g., centrifuge, separate, label)
      5. Store specimens appropriately (e.g., time, temperature, light, packaging, and off-site transport)
      6. Follow chain-of-custody procedures

Clinical Laboratory Scientist Content Outline

	R	AP	AN
1. CHEMISTRY/URINALYSIS	9	16	23
A. Chemistry	8	13	17

1. CHEMISTRY/URINALYSIS
   A. Chemistry
      1. Determine specimen suitability considering patient preparation; type of specimen; collection, handling, and storage of specimen; presence of interfering substances
      2. Preparation for a test run, including sample and reagent preparation; use of standards and controls; instrument calibration, performance, and maintenance checks; malfunction identification and troubleshooting
      3. Perform analytical procedures recognizing method and instrument limitations; prepare and read manual or computer calculations; prepare and read data from a calibration curve

	R	AP	AN

4. Interpret and report results, including identification of analyte reference values; recognize normal/abnormal results; identify values that are significantly different (e.g., risk values, panic values, analytical errors) and action required; correlate laboratory results with patient information

5. Quality assurance, including performance of method selection and evaluation studies; calculation and evaluation of method-comparison data (e.g., linear regression analysis, F test, paired t-test)

B. Urinalysis   1   3   6

1. Preparation for testing including instrument set up, calibration, and maintenance; evaluation of reagent/dipstick acceptability; specimen collection, handling, and storage; quality control procedures

2. Performance of macroscopic examination of urine, including physical and chemical tests, identification of normal/abnormal values, corrections for abnormal constituents or temperature, definition of method limitation(s)

3. Performance of microscopic examination of urine, including selection of appropriate microscopy, preparation of reagents and controls, identification and enumeration of casts and other formed elements (e.g., cells, bacteria, crystals, artifacts)

4. Performance of confirmatory test(s) and quantitative 24-hour test(s), including specimen collection and preparation of reagents and controls, determination of analyte concentration by calculation or reading of charts and graphs, identification of interfering substances or analytical interference, determination of method limitation(s)

5. Interpretation and reporting of results including identification of questionable or contradictory results, correlation of laboratory data with normal/abnormal physiologic conditions, identification of values that are significantly different (e.g., risk values, panic values) and action required

2. HEMATOLOGY   8   21   9

A. Hematology   5   13   6

1. Determine specimen acceptability by evaluating type and age of specimen, additive, ratio of blood to additive, proper mixing, and proper labeling

2. Prepare specimen for analysis by mixing specimen or checking for clots

3. Prepare acceptable peripheral blood films (as described by NCCLS) considering size/width, thickness, feather edge (straight and free of streaks), homogeneity, and labeling

4. Properly stain blood films with Romanowsky's stain

5. Perform manual cell counts for leukocytes, platelets, and eosinophils

6. Perform a microhematocrit

7. Perform manual hemoglobin determinations

8. Calculate erythrocyte indices (MCV, MCH, MCHC)

9. Perform erythrocyte sedimentation rates (Wintrobe, Westergren, or their modifications) by making the appropriate blood dilution, if necessary; filling the ESR tube; and accurately reading the results

10. Perform reticulocyte counts

11. Perform manual peripheral blood differentials

12. Perform screening solubility tests

13. Perform tests related to hemolytic anemias

14. Perform cytochemical procedures

	R	AP	AN

15. Perform physical and quantitative analysis of body fluids
16. Process bone marrow aspirates and biopsies
17. Examine bone marrow preparations
18. Instrumentation

B. Hemostasis   3   8   3

1. Determine specimen acceptability by considering collection techniques, transport conditions, time, temperature, what (if any) additives are present, blood-to-anticoagulant ratio, as well as patient hematocrit
2. Prepare specimen for analysis by checking for clots or hemolysis; centrifuging (if necessary); and maintaining specimen acceptability relative to time, temperature, and pH
3. Perform routine procedures
4. Perform specialized hemostasis procedures
5. Perform quality control on procedures; recognize out-of-range values
6. Correlate results of various hemostasis determinations and recognize discrepant results, interfering substances, or other sources of error
7. Take appropriate action when quality-control specimens are out of range, when results do not correlate, or when a known source of error is recognized
8. When requested, determine what additional testing should be performed when unexpected abnormalities are detected
9. Set up, calibrate, maintain, and shut down instruments used in hemostasis testing
10. Operate instruments used in hemostasis testing
11. Perform platelet aggregation tests using platelet aggregometers

3. IMMUNOHEMATOLOGY   6   18   14

A. Donors and donor blood   2   3   0

1. Select suitable donors
2. Collect single unit of blood from donor
3. Collect products by hemapheresis
4. Process donor blood
5. Harvest components from single donor units
6. Package and ship products

B. Basic techniques in blood group serology   3   13   13

1. Prepare saline suspensions of red blood cells to specified concentrations (e.g., 2%, 4%)
2. Read and grade tube agglutination tests
3. Use a cell washer for antiglobulin testing
4. Wash cells manually for antiglobulin testing
5. Perform antiglobulin test procedures, including use and interpretation of Coombs' control (check) cells
6. Balance and use a serologic centrifuge
7. Determine suitability of specimens for any given test, including analysis of relevant factors
8. Perform elution
9. Perform absorption/adsorption
10. Perform neutralization techniques according to protocols
11. Perform antibody titration and interpret results
12. Perform microtiter testing
13. Perform antigen typings
14. Perform antibody screening and identification

	R	AP	AN
15. Perform routine pretransfusion testing			
16. Perform and interpret direct antiglobulin testing, including use of polyspecific and monospecific reagents			
17. Perform routine testing for administration of Rh immune globulin			
18. Investigate suspected transfusion reactions			
19. Investigate hemolytic disease of the newborn			
C. Issue blood and blood products	1	2	1
1. Maintain adequate supply of blood and blood products			
2. Issue blood and blood products			
3. Receive unused or returned blood components			
4. MICROBIOLOGY	**8**	**23**	**7**
A. Bacteriology	5	15	5
1. Basic principles of diagnostic bacteriology			
2. Laboratory examinations of specimens for bacteriology			
B. Mycology	1	2	1
1. General mycology			
2. Laboratory examination of specimens for fungi			
3. Procedures and techniques in diagnostic mycology			
4. Clinically important fungal agents and infectious diseases			
5. Quality control			
C. Parasitology	1	3	1
1. Process, collect, handle preservation of specimens, and examine macroscopically			
2. Calibration of ocular micrometer			
3. Direct microscopic examination			
4. Concentration methods, permanent staining techniques			
5. Preparation, staining, and examination of thick and thin smears, and concentration procedures for blood parasites			
6. Detection and identification of parasites			
D. Virology	1	2	0
1. Selection, collection, and transport of specimens			
2. Processing—inoculation and maintenance of cultures			
3. Recognition of viral growth, identification and interpretation of results			
E. Infection Control	0	1	0
1. Surveillance—confirmation of nosocomial cases and epidemics			
2. Surveillance—handling and disposal of biohazardous wastes			
5. IMMUNOLOGY	**2**	**18**	**0**
A. Serology	1	15	0
1. Perform radical immunodiffusion			
2. Perform electrophoretic procedures			
3. Perform flocculation tests (e.g., VDRL, RPR)			
4. Perform agglutination assays (e.g., latex, red cell, bacterial)			
5. Perform immunofluorescence assays (e.g., ANA, FTA-ABS)			
6. Perform ligand assays			
7. Perform neutralization assays (e.g., ASO, Anti-DNAse B)			
B. Miscellaneous serologic assays	0	3	0
1. Perform differential absorption test (i.e., heterophil antibody) for infectious mononucleosis			
2. Perform titrations (e.g., ASO, cold agglutinin)			

	R	**AP**	**AN**
C. Cellular assays	1	0	0
1. Enumerate and differentiate subsets of immunocompetent cells			
6. LABORATORY PRACTICE	**2**	**7**	**9**
A. Safety	0	1	2
1. Establish and conform to guidelines for safety			
2. Enforce established guidelines for safety			
B. Management	1	2	0

    1. Comply with laws, regulations, and guidelines: federal, state, and local (e.g., HHS, CDC, OSHA, EEOC, CLIA, OPA)

    2. Voluntary accrediting and inspection agency requirements (e.g., CAP, JCAHO)

    3. Supervise laboratory personnel and operations

    4. Communicate/coordinate laboratory services to physician, institution, suppliers, and client

    5. Evaluate equipment

    6. Perform quality assessment activities

    7. Develop and maintain procedure manuals

C. Information management	0	1	0

    1. Record and retrieve laboratory data from work produced on site and from reference laboratories

D. Education	1	1	0

    1. Provide clinical instruction to staff, students, and others

    2. Assist with development of continuing education program

E. Reagent preparation	0	1	2

    1. Prepare and label reagents

    2. Store stock and working reagents properly

F. Instrumentation and equipment	0	0	3

    1. Operate and perform preventive maintenance

    2. Calibrate and monitor instruments

G. Specimen collection and handling	0	1	2

    1. Identify specimen-collection procedures for venous blood, arterial blood, capillary blood, blood cultures, throat cultures, and other cultures

    2. Instruct patients and healthcare providers on the proper procedure for collection of semen, urine, feces, and other body fluids

    3. Evaluate acceptability of specimens

    4. Processing and preanalytic preparation of specimens (e.g., centrifuge, separate, label)

    5. Store specimens appropriately (e.g., time, temperature, light, packaging, and off-site transport)

    6. Follow chain-of-custody procedures

Examination Format

The NCA examinations are comprehensive, job-related, objective, written tests. The test items are in a multiple choice format similar to the examples in this book. The "stem" of the item will contain a statement or a question; after the stem, four alternative answers will be presented. The one best answer should be chosen.

The distribution of items for the CLT and CLS generalist examinations are as follows.

Content area	No. of questions
Chemistry	38
Urinanalysis	10
Hematology	24
Hemostasis	14
Immunohematology	38
Immunology	20
Microbiology	38
Laboratory practice	18
Total	200

Categorical examinations are offered at the CLS level in Chemistry, Hematology, Immunohematology, and Microbiology. The distribution of items for the categorical examinations is as follows.

Specialty	Questions in specialty	Laboratory practice questions	Total
Chemistry/urinalysis	48	18	66
Hematology	38	18	56
Immunohematology	38	18	56
Microbiology	38	18	56

Scoring the Examination

In determining the passing score for the NCA examination, the NCA seeks to reflect the minimum skill level required for competent job performance. The passing score separates the individuals who are minimally competent to practice from the individuals who are not competent to practice. This method of scoring is very different from the norm-referenced scoring used in many educational programs. The criterion-referenced NCA examinations do not compare candidates with one another but with a predetermined score that reflects minimal competence. To determine the passing score, the NCA conducts a cut-score study. Raters who are experts in the field are asked to evaluate the questions on the examinations and to determine the percentage of minimally competent candidates who would be likely to answer each question correctly. The estimates of eight to ten raters are averaged for each question. The minimum passing score on an examination is determined by averaging the probabilities for all the items on the examination.

Each item contributes equally to the final test score. The candidate is not required to answer a specific number of items correctly in each section to pass the examination. For example, if 120 correct answers were required to pass a 200 item CLT examination, the candidate could correctly answer any combination of items on that test provided that at least 120 of them were answered correctly. Only correct answers contribute to the total score; points are not subtracted for incorrect answers or unanswered items.

Scaled Scores

The raw-cut score (passing score) will vary somewhat from one examination administration to the next because the items on each examination will vary slightly in difficulty. To ensure that test scores are comparable, the NCA converts raw scores to scaled scores using a linear equation with the raw-cut score set at a scaled score of 75. It is possible that a raw score of 120 on two examinations could result in two different scaled scores. For example, a score of 120 on examination A might result in a scaled score of 75, while a scaled score of 120 on examination B, a slightly less difficult examination, might result in a scaled score of 74.

Tips for the Day of the Examination

Arrive on Time

Give yourself plenty of time to find the test center, park your car, and check in with the test supervisors. Arriving with time to spare will help you feel more relaxed and less rushed when you begin the examination. Anyone who arrives after the testing begins will not be admitted.

Items to Bring with You

- Your admission ticket and an official form of identification such as a driver's license.
- Several sharpened No. 2 pencils. Pencils and erasers will not be furnished at the examination, and ball point pens, colored pencils or felt tip pens will not be permitted.
- A watch. The test center supervisor will keep the official time, but you may wish to use your watch to pace yourself on the test.
- A silent, hand-held, solar or batter-operated calculator without paper-tape printing or alphabetic memory may be used during the examination.

Review the Test Instructions

Listen to the instructions given by the supervisor and read all directions in the test booklet. Take a minute to look over the entire examination. This will serve as an overview of what to expect as well as a check for missing pages in the examination booklet.

Test Taking Strategies

Study!

There is no substitute for knowing the subject material. Review and study all the resources from your educational program. The notes and charts that you prepared as a student or that you make as you study are particularly helpful because they reflect your learning style and organization schemes. After you have studied a section, use this book to test your knowledge and understanding of the material. Remember that items in this book are only samples of the subject matter. Your review must be comprehensive.

Study the content outline. This provides an important guide to the content of the examinations and the amount of coverage given to each area. Make a special effort to review areas on the content outline that are unfamiliar to you.

Organize Your Time

If you are taking the generalist examination, you will have 4 hours to complete it. Periodically note the time as you work through the examination so that you give yourself sufficient time for each part. Use the practice tests in this book to estimate the time it will take you to complete a 200-point exam.

Stay Calm

Do not let frustration over any one item or section influence your performance on the rest of the examination. If you have a question about an item, write your comments on the form provided. Your comments will be reviewed by the NCA before the test is scored. Do not panic if you are stumped by an item. It is possible that items will be difficult for you or will contain unfamiliar or unknown information. Everyone misses some questions on a national certification exam. If you stay calm, you will be more confident as you continue to work through the exam. Remember that all items are equally weighted, so it is in your best interest to proceed to an easier question if you are having difficulty.

Be Careful Not to Skip Answers on the Answer Sheet

Mark each answer on the correct line of the answer sheet. You do not want to finish the test and find that you have been off one line for an undetermined amount of time. As you work through the test, record each answer on the answer sheet and double-check that your answer sheet and test questions match. Avoid leaving items unanswered to prevent incorrect marking on your answer sheet. Some people prefer to fill in the answer sheet at the end of the examination. If you choose to complete the answer sheet in one step at the end of the test, it is essential that you leave sufficient time to do a careful job. If you are rushed when completing the answer sheet, you risk making errors.

Changing Your Answers

In general, it is better not to change an answer, because your first impression is usually best. However, if you find that you misread a question the first time or if you recall some information after working through the examination, you may improve your score by changing the answer to an item.

Multiple-Choice Questions

Most candidates have answered thousands of multiple choice questions by the time they take the NCA exam and are comfortable with this format. Many candidates like multiple-choice questions because the correct answer is provided and they always have a 25% chance of guessing the right answer.

Other candidates have difficulty with multiple choice questions, however, because they read too much into the question or because they read too quickly and miss a key word or number. The multiple choice items used on the NCA examinations have been carefully written and reviewed. In answering the questions, remember that they are straightforward and are not intended to "trick" the candidate but to assess the candidate's knowledge in a particular area.

Performance on multiple-choice items cam be improved by following a few guidelines.

- Read the stem carefully. After reading the stem, think of the correct answer before you look at the alternatives. Some people cover the alternatives while reading the stem to force themselves to come up with the answer. After deciding on the right answer, read the alternatives. If you are correct, your answer should be one of the choices.
- In some cases, you may not be sure of the right answer immediately after reading the stem. In this case, read each alternative. Cross out any alternatives that are obviously incorrect. Select the best answer from the plausible alternatives. If you have no idea what the correct answer is, make a guess and go on to the next question. Remember that you have a 25% chance of guessing correctly and that there is no penalty for guessing incorrectly.
- Do not spend too much time on any one question. If you are having difficulty with an item, make a guess and proceed to the next item. The more items you answer, the better your chances of achieving a passing score.

Summary

Study the material that you have been given in your educational program. Use the content outline as a study guide and this book to test your performance. Review all the material in the candidate handbook regarding test administration so that there will be no surprises on the day of the exam. Stay calm and pace yourself as you work through the examination.

NCA Review for the Clinical Laboratory Sciences

Clinical Chemistry

1

Section Editor   **Sharon M. Miller**

CLT Review Questions

Contributors

Shauna C. Anderson
Nancy A. Brunzel
Susan Cockayne
Joan E. Polancic
Joan A. Radtke
Patricia Etnyre-Zacher

1. In an adult, a blood glucose level of 35 mg/dL is

A. dangerously high
B. dangerously low
C. normal
D. physiologically impossible

The answer is B. True hypoglycemia of this magnitude can cause neurologic symptoms and may result in irreversible damage. A very low serum glucose value also may be an artifact caused by cellular metabolism or bacterial contamination if serum is not separated from cells promptly. (Kaplan and Pesce, p. 602; Bishop et al., p. 307)

2. The hexokinase reaction for serum glucose

A. reduces cupric ions to cuprous ions
B. measures the amount of hydrogen peroxide produced
C. uses a glucose-6-phosphate dehydrogenase (G-6-PD)–catalyzed indicator reaction
D. produces a green condensation product with *o*-toluidine

The answer is C. Hexokinase catalyzes the phosphorylation of several monosaccharides using ATP as the phosphate donor and producing the corresponding sugar-6-phosphate. The G-6-PD–catalyzed indicator reaction uses only glucose-6-phosphate as substrate. The high specificity of this latter reaction prevents interference from other monosaccharides. (Bishop et al., pp. 308–309)

3. Which of the glucose tolerances shown in the figure on p. 2 meet NDDG (National Diabetes Data Group) criteria for the diagnosis of diabetes mellitus?

A. Curves 1 and 2
B. Curves 1 and 4
C. Curves 3 and 4
D. Only curve 4

The answer is C. NDDG criteria for the diagnosis of diabetes mellitus include either (1) fasting serum glucose level greater than 140 mg/dL on more than one occasion, or (2) two or more serum samples with glucose levels greater than 200 mg/dL following a meal. Curve 3 meets the latter criterion and curve 4 meets both criteria. (Bishop et al., p. 311)

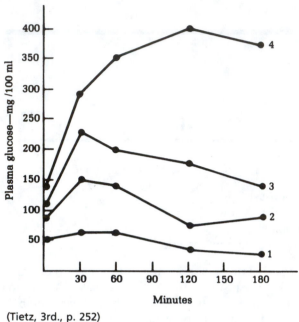

(Tietz, 3rd., p. 252)

4. A lipemic serum will have a turbid appearance due to an elevated level of

A. cholesterol
B. HDL
C. phospholipid
D. triglycerides

The answer is D. Lipemia is due to the presence of large fat-containing micelles. Both chylomicrons and VLDL particles have large enough diameters to scatter light, giving the specimen a turbid appearance. Both particles contain a high proportion of triglycerides. (Kaplan and Pesce, p. 811; Bishop et al., pp. 358–359)

5. An enzymatic method for measuring cholesterol in serum uses the reduced form of a dye and all of these reagents *except*

A. cholesterol esterase
B. cholesterol oxidase
C. NADH
D. peroxidase

The answer is C. The enzymatic method for measuring total cholesterol incubates serum with cholesterol esterase (to release free cholesterol), cholesterol oxidase (to oxidize cholesterol and produce hydrogen peroxide), and a reduced dye which is oxidized to a chromogen by hydrogen peroxide and peroxidase. (Kaplan and Pesce, p. 975; Bishop et al., p. 360)

6. pH 8.6 is used for serum protein electrophoresis so that

    A. all serum proteins will have a net negative charge
    B. all serum proteins will have a net positive charge
    C. electroendosmosis is avoided
    D. heat production is minimized

The answer is A. Proteins are ampholytes whose terminal amino and carboxyl groups, as well as ionizable side groups on component amino acids, change their charges with change in pH. At a pH higher than the pK of these ionizable groups, dissociable hydrogen ions are lost to the medium resulting in no charge on each amino group and a negative charge on each carboxyl group. The net charge on the protein therefore becomes negative. The amount of heat produced and the buffer migration (electroendosmosis) which occur are determined in large part by the concentration of the buffer. (Kaplan and Pesce, pp. 145, 1055; Bishop et al., pp. 192–193)

7. Biuret reagent reacts with

    A. ammonia released from proteins
    B. free amino groups in proteins
    C. peptide bonds in proteins
    D. tyrosine residues in proteins

The answer is C. In alkaline solution, cuprous ions in biuret reagent form coordinate bonds with the carbonyl groups of peptide bonds resulting in a colored complex. (Kaplan and Pesce, p. 1058; Bishop et al., p. 189)

8. Which one of these protein bands, when separated from serum by electrophoresis on cellulose acetate, contains only one protein?

    A. Albumin
    B. Alpha₁-globulin
    C. Alpha₂-globulin
    D. Beta-globulin

The answer is A. The large peak of albumin seen on a serum electropherogram is virtually pure albumin. Since electrophoresis on cellulose acetate separates proteins according to their net charges, the other peaks seen are mixtures of the proteins which share approximately the same net charge. (Kaplan and Pesce, pp. 1054–1056; Bishop et al., pp. 193–194)

9. Which serum isoenzyme result may be falsely increased if a hemolyzed sample is analyzed?

    A. CK-MB (CK-2)
    B. CK-MM (CK-3)
    C. LD isoenzyme 1 (HHHH)
    D. LD isoenzyme 2 (MMMM)

The answer is C. Erythrocytes are rich in LD isoenzyme 1. Hemolysis, whether artifactual or in vivo, can cause LD isoenzyme 1 to be increased and the LD-isoenzyme-1–to–LD-isoenzyme-2 ratio to exceed 1.0. The data then may be indistinguishable from those obtained following myocardial infarction. Erythrocytes do not contain a discernible amount of LD isoenzyme 5. RBCs contain virtually no CK. However, since adenylate kinase in the cells may interfere with electrophoretic methods, it is undesirable to use hemolyzed specimens in serum isoenzyme assays. (Kaplan and Pesce, pp. 924–929; Bishop et al., pp. 228–229)

10. Which enzyme catalyzes this reaction?

L-alanine + alpha ketoglutarate → glutamate + pyruvate

A. Alkaline phosphatase (ALP)
B. Alanine aminotransferase (ALT)
C. Aspartate aminotransferase (AST)
D. Gamma-glutamyl transpeptidase (GGT)

The answer is B. The rules for trivial enzyme names state that the first name of an enzyme indicates its substrate and the second name indicates the type of reaction catalyzed. Thus, in this case, alanine is the principal substrate and transamination between alanine and the general substrate ketoglutarate is the reaction catalyzed by ALT. (Kaplan and Pesce, p. 895)

11. Which of these serum samples is satisfactory for acid phosphatase measurement?

A. Acidified to pH 5
B. Heated to 56°C for 30 min
C. Hemolyzed
D. Refrigerated for 18 h

The answer is A. Acid phosphatase in serum is very unstable. At a pH below 5.4 or when frozen, the enzyme activity is stabilized. Erythrocytes contain large amounts of acid phosphatase and make a hemolyzed sample unsatisfactory for the analysis. (Kaplan and Pesce, p. 891; Bishop et al., p. 234)

12. Turbidimetric assays for serum lipase measure the

A. amount of bile acid produced
B. amount of titratable acid produced
C. rate of degradation of triglycerides
D. rate of production of NADH

The answer is C. Lipase acts at the surface of nonwater-soluble triglyceride micelles, hydrolyzing terminal fatty acids from glycerol. As the micelles become smaller they scatter less light and the substrate suspension becomes less turbid. The rate of clearing of turbidity reflects the amount of lipase activity. (Kaplan and Pesce, p. 931; Bishop et al., p. 237)

13. Serum is evaluated for urea to

A. assess renal function
B. diagnose diabetes
C. monitor treatment for coronary artery disease
D. diagnose rheumatoid arthritis

The answer is A. Urea is the major excretory product of protein metabolism. It is synthesized in the liver, transported in the plasma to the kidney, and readily filtered by the glomeruli. Most of the urea in the glomerular filtrate is excreted in the urine. (Bishop et al., pp. 436–437)

14. Increased serum uric acid is found in all *except*

A. gout
B. hypothyroidism
C. Lesch-Nyhan syndrome
D. renal failure

The answer is B. Thyroid hormones have no specific effect on formation of uric acid. Gout is the disease caused by deposition of excessive uric acid in body spaces, e.g., joints. Lesch-Nyhan syndrome is a rare inborn error of metabolism in which the salvage enzyme of purine catabolism is deficient. This results in excessive production of the purine catabolite uric acid. Renal failure results in inability to clear the blood of waste products including uric acid. (Bishop et al., p. 442)

15. Ionized calcium should be measured using a sample which is

A. anticoagulated with EDTA
B. deproteinized
C. protected from oxidation
D. the same pH as the patient's blood

The answer is D. Calcium is present in blood in three forms: free ions, protein-bound, and combined with anions such as bicarbonate, citrate, and lactate. Only the free ionized form is physiologically active. The dissociation of calcium from its complexed forms depends on pH. This is particularly true of protein-bound calcium, since hydrogen ions and calcium ions, both being cations, compete for binding sites on protein. A change in the pH of the blood sample would alter the amount of calcium bound to protein and therefore alter the amount of free ionized calcium measured. If this occurs, the concentration of free ionized calcium measured in the specimen will not coincide with the actual in vivo level of the analyte. (Kaplan and Pesce, p. 867; Bishop et al., p. 285)

16. Identify the results that are *not* in electrolyte balance. (Results are in mmol/L.)

	Na^+	K^+	Cl^-	CO_2 content
A.	125	4.5	100	10
B.	135	3.5	95	28
C.	145	4.0	90	15
D.	150	5.0	110	30

The answer is C. Electrolyte balance is judged by calculating the anion gap: $(Na + K) - (CL + CO_2$ content). The difference reflects the net concentration of anions that have not been included in the equation. Anion gap is normally 10 to 20 mmol/L. (Kaplan and Pesce, pp. 859–860; Bishop et al., p. 294)

17. A serum or urine osmolality is ordered to measure the

A. activity of ions per kilogram of solvent

B. grams of solute per kilogram of solvent
C. osmoles of dissolved solutes per kilogram of solvent
D. equivalents of solute per kilogram of solvent

The answer is C. Osmolality expresses the total effective concentration of all solutes. The osmotic pressure of a solution is determined by the total number of solute particles per volume of solvent irrespective of whether the particles are ions or nonionized solutes. (Kaplan and Pesce, pp. 879–881; Anderson and Cockayne, p. 387)

18. Sample pretreatment is required for the determination of serum sodium, potassium, and lithium using flame emission spectrophotometry. Specimens, controls, and standards are diluted with a cesium solution for all of the following reasons *except*

    A. to ionize sodium, potassium, and lithium
    B. to compensate for changes in the aspiration rate
    C. because cesium is excited and emits light under the same thermal conditions as Na, K, and Li
    D. to minimize error due to mutual excitation

The answer is A. Sodium, potassium, and lithium ionize spontaneously in aqueous solution. Cesium is added to samples for flame emission analysis if the patient is receiving lithium therapeutically so that it can act as an internal standard and a radiation buffer. These functions are defined by answers B, C, and D. (Bishop et al., p. 111; Anderson and Cockayne, p. 87)

19. A patient admitted to the emergency room is suspected of having ingested some type of volatile substance. Which of the following formulas would be used to support this theory?

    A. $2.5 \times Na^+$
    B. $Na^+ + K^+ + Cl^- + CO_2$ content
    C. $(1.86 \times Na^+) + (1/18 \times glucose) + (1/2.8 \times BUN) + 9$
    D. $(Na^+ + K^+) - (Cl^- + HCO_3^-)$

The answer is C. This formula, using routine serum determinations of Na, glucose, and BUN, can be utilized to **estimate** serum osmolality. Sodium is by far the major cation in serum, and each cation is matched with an anion. Thus, two (or more accurately, 1.86) × Na (in mmol/L) accounts for most ions present. Glucose and BUN are also major contributors to serum osmolality. Dividing glucose (in mg/dL) by 18 and BUN (in mg/dL) by 2.8 converts these values to their millimolar equivalents. The unmeasured particles that contribute to the osmolality in serum normally amount to 9 mmol/L. The osmolal gap is calculated by subtracting the **estimated** serum osmolality from the **measured** value. An abnormally high osmolal gap may be due to the ingestion of a volatile substance such as ethanol, methanol, or ethylene glycol. Response D is another useful calculated parameter known as the anion gap. (Bishop et al., p. 272; Anderson and Cockayne, pp. 387 and 460)

20. The normal ratio of bicarbonate ion to carbonic acid in arterial blood is

    A. $0.03 : 1$
    B. $1 : 1.8$

C. 20 : 1
D. 6.1 : 7.4

The answer is C. The Henderson-Hasselbalch equation defines the ratio of base to acid that is required for a given pH. At normal arterial pH the ratio of concentrations of bicarbonate ion to carbonic acid is 20 : 1. The pKa of this buffer system in whole blood at 37°C is 6.1. (Kaplan and Pesce, p. 334; Bishop et al., p. 254)

21. Which of these patients has respiratory acidosis?

	Arterial blood pH	Arterial pCO_2
A.	Decreased	Decreased
B.	Decreased	Increased
C.	Increased	Decreased
D.	Increased	Increased

The answer is B. Respiratory acidosis is defined as decreased blood pH caused by an absolute excess of carbonic acid. The carbonic acid concentration can be calculated from the pCO2 ($0.03 \times pCO2 = H_2CO_3$). The excess carbonic acid relative to bicarbonate concentration causes blood pH to decrease. (Anderson and Cockayne, p. 421; Bishop et al., p. 255)

22. The toxic effects of carbon monoxide are caused by

A. displacement of oxygen from heme
B. formation of methemoglobin
C. oxidation of heme iron
D. a right-shifted oxyhemoglobin dissociation curve

The answer is A. Carbon monoxide strongly binds to heme at the same site that oxygen does and prevents formation of oxyhemoglobin. The iron in the heme pocket remains in its active ferrous state. When oxygen gradually displaces carbon monoxide from carboxyhemoglobin, the function of the hemoglobin molecule is restored. (Kaplan and Pesce, p. 515; Bishop et al., p. 608)

23. The trough blood sample for routine therapeutic drug monitoring is usually obtained

A. at the calculated peak time after a dose
B. just after a dose is administered
C. just before the next scheduled dose
D. one half-life after a dose is administered

The answer is C. Individuals differ markedly in their rates of clearance of drugs due to differences in absorption, distribution, metabolism, and excretion. Factors such as age, liver and kidney status, protein binding, and the presence of other drugs influence serum drug levels. The trough level, obtained immediately before administering a dose, is frequently used to monitor serum drug concentrations and adjust drug dosage regimens. (Anderson and Cockayne, p. 440; Kaplan and Pesce, p. 796)

24. Measurement of urinary vanillylmandelic acid (VMA) indicates the amount of hormone secreted by the

A. adrenal cortex
B. adrenal medulla
C. gonads
D. pituitary gland

The answer is B. Vanillylmandelic acid (VMA) is a metabolite of the catecholamines: epinephrine, norepinephrine, and dopamine. Epinephrine is mainly secreted by the adrenal medulla, whereas norepinephrine is primarily released by sympathetic neurons. High catecholamine secretion demonstrated by increased urinary VMA is associated with two types of tumors: pheochromocytomas in adults and neuroblastomas in children. (Kaplan and Pesce, pp. 674–679; Anderson and Cockayne, p. 327)

25. Urinary human chorionic gonadotropin (HCG) is commonly used to

A. detect excessive estrogen secretion
B. evaluate fetal lung function
C. diagnose hypogonadism
D. confirm pregnancy

The answer is D. HCG is produced by placental trophoblastic tissue, absorbed into the maternal plasma and excreted in the mother's urine. In a normal pregnancy, maternal serum and urine HCG levels rise soon after implantation of the fertilized ovum and double approximately every two days during the first trimester. HCG levels slowly decline in the second and third trimester. In addition to the detection of pregnancy, HCG is frequently used as a tumor marker to detect or monitor cancers of the ovary, testes, and placenta. (Kaplan and Pesce, pp. 572, 735; Bishop et al., p. 344)

26. Elevated serum cortisol may indicate

A. Addison's disease
B. Cushing's syndrome
C. Graves' disease
D. Paget's disease

The answer is B. Cushing's syndrome describes the signs and symptoms associated with excessive levels of cortisol. Hypercortisolism may be due to tumors of the pituitary or adrenal glands or ectopic ACTH-secreting tumors. Exogenous administration of glucocorticoids or ACTH will also result in Cushing's syndrome symptoms. Addison's disease is adrenal hypofunction demonstrated by low cortisol levels, Graves' disease is a type of hyperthyroidism, and Paget's disease is a progressive skeletal disorder that involves excessive bone destruction and repair. (Kaplan and Pesce, p. 679; Anderson and Cockayne, p. 541)

27. The direct fraction of the total serum bilirubin is produced primarily in the

A. common bile duct
B. hepatocytes
C. intestinal lumen
D. renal tubules

The answer is B. Bilirubin is formed in reticuloendothelial cells by the degradation of heme and circulates in the plasma bound chiefly to albumin. Hepatocytes efficiently take up this bilirubin, trap it intracellularly by protein binding, conjugate it with glucuronic acid, and excrete it into the biliary tract. (Kaplan and Pesce, p. 508; Bishop et al., p. 475)

28. A clay-colored stool is frequently associated with an obstructive type of jaundice. The dark brown color of a normal stool is due to the presence of intestinal

A. bilirubin
B. porphobilinogen
C. urobilinogen
D. δ-aminolevulinic acid

The answer is C. Hepatocytes excrete conjugated bilirubin into the bile duct for passage to the intestine. Intestinal bacteria degrade the molecule into derivatives which are collectively called urobilinogen. Urobilinogen is quickly oxidized to urobilin, which gives the stool its normal dark brown color. If the common bile duct is obstructed by a stone or neoplasm, the flow of conjugated bilirubin will be reduced and the stool will appear very light. (Bishop et al., p. 482; Anderson and Cockayne, p. 297)

29. Xanthochromic cerebrospinal fluid is an indicator of

A. bacterial meningitis
B. increased pressure of cerebrospinal fluid
C. increased protein concentration in cerebrospinal fluid
D. cerebral hemorrhage

The answer is D. Xanthochromia in spinal fluid is yellow pigmentation caused by the presence of bilirubin. The bilirubin results from breakdown of heme released from erythrocytes after bleeding into the brain or spinal column such as occurs in cerebral hemorrhage. (Kaplan and Pesce, p. 604; Bishop et al., p. 534)

30. The lecithin-sphingomyelin (L/S) ratio in amniotic fluid is used to indicate functional maturity of the fetal

A. kidneys
B. liver
C. lungs
D. muscles

The answer is C. Increased synthesis of lecithin by fetal lungs begins in the 34th to 36th week of pregnancy. The alveolar lining becomes coated with this surface-active phospholipid, which then appears in the amniotic fluid. An L/S ratio higher than 2.0 is associated with decreased risk of respiratory distress syndrome in the newborn period. (Kaplan and Pesce, pp. 577–579; Bishop et al., p. 530)

31. Samples for calcium analysis by atomic absorption spectrophotometry should be diluted with a lanthanum solution because lanthanum ions

A. blank for variations in flame temperature
B. blank for variations in lamp intensity
C. emit light used as the internal standard
D. enhance dissociation of calcium phosphate

The answer is D. Because of the requirement of a cool flame in atomic absorption spectrophotometry, some calcium salts are not broken into their component atoms; calcium phosphate is an example. The electrons in these anion-bound calcium atoms are then unable to absorb the incident wavelength of light and are not measured. Lanthanum binds the same anions more tightly than does calcium, which releases calcium from these salts. This allows the calcium electrons to achieve their ground state, absorb light energy, and be measured. (Kaplan and Pesce, p. 62; Bishop et al., p. 283)

32. A fluorometer measures light that is

A. absorbed by excited electrons as they return to the ground state
B. emitted by excited electrons as they return to the ground state
C. polarized by the chemical reaction
D. scattered by insoluble particles produced by the reaction

The answer is B. The ground-state electrons of a fluorescent analyte absorb light of specific wavelengths, become excited for a few nanoseconds, and then reemit their remaining energy as light of longer wavelengths. (Kaplan and Pesce, p. 63; Bishop et al., p. 112)

33. When an ion-selective electrode interacts with its analyte, it produces a change in the electrode's

A. conductance
B. current
C. resistance
D. voltage

The answer is D. In an ion-selective electrode, ionic analyte reacts with an electrode surface producing a change in potential (voltage) across the selective membrane. No current is allowed to flow. The membrane potential (analyte voltage) is then compared to a known stable voltage, and the meter expresses the difference between them as the concentration of analyte. (Kaplan and Pesce, pp. 215–216; Bishop et al., pp. 117–118)

34. Electrophoretic separation of proteins on cellulose acetate depends on the proteins differing in

A. concentration
B. molecular weight
C. net charge
D. number of peptide bonds

The answer is C. Electrophoresis is movement of an ion in an electrical field. The rate of movement is directly proportional to the net charge of the ion. This principle is the basis for electrophoretic separation of serum proteins. The size of the ion also influences its mobility, but this is not a major determinant when using cellulose acetate. (Bishop et al., pp. 120–121)

35. In an automated instrument, the amount of carryover between consecutive samples is *not* affected by

    A. rinsing the probe between samples
    B. separating consecutive samples in a tubing by air segments
    C. using a separate reaction chamber for each sample
    D. using a serum blank

The answer is D. Carryover is the percent error produced by interaction or cross-contamination between adjacent samples. All techniques that rinse the components which touch adjacent samples or that increase the physical separation between adjacent samples decrease carryover. (Kaplan and Pesce, p. 232; Bishop et al., p. 139)

36. Chromatographic separation of a mixture of compounds depends on

    A. some compounds being degraded by the mobile phase
    B. some compounds being more strongly attracted to the stationary phase than others
    C. some compounds being undetectable
    D. some compounds being insoluble in the mobile phase

The answer is B. Chromatography separates solutes by competition between adsorption of solute to the support and dissolving it in the mobile phase. Thus, compounds that differ in their attraction to the stationary phase can be separated from one another. (Kaplan and Pesce, pp. 74–76; Bishop et al., pp. 122–123)

37. In double-beam spectrophotometry, the beams referred to are

    A. matched cuvettes
    B. separate light paths
    C. supports for the instrument
    D. the spectrum from a diffraction grating

The answer is B. The second (reference) light beam in a double-beam spectrophotometer continuously monitors the amount of light transmitted in the absence of sample chromogen. By expressing the absorbance of a sample as the ratio between its measuring light beam and the reference light beam, variation in lamp intensity or detector sensitivity are blanked. (Tietz, 3rd ed., p. 51)

38. If serum protein electrophoresis is performed using higher voltage than the method calls for, which one of the following is *least* likely?

    A. Proteins migrate at a faster rate
    B. Greater distance separates adjacent bands of protein
    C. Less wick flow occurs
    D. More heat is generated

The answer is C. Higher voltage causes increased heat production, which leads to drying of the support. Capillary action then draws buffer from the reservoirs onto the unsaturated support. This buffer movement is referred to as wick flow. The greater voltage also will cause the proteins to migrate more rapidly and to separate more from each other. (Tietz, 3rd ed., p. 84)

39. For the examination of an unstained urine sediment, which type of microscopy provides the maximum contrast, optimal resolution and best visualization of elements without haloing?

A. Darkfield microscopy
B. Phase-contrast microscopy
C. Polarizing microscopy
D. Interference-contrast microscopy

The answer is D. In interference-contrast microscopy, the microscope converts differences in the optical path through the specimen to intensify differences in specimen image. The image achieved has high contrast and resolution without haloing and is superior to all other types of microscopy listed above for detailed viewing of unstained specimens. (Brunzel, pp. 16–17, 22)

40. To assess the permeability of the blood/brain barrier, the cerebrospinal fluid (CSF) level of which of the following proteins will be measured by the laboratory?

A. Albumin
B. IgG
C. Transferrin
D. Prealbumin

The answer is A. Albumin is usually employed as the reference protein for permeability because it is *not* synthesized to any extent in the CNS. In CSF uncontaminated by blood, any albumin present must have come from plasma through the blood/brain barrier. The permeability of the blood/brain barrier to plasma proteins is increased by high intracranial pressure due to brain tumor or intracerebral hemorrhage, or by inflammation, especially bacterial meningitis. (Brunzel, pp. 375–376)

41. Which of these cells found in increased numbers in urinary sediment are indicative of kidney disease and not just lower urinary tract disease?

A. Erythrocytes
B. Squamous epithelial cells
C. Polymorphonuclear leukocytes
D. Tubular epithelial cells

The answer is D. Blood cells may pathologically enter the urinary tract at any point. Squamous epithelium only occurs in the lower urinary tract. Renal tubular cells are only found in the upper urinary tract. (Brunzel, p. 227)

42. Urinary sediment that contains red blood cells, red blood cell casts, and protein is characteristic of

A. acute glomerulonephritis
B. bladder infection
C. nephrotic syndrome
D. prostatic hypertrophy

The answer is A. In acute glomerulonephritis, injury to the glomeruli allows blood components, including erythrocytes and proteins, to enter the renal tubules. Subsequent concentration of the filtrate in the distal tubules results in formation of tubular casts which envelope the red blood cells present. (Brunzel, p. 277)

43. The dipstick that contains ferric ion produces a blue-green color on reaction with urine from a patient who has untreated

    A. cystinuria
    B. galactosemia
    C. maple syrup urine disease
    D. phenylketonuria

The answer is D. Phenylketones, which are excreted in high concentration in the urine of patients with untreated phenylketonuria. One of these catabolites, phenylpyruvic acid, reacts with ferric ions in an acid medium to produce a blue-green chromogen. (Brunzel, p. 297)

44. In which of the glucose tolerances shown in the figure on p. 2 would you expect to find concurrent glycosuria?

    A. Curves 1 and 2
    B. Curves 1 and 3
    C. Curves 3 and 4
    D. Only curve 4

The answer is C. The normal renal threshold for glucose is a plasma level of 160 to 180 mg/dL. There is a limited amount of reabsorption mechanism in the proximal convoluted tubules. At blood glucose levels higher than the renal threshold, the limited reabsorption allows excretion of the excess glucose in the urine. Both curves 3 and 4 exceed this renal threshold value. Individuals with renal disease, which includes many diabetic patients, may have even lower renal thresholds for glucose. (Brunzel, p. 172)

45. Hyaline casts are found in urinary sediment

    A. following strenuous exercise
    B. in an alkaline urine
    C. whenever an abnormal amount of protein is present
    D. when examined using bright light

The answer is A. Hyaline casts are not considered pathologic when they are the only abnormal finding following exercise. In these cases they are probably the result of temporary minor dehydration and consequent stagnation of renal filtrate. (Strasinger, p. 88)

46. Which of these sugars *cannot* be detected in urine using the copper reduction test?

    A. Fructose
    B. Galactose
    C. Arabinose
    D. Sucrose

The answer is D. The copper reduction test detects carbohydrates by the reducing power of their free aldehyde groups. Sucrose is a disaccharide that has no free aldehyde group and does not produce the yellow-orange salts of oxidized copper. Sucrose is not absorbed or produced by the body. It only appears in urine as an artifact. (Brunzel, p. 176)

47. Which protein test is *not* able to detect immunoglobulin light chains (i.e., Bence Jones proteins) in urine?

    A. Immunoelectrophoresis
    B. Protein precipitation between 40 and 60°C
    C. Sulfosalicylic acid (SSA) precipitation test
    D. Reagent strip test based on the protein error of indicators

The answer is D. Bence Jones protein was originally recognized by its reversible precipitation between 40 and 60°C. Sulfosalicylic acid is a general protein precipitant and will precipitate Bence Jones protein. Immunoelectrophoresis is the definitive method for identifying the specific types of immunoglobulin polypeptides (Bence Jones protein) that are being excreted. Bence Jones protein is not usually detectable using the dipstick method. (Brunzel, pp. 169–172)

48. False-positive reagent strip ketone results can occur when drugs containing free sulfhydryl groups are excreted in the urine. These compounds will react with which of the following reagent test-strip chemicals?

    A. Potassium iodide
    B. Sodium nitroprusside
    C. Diazotized sulfanilic acid
    D. p-dimethylaminobenzaldehyde

The answer is B. Compounds that contain free sulfhydryl groups can react with sodium nitroprusside (nitroferricyanide) to produce a false-positive reagent test-strip test for ketones. Examples of drugs containing free sulfhydryl groups include penicillamine, a chelating agent, and captopril, an antihypertensive drug. (Brunzel, p. 179)

49. Calculate the creatinine clearance using these data obtained from a person with 1.73 m² body surface area:

    Serum creatinine: 1.8 mg/dL
    Urine creatinine: 54 mg/dL
    Urine volume: 640 mL/1440 min

    A. 3 mL/min
    B. 13 mL/min
    C. 21 mL/min
    D. 68 mL/min

The answer is B. The formula for calculating creatinine clearance is

$$\frac{\text{urine creatine concentration}}{\text{serum creatine concentration}} \times \frac{\text{urine volume}}{\text{urine collection time}} \times \frac{1.73 \text{ m}^2}{\text{BSA}} = C_{cr}$$

where urine and serum concentrations are both expressed in the same units, volume is milliliters, time is minutes, and BSA is body surface area in square meters. The calculated value has the units mL/min. (Strasinger, pp. 21–24)

50. A creatinine clearance result below the normal reference range indicates a decrease in

A. hepatic blood flow
B. hepatic creatinine synthesis
C. renal blood flow
D. renal glomerular filtration

The answer is D. Creatinine is filtered by glomeruli and excreted with little or no tubular reabsorption or secretion. Calculation of creatinine clearance essentially solves an equation for the amount of creatinine-containing plasma which must have been filtered in order to account for the amount of creatinine excreted in the urine. (Brunzel, pp. 106–109)

CLS Review Questions

1. Select the finding that is *not* a criterion for a diagnosis of diabetes mellitus:

A. on at least two separate occasions, a fasting glucose ≥ 140 mg/dL
B. within 3h after an oral dose of glucose, a serum glucose ≤ 40 mg/dL
C. glucosuria within 2h after an oral glucose dose in the absence of renal disease
D. on at least two separate occasions, a serum glucose ≥ 200 mg/dL within 2h after an oral glucose dose

The answer is B. NDDG criteria for the diagnosis of diabetes mellitus include either (1) a fasting serum glucose level greater than 140 mg/dL on more than one occasion or (2) two or more serum samples with glucose levels greater than 200 mg/dL following a meal. The latter values exceed the renal threshold for glucose and result in glycosuria. (Tietz, 3rd ed., p. 433)

2. The purpose of hemoglobin A_{1c} determinations is to

A. identify individuals who have diabetes mellitus
B. predict the current plasma glucose level in diabetic individuals
C. monitor the long-term plasma glucose level in diabetic individuals
D. assist in the adjustment of insulin dosage for diabetic individuals

The answer is C. Hemoglobin A_{1c} is slowly produced by a nonenzymatic reaction during the life span of a circulating erythrocyte. It is the condensation product of glucose and the *N*-terminal amino group of beta-globin of hemoglobin. (Kaplan and Pesce, p. 451)

3. Each of these enzymes can be used in a method to quantitate serum glucose. Select the enzyme that catalyzes the conversion of glucose to hydrogen peroxide and gluconic acid.

A. G-6-PD
B. Glucose oxidase
C. Hexokinase
D. Peroxidase

The answer is B. Glucose oxidase catalyzes the oxidation of glucose by molecular oxygen. The products are gluconic acid and hydrogen peroxide. There are several indicator reactions available for measuring the hydrogen peroxide. (Kaplan and Pesce, pp. 850–853)

4. If LDL receptors are nonfunctional due to disease, the plasma level of which lipid would increase the most?

A. Fatty acids
B. Cholesterol
C. Cholesterol esters
D. Triglycerides

The answer is B. Lipoprotein lipases remove triglycerides from triglyceride-rich VLDL and chylomicrons and successively produce IDL (intermediate-density lipoproteins) and then cholesterol-rich LDL particles. The apoliprotein B moiety in LDL binds to specific receptors in the liver, and the hepatocytes then internalize the particle and catabolize it. (Kaplan and Pesce, p. 474)

5. LDL cholesterol can be estimated using the Friedewald formula:

$$LDL = \text{Total cholesterol} - HDL - \frac{\text{triglycerides}}{5}$$

This calculation should *not* be used when the

A. HDL cholesterol is greater than 40 mg/dL
B. triglyceride level is greater than 400 mg/dL
C. plasma shows no visible evidence of lipemia
D. total cholesterol is elevated based on the age and sex of the patient

The answer is B. The formula estimates cholesterol contained in LDL particles by subtracting cholesterol in other lipoprotein particles from total cholesterol. An essential assumption is that 20% ($^1/_5$) of VLDL particles is cholesterol and that measured triglyceride accurately estimates the amount of VLDL. When the triglyceride result is excessively high (>400 mg/dL) this assumption is not valid. (Tietz, 3rd ed., p. 469)

6. The serum protein electrophoresis pattern typical of nephrotic syndrome is

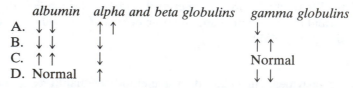

The answer is A. In nephrotic syndrome, increased permeability of the glomerular membrane allows proteins of small molecular weight to escape into the urine in large quantities. Albumin and IgG, having relatively low molecular

weights, are lost and the larger proteins, which remain in the plasma, appear to be present in increased concentration. (Kaplan and Pesce, p. 352)

7. Select the method of protein quantitation that is *least* specific for albumin.

   A. Immunonephelometry
   B. Electrophoresis at pH 8.6
   C. Sulfosalicylic acid (SSA) precipitation test
   D. Dye-binding method using bromcresol green

The answer is C. Bromcresol green, under appropriate conditions of pH and ionic strength, binds specifically to albumin. This shifts the wavelength of light absorbed by the dye. Electrophoresis of serum proteins results in a virtually pure band of albumin, in contrast to the other bands which are mixtures of proteins. Immunonephelometry is specific for an individual protein by virtue of antigen-antibody recognition. Sulfosalicylic acid is a general protein precipitant and is not specific for albumin. (Kaplan and Pesce, p. 1030)

8. The use of a moderately hemolyzed serum specimen for protein electrophoresis can elevate which protein fraction?

   A. albumin
   B. alpha$_1$ globulin
   C. beta globulin
   D. gamma globulin

The answer is C. Haptoglobin binds a small amount of hemoglobin in serum; the remaining free hemoglobin migrates electrophoretically with serum beta globulins. (Henry, pp. 648–649)

9. Which enzyme is *least* likely to be elevated in a specimen drawn 72 hours after an uncomplicated myocardial infarction?

   A. CK-MB (CK-2)
   B. CK-MM (CK-3)
   C. LD$_1$ (HHHH)
   D. AST

The answer is A. For the remaining cardiac enzymes, preinfarction levels are not reestablished as quickly. CK-MM requires 3–4 days, AST, 4–5 days and LD, 7–12 days following the event to decline to pre-AMI values. (Kaplan and Pesce, p. 420)

10. Which ratio of enzymes provides the *best* indication of hepatitis?

   A. ALT/AST
   B. Amylase/lipase
   C. CK-MB/total CK
   D. LD$_1$/LD$_5$

The answer is A. Hepatocytes are rich in both of these transaminases. The ratio of ALT to AST characteristically exceeds 1.0 in toxic or viral hepatitis. The other enzymes and isoenzymes listed are not found in significant quantities in hepatocytes. (Kaplan and Pesce, pp. 368–370)

11. The following kinetic enzyme data is obtained from a serum specimen:

Time (min)	Absorbance
0	0.020
1	0.200
2	0.315
3	0.395
4	0.435
5	0.480

Select the statement that *best* summarizes the enzyme assay results obtained.

A. Readings are satisfactory; calculate the result
B. Substrate depletion; repeat assay using a serum dilution
C. The 0–3min readings are satisfactory; use these for result calculation
D. The 3–5min readings are satisfactory; use these for result calculation

The answer is B. The rate of change of absorbance (change in absorbance per minute) is not constant for any of the data given. This indicates that there is insufficient substrate present for all of the enzyme molecules to be continuously active during the analysis, a condition referred to as substrate exhaustion. The rate of change of absorbance is therefore dependent on both enzyme concentration and substrate concentration. Use of less enzyme-containing serum will allow sufficient substrate for zero-order kinetics and still produce a measurable change in absorbance. (Kaplan and Pesce, pp. 776–780)

12. Significantly elevated serum amylase with normal urine amylase indicates

A. acute pancreatitis
B. chronic pancreatitis
C. macroamylasemia
D. salivary gland inflammation

The answer is C. Amylase is a sufficiently small protein to be filtered through normal renal glomeruli. This accounts for its rapidly increasing level in urine following a rise in serum value as is found in acute inflammation of the pancreatic or salivary glands. Macroamylasemia is a benign finding in which the small amount of amylase normally released into plasma is bound to an immunoglobulin, which results in a molecule too large for glomerular filtration. This enzyme-immunoglobulin complex is reactive in assays for amylase activity. Typical results are several times normal in serum but are not associated with any pathologic disorder. Chronic pancreatitis is not commonly associated with elevated amylase. (Bishop et al., p. 236)

13. A cancer patient responding favorably to chemotherapy is most likely to have an elevated serum level of which substance due to rapid turnover of cells?

A. Creatinine
B. Uric acid
C. Blood urea nitrogen
D. Potassium

The answer is B. During degradation of purines (adenine and guanine), the ring structure is largely salvaged for reuse. That amount which escapes salvage is converted to uric acid and excreted into the urine. (Anderson and Cockayne, p. 371)

14. Urea can be measured by incubation with urease followed by all *except*

   A. formation of a colored product by reaction with diacetyl
   B. measurement of increased conductivity
   C. ion-selective electrode measurement of the ammonia produced
   D. NADH consumption in a reaction catalyzed by glutamate dehydrogenase

The answer is A. Diacetyl condenses with urea in acid conditions producing a colored diazine. However, the urea molecule is broken down by urease into ammonium and carbonate ions. These ions increase the conductivity of the reaction mixture. Alternatively, the ammonium ions produced can be measured by an ion-selective electrode or by using them as substrate for glutamate dehydrogenase. (Anderson and Cockayne, p. 368)

15. Which one of these serum electrolyte results (mmol/L) is *most likely* in a serum with elevated lactate level?

	Na^+	K^+	Cl^-	CO_2 content
A.	125	4.5	100	10
B.	135	3.5	95	28
C.	145	4.0	90	15
D.	150	5.0	110	30

The answer is C. Excessive production of H^+ from lactic acid causes metabolic acidosis by depleting bicarbonate, the major component of CO_2 content. The total number of anions present is unchanged even though their relative amounts are abnormal. Therefore the concentrations of Na^+ and Cl^- do not become abnormal despite the increased anion gap. (Anderson and Cockayne, p. 422)

16. For the best indication of neuromuscular irritability, which of the following could be assayed in the extracellular fluid?

   A. Complexed calcium
   B. Free ionized calcium
   C. Protein-bound calcium
   D. Total calcium

The answer is B. The functional form of calcium is the free ionized form. These functions include muscle contraction and neurotransmission as well as enzyme activation and its presence as a component of hydroxyapatite (the mineral deposit in bones and teeth). (Anderson and Cockayne, p. 526)

17. Which of these serum constituents has the largest effect on osmolality?

   A. Glucose
   B. Protein

C. Sodium
D. Urea

The answer is C. Osmolality is a measure of the molal activity of total solutes. In serum the molal concentration of sodium approximates its molar concentration and far exceeds that of any other serum solute. A glucose level of 100 mg/dL, e.g., is only 5.5 mmol/L, a urea nitrogen level of 15 mg/dL is only 2.5 mmol/L, and the molal concentration of 7 g/dL total proteins is very low due to the large molecular weights of proteins. (Anderson and Cockayne, p. 403)

18. Calculate the blood pH from these arterial blood results.

PCO_2	45 mm Hg
PO_2	95 mm Hg
Carbonic acid	1.35 mmol/L
Bicarbonate ion	27 mmol/L
CO_2 content	28 mmol/L

A. 6.62
B. 7.40
C. 7.51
D. 7.62

The answer is B. Of the values given, only the bicarbonate and carbonic acid concentrations are needed to solve the Henderson-Hasselbalch equation for pH. The pK_a for this buffer system is 6.1 in blood at 37°C:

$$pH = 6.1 + \log \frac{HCO_3^-}{H_2CO_3}$$

(Anderson and Cockayne, p. 415)

19. In a patient with metabolic acidosis, one would expect to see

A. a decreased rate of breathing
B. a decreased reabsorption of renal bicarbonate
C. an increased metabolic production of CO_2
D. hyperventilation

The answer is D. Low blood pH caused by metabolic acidosis stimulates respiration. This decreases the blood PCO_2 which shifts the ratio of bicarbonate to carbonic acid toward the normal, 20 : 1, and therefore shifts blood pH toward normal. At the same time, renal compensatory mechanisms conserve bicarbonate which also helps to restore the ratio of base to acid. (Anderson and Cockayne, p. 422)

20. An elderly man, previously treated for depression but with no history of alcohol abuse, is brought to the emergency room (ER). He was found staggering outside his home, extremely confused. In the ER, he became progressively drowsy and unaware of his surroundings. Laboratory results reveal a large osmolal gap (110 mOsm/kg) and increased anion gap (42 mmol/L). Urinalysis is positive for glucose, but negative for ketones. Other laboratory results include:

glucose, serum	85 mg/dL	urea nitrogen,	16 mg/dL
creatinine, serum	0.93 mg/dL	serum sodium, serum	139 mmol/L

These findings are MOST consistent with:

A. ethylene glycol ingestion
B. chronic renal failure
C. diabetic ketoacidosis
D. insulin overdose

The answer is A. The osmolal gap is the difference between measured (actual) and calculated plasma osmolality. Calculated osmolality is determined by measuring concentrations of sodium, glucose and urea. The value of the plasma osmolal gap is increased in hyperosmolal states. Moderate increases (up to 10 mOsm/kg) are seen in ketoacidosis, renal acidosis and lactic acidosis. A large osmolal gap suggests poisoning with nonelectrolytes such as ethanol, methanol, acetone or ethylene glycol. Accumulation of various types of inorganic acids such as phosphate or sulfate that occurs in renal failure, as well as the accumulation of organic acids from ketoacidosis are the most common cause of an increased anion gap. Ingestion of such toxic substances as methanol, ethylene glycol and salicylates leads to accumulation of organic acid metabolites that increase the anion gap. Large anion and osmolal gaps, in the absence of elevated serum levels of glucose, urea nitrogen and/or creatinine, and without ketonuria are consistent with the possible ingestion of a toxic, osmotically active substance such as ethylene glycol. (Bishop, 2nd ed, p. 272; Anderson and Cockayne, pp. 387, 460)

21. Lead poisoning may be detected by elevated levels of all *except*

A. δ-aminolevulinate (ALA) dehydratase (porphobilinogen synthase) activity
B. free erythrocyte protoporphyrin
C. 24-hr urinary lead
D. whole blood lead

The answer is A. Delta-ALA dehydratase (porphobilinogen synthase), an enzyme in the pathway of heme synthesis, is inhibited by lead. Lead also inhibits incorporation of iron into protoporphyrin IX, which results in accumulation of free protoporphyrin in erythrocytes. Whole blood is a good sample for detection of lead poisoning since lead tends to be sequestered and concentrated in erythrocytes. The small amount of excess lead that is free in plasma is excreted in the urine. (Anderson and Cockayne, pp. 461–463)

22. Calculate the half-life of this drug in the circulation.

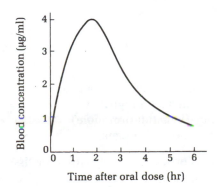

Time after oral dose (hr)

A. $^{1}/_{2}$ hr
B. $1^{1}/_{2}$ hr
C. $2^{1}/_{2}$ hr
D. 4 hr

The answer is B. The biologic half-life of a drug is the length of time required for any blood level to decay to half that level. In the diagram, the blood concentration is approximately 4 μg/mL at 2 hr and approximately 2 μg/mL at $3^{1}/_{2}$ hr; thus the level has dropped to one-half value in $3^{1}/_{2} - 2 = 1^{1}/_{2}$ hr. (Bishop et al., p. 582; Anderson and Cockayne, p. 440)

23. A patient with intermittent hypertension has an elevated value for urinary catecholamine metabolites (e.g., vanillylmandelic acid [VMA]). This result may indicate

A. hyperaldosteronism
B. hypercortisolism
C. idiopathic hypertension
D. pheochromocytoma

The answer is D. Pheochromocytoma is a catecholamine-secreting tumor of the adrenal medulla. Epinephrine and norepinephrine are catecholamines. Most pheochromocytomas produce a mixture of the two. The release of catecholamines by the tumor accounts for the patient's hypertension. Catecholamine metabolites, including VMA, are excreted in the urine. (Anderson and Cockayne, p. 550)

24. Blood from a newborn has low thyroxine (T_4) and elevated thyroid-stimulating hormone (TSH) compared to reference ranges for that age. These results indicate

A. congenital hypopituitarism
B. congenital primary hypothyroidism
C. congenital secondary hypothyroidism
D. normal response to pregnancy-induced changes in maternal thyroid function

The answer is B. Production of T_4 by the thyroid gland has a negative feedback relationship with thyrotropin (TSH) produced by the anterior pituitary gland. Congenital abnormalities which prevent adequate production of T_4 result in a high level of TSH through this feedback loop. The elevated T_4 values seen in maternal serum are an artifact caused by estrogen-induced increase in synthesis of thyroxine-binding globulin. (Bishop et al., p. 519; Anderson and Cockayne, pp. 512–513)

25. Urinary HCG concentration is higher than nonpregnant values in all of these cases *except*

A. ten days following spontaneous abortion
B. the 10th week of normal pregnancy
C. molar pregnancy (hydatidiform mole)
D. third trimester of normal pregnancy

The answer is A. HCG is produced by trophoblastic tissue, absorbed into the maternal plasma, and then excreted in the urine. Loss of trophoblastic tissue, such as happens in spontaneous abortion, results in rapid urinary clearance of the hormone resulting in values that are less than expected for the presumed period of gestation. Trophoblastic tumors, such as molar pregnancy, are associated with elevated values in the absence of pregnancy. In a normal pregnancy, HCG rises in maternal blood soon after implantation of the fertilized ovum and doubles approximately every two days during the first trimester. A very slow decline then occurs through the rest of the gestation period. (Bishop et al., pp. 547–548; Anderson and Cockayne, pp. 659–660)

26. A patient whose admission diagnosis is biliary obstruction has these laboratory results:

	Test	Result
Serum:	Conjugated bilirubin	Increased
	Total bilirubin	Increased
Urine:	Bilirubin	Positive
	Urobilinogen	Increased

Which result is *inconsistent* with the admission diagnosis?

A. Serum conjugated bilirubin
B. Serum total bilirubin
C. Urinary bilirubin
D. Urinary urobilinogen

The answer is D. Urobilinogen is formed in the intestinal lumen by bacteria acting on excreted bile. A significant portion of the urobilinogen is then reabsorbed into the portal blood from which it is extracted and reexcreted on passage through the liver. Only the urobilinogen which escapes this hepatic removal reaches the kidneys for filtration into urine. A patient with obstructive liver disease would be expected to excrete less bilirubin into the intestine. Thus less urobilinogen would be formed, less would be reabsorbed, less would escape hepatic removal, and less would appear in the urine. Urinary bilirubin, on the other hand, is the water-soluble conjugated form. Regurgitation from canaliculi, caused by biliary obstruction results in increased serum levels and filtration into urine. (Anderson and Cockayne, pp. 284–286)

27. When measuring serum bilirubin, the purpose of adding caffeine–sodium benzoate or methanol to the reaction mixture is to

A. accelerate the reaction with conjugated bilirubin
B. accelerate the reaction with unconjugated bilirubin
C. destroy excess diazo reagent
D. shift the wavelength absorbed by azobilirubin

The answer is B. Unconjugated bilirubin is poorly soluble in aqueous solution. It reacts very slowly with aqueous solution of the diazotizing color reagent unless an accelerating reagent, such as caffeine–sodium benzoate (Jendrassik-Grof method) or methanol (Evelyn-Malloy method), is added. (Bishop et al., p. 480; Anderson and Cockayne, p. 289)

28. Which of these vitamin levels would be expected to be abnormal due to poor absorption in a patient with pancreatic insufficiency?

A. Vitamin A
B. Vitamin B$_1$ (thiamine)
C. Vitamin B$_{12}$
D. Vitamin C

The answer is A. Vitamin A, a fat-soluble compound, is a nonpolar derivative of isoprene which is poorly soluble in water. Without the assistance of bile acids and the action of pancreatic lipase, vitamin A is minimally solubilized and therefore is not efficiently absorbed from the intestine. (Bishop et al., p. 381)

29. Amniotic fluid from an expectant mother in the 39th week of gestation gives these laboratory results:

L/S ratio: 4.0
Creatinine: 2.8 mg/dL
Delta A$_{450}$: 0.008 (Liley zone I)

These results indicate

A. inadequate fetal kidney function
B. intrauterine hemolysis
C. mature fetal lungs
D. small fetal body size

The answer is C. Increased synthesis of lecithin by fetal lungs begins in the 34th to 36th week of pregnancy. The alveolar lining becomes coated with this surface-active phospholipid which then appears in the amniotic fluid. An L/S ratio higher than 2.0 in amniotic fluid is associated with maturation of the pulmonary lining and decreased risk of respiratory distress syndrome in the newborn period. Intrauterine hemolysis results in release of bilirubin, which absorbs light of 450-nm wavelength, into the amniotic fluid. Creatinine in amniotic fluid is a product of fetal muscle mass and correlates with fetal body weight. (Bishop et al., pp. 528–529)

30. When iontophoresis is used to collect sweat for chloride analysis, pilocarpine is used to

A. clean the skin area
B. complex with chloride
C. complete the circuit
D. induce sweat secretion

The answer is D. Pilocarpine is driven into the skin surface by iontophoresis (the migration of ions induced by direct current). It stimulates the production of sweat which is subsequently collected on preweighed filter paper or gauze for analysis of chloride or sodium. (Bishop et al., p. 536)

31. These blood and cerebrospinal fluid (CSF) samples were collected within 30 min of each other. Which of the pairs of glucose results indicates possible bacterial meningitis?

	Blood	CSF
A.	60 mg/dL	40 mg/dL
B.	100 mg/dL	60 mg/dL

C. 200 mg/dL   30 mg/dL
D. 200 mg/dL   120 mg/dL

The answer is C. In the absence of bacteria or increased numbers of leukocytes, the glucose concentration in CSF should be 60 to 80% of the concurrent concentration in blood. (Bishop et al., p. 307)

32. A fuel-rich flame is used in atomic absorption spectrophotometry in order to

A. avoid interference from other metals in the sample
B. maximize production of oxide and hydroxide radicals
C. minimize excitation of the analyte by heat
D. prevent damage to the burner

The answer is C. A fuel-rich flame is cooler than an oxidant-rich flame. In order to absorb the incident wavelength of light efficiently, the electrons of the metallic analyte must be in their ground state. Excessive energy from a too-hot flame tends to excite some of these electrons and results in fewer ground-state electrons capable of light absorption. (Bishop et al., pp. 109–110)

33. Ion-selective electrodes compare the voltage of the measuring electrode to

A. a known stable reference voltage
B. the conductivity of the sample
C. the current required to establish the voltage
D. the resistivity of the sample

The answer is A. Potentiometric electrodes require two half-cells. One of them (the measuring electrode) produces a voltage which depends on the amount of the analyte being measured, and the other (the reference electrode) is a source of known stable voltage. The meter then expresses the difference between these voltages which correlates with analyte concentration. (Bishop et al., pp. 115–117)

34. A nonhemolyzed, nonlipemic serum specimen was collected in a doctor's office. The instructions indicated that the specimen for the analyte should be protected from light following collection. If these instructions are *not* followed, what analyte can not be accurately measured?

A. Glucose
B. AST
C. Calcium
D. Bilirubin

The answer is D. Bilirubin degrades in the presence of light. Nonhemolyzed, nonlipemic serum specimens should be stored in the dark and refrigerated unless analyzed within three hours. (Bishop et al., p. 480)

35. Which of these characteristics is desired for a substance to be used as an internal standard?

A. Does not change when instrument variables change
B. Is more soluble in sample than the analyte is

    C. Is present in normal serum sample
    D. Produces a reaction detectable using the same type of detector as the
        analyte reaction

The answer is D. An internal standard is a substance added to all samples in
constant concentration. The analyte and internal standard are then measured
simultaneously, and any variation measured in the internal standard is assumed
to have occurred also to the analyte. The measured signal from the internal
standard is then used to correct the analyte signal to what it would have been
had there been no variation. This correction assumes that the substance chosen
for the internal standard reacts to all variables in the same way and to the
same extent as the analyte. (Bishop et al., p. 111)

36. The PO_2 electrode measures

    A. H^+ generated by reaction at the electrode surface
    B. the amount of O_2 oxidized to hydrogen peroxide
    C. the number of electrons used to reduce O_2
    D. voltage between the measuring half-cell and the reference half-cell

The answer is C. The PO_2 electrode differs from other commonly used electrodes in that it is amperometric instead of potentiometric. A known stable
voltage is maintained between the anode and the platinum cathode. Oxygen
diffuses through the membrane to the cathode where it is reduced by electrons
furnished by the anode. The amount of current (electron flow) is measured
and expressed as concentration of O_2. (Bishop et al., p. 260)

37. Thin-layer chromatography on silica gel uses solvent which is

    A. more polar than silica gel
    B. less polar than silica gel
    C. more acidic than silica gel
    D. more basic than silica gel

The answer is B. Silica gel chromatography separates a mixture of solutes by
differential competition between adsorption of each solute to the support and
its solubility in the mobile phase. Since silica gel is polar, the solvent used
with it is relatively nonpolar in order to maximize separation of the mixture.
(Tietz, p. 105)

38. You obtain the following data on a cholesterol assay:

Sample	Absorbance 530 nm	Concentration (mg/dL)
Standard	0.2	150
Normal control	0.2	100–200 (expected)
Abnormal control	0.4	250–300 (expected)
Patient	0.5	

H = flag for elevated values
L = flag for low values

Assuming the test results could be reported, the patient's cholesterol
would be reported as

A. 60 mg/dL L
B. 150 mg/dL
C. 375 mg/dL H
D. 500 mg/dL H

The answer is C. Beer's law holds and the analyte concentration is directly proportional to the solution absorbance. The reference ranges for cholesterol are influenced by age and gender. The National Cholesterol Education Program recommends that desirable levels should be less than 200 mg/dL. A cholesterol value of 375 mg/dL falls within the high-risk range and the physician should be notified immediately. (Bishop et al., p. 356)

39. The ratio of serum urea nitrogen to serum creatinine is elevated by

A. decreased flow of renal tubular filtrate
B. decreased renal tubular reabsorption
C. increased blood pressure
D. increased hepatic blood flow

The answer is A. A significant amount of filtered urea is reabsorbed from renal tubules, especially when the flow rate of the filtrate is decreased. Under the same conditions there is little or no change in the reabsorption of creatinine. This circumstance will cause less urea than creatinine to be cleared from the plasma. Thus the serum level will be elevated more than serum creatinine. (Tietz, 3rd ed., p. 676)

40. The urine of a patient with light, clay-colored feces is *unlikely* to have

A. positive bilirubin
B. elevated urobilinogen
C. positive dipstick nitrite test
D. positive test for porphobilinogen

The answer is B. The normal color of stool is largely due to urobilins, the oxidation products of urobilinogens. Light clay-colored stools lack this pigmentation, often because of obstruction of the bile duct. This obstruction prevents entry of bilirubin glucuronide into the intestine and subsequent degradation of bilirubin into urobilinogens. The amount of urobilinogens reabsorbed into plasma is then decreased, and this in turn decreases the amount filtered from plasma into the urine. (Kaplan and Pesce, p. 365)

41. Given the following laboratory results, what is the most likely cause for the patient's condition?

Serum results: BUN 35 mg/dL, creatinine 2.0 mg/dL, uric acid 9.5 mg/dL
Urine macroscopic results: Glucose negative, blood positive, WBC negative, pH 6.0, protein positive, SSA 2+
Urine microscopic results: 25–50 RBCs/hpf, 0–2 WBCs/hpf, 2–5 RBC casts, 3–5 hyaline casts, 0–2 granular casts, few uric-acid crystals

A. Gout
B. Glomerulonephritis
C. Pyelonephritis
D. Urinary-tract obstruction

The answer is B. Glomerulonephritis is an inflammatory condition of the glomerulus that allows protein and blood to enter the urine filtrate. Classic urinalysis findings are hematuria, RBC casts, proteinuria, hyaline casts, granular casts, and WBCs. (Strasinger, p. 32)

42. The presence of granular casts in urinary sediment may indicate any of these diseases *except*

A. cystitis
B. glomerular nephritis
C. pyelonephritis
D. renal failure

The answer is A. A cast is a mold of the renal tubule in which it has gelled. Cells that are trapped in the cast undergo degenerative changes producing granular casts. Cystitis is an infection of the lower urinary tract (e.g., the urinary bladder) and does not involve the kidney tubules. (Kaplan and Pesce, p. 846)

43. A urine sample that tests positive for ketones but negative for glucose is *most likely* from a patient suffering from

A. diabetes insipidus
B. diabetes mellitus
C. polydipsia
D. starvation

The answer is D. Ketones are the product of lipid catabolism producing acetoacetate in excess of the body's ability to catabolize it. This excessive lipid catabolism may occur in any state in which there is insufficient glucose metabolism for cellular energy requirements. (Strasinger, pp. 62–63)

44. The following results are obtained from a 28-year-old diabetic patient:

Glucose:	210 mg/dL (70–105)	Na⁺	140 mmol/L (136–145)
BUN:	25 mg/dL (10–20)	K⁺	3.8 mmol/L (3.5–5.0)
Serum Osmolality:	312 mOsmol/kg (275–295)	Cl⁻	101 mmol/L (99–109)

Based on this data, the patient's osmolal gap is

A. 31 mOsmol/kg
B. 96 mOsmol/kg
C. 203 mOsmol/kg
D. 301 mOsmol/kg

The answer is A. One formula used to calculate osmolality is

$$1.86 \times Na^+ \ (mmol/L) + \frac{Glucose \ (mg/dL)}{18} + \frac{BUN \ (mg/dL)}{2,8}$$

The calculated value has the units mOsmol/kg. The osmolal gap is then calculated by Osmolal Gap (mOsmol/kg) = osmolality (measured) − osmolality (calculated)

(Kaplan & Pesce, p. 209; Bishop et al., p. 272; Anderson and Cockayne, p. 461)

45. These results are obtained on a sample for routine urinalysis:

Appearance:	cloudy, dark-colored
Dipstick for hemoglobin:	negative
Microscopy:	25–50 RBCs per high-power field

Plausible explanations of these results include all *except*

A. the hemoglobin test may be falsely negative due to bleach
B. the hemoglobin test may be falsely negative due to ascorbic acid
C. the apparent RBCs may be truly yeast
D. the apparent RBCs may be truly WBCs

The answer is B. Bleach is an oxidant which can cause the dipstick for hemoglobin to be artifactually positive. Ascorbic acid is a reducing substance which, in excessive amounts, can cause it to be falsely negative. Even though the dipstick is less sensitive to intracellular hemoglobin than it is to free hemoglobin, it should be positive in the presence of this large number of RBCs. The identification of the cells can be confirmed by addition of weak acetic acid which will lyse RBCs but not yeast or WBCs. (Strasinger, p. 65)

46. Each of these crystals is found in urinary sediment of an acidic urine *except*

A. cystine
B. calcium oxalate
C. triple phosphate
D. sodium urate

The answer is C. Triple phosphate is magnesium-ammonium phosphate, a salt that is poorly soluble at alkaline pH. At acid pH it dissociates into its soluble component ions. The other crystals listed are less soluble at acid pH than at alkaline pH. (Strasinger, pp. 92–95)

47. All of the following may interfere with glucose detection in an unpreserved urine specimen *except*

A. galactose
B. ascorbic acid
C. bleach
D. sample at room temperature for > 4 h

The answer is A. Urine dipsticks utilize the glucose oxidase enzyme, which is specific for glucose; other sugars will not react. The greatest source of a false-negative urine glucose result is due to an unpreserved sample being allowed to sit at room temperature for a prolonged period of time; glucose rapidly undergoes glycolysis. Excessive amounts of ascorbic acid can cause a falsely decreased result and bleach causes a false-positive result. (Strasinger, pp. 60–61)

48. Creatinine clearance assesses the rate of

   A. glomerular filtration
   B. renal blood flow
   C. renal tubular reabsorption
   D. renal tubular secretion

The answer is A. Creatinine is filtered by glomeruli and then excreted with little or no tubular reabsorption or secretion. Calculation of creatinine clearance essentially is solving an equation for the amount of creatinine-containing plasma which must have been filtered in order to account for the amount of creatinine excreted in the urine. (Kaplan and Pesce, p. 354)

49. Calculate the creatinine clearance using these data:

   Serum creatinine: 1.8 mg/dL
   Urine creatinine: 54 mg/dL
   Urine volume: 640 mL/24h
   Body surface area: 1.25 m^2

   A. 1.1 mL/min
   B. 5 mL/min
   C. 13 mL/min
   D. 18 mL/min

The answer is D. The formula for calculation of creatinine clearance is

$$\frac{\text{urine creatine concentration}}{\text{serum creatine concentration}} \times \frac{\text{urine volume}}{\text{urine collection time}} \times \frac{1.73 \text{ m}^2}{\text{BSA}}$$

where urine and serum concentrations are both expressed in the same units, volume is milliliters, time is minutes, and BSA is body surface area in square meters. The calculated value has the units mL/min. (Kaplan and Pesce, p. 354; Anderson and Cockayne, p. 373)

50. Each of these urine tests measures the concentrating ability of the kidney *except* the

   A. number of casts per low-power field
   B. refractive index
   C. osmolality
   D. specific gravity

The answer is A. Refractive index, osmolality, and specific gravity are all influenced by the concentration of dissolved solutes in urine. On the other hand, casts are produced when Tamm-Horsfall protein congeals during stagnant flow of filtrate in renal tubules. (Strasinger, p. 44)

References

Anderson SC, Cockayne A. *Clinical Chemistry.* Philadelphia: Saunders, 1993.

Bishop ML, Duben-von Laufen JL, Fody EP (eds). *Clinical Chemistry Principles, Procedures, Correlations* (2nd ed). Philadelphia: Lippincott, 1992.

Brunzel NA. *Fundamentals of Urine and Body Fluid Analysis.* Philadelphia: Saunders, 1994.

Henry JB. *Clinical Diagnosis and Management by Laboratory Methods* (18th ed). Philadelphia: Saunders, 1991.

Kaplan LA, Pesce AJ. *Clinical Chemistry: Theory, Analysis, and Correlation* (2nd ed). St. Louis: Mosby, 1989.

Strasinger SK. *Urinalysis and Body Fluids* (3rd ed). Philadelphia: FA Davis, 1994.

Tietz NW (ed). *Fundamentals of Clinical Chemistry* (2nd ed). Philadelphia: Saunders, 1976.

Tietz NW (ed). *Fundamentals of Clinical Chemistry* (3rd ed). Philadelphia: Saunders, 1987.

Hematology and Hemostasis

Section Editors **Bernadette F. Rodak and Susan J. Leclair**

CLT Review Questions—Hematology

1. The internationally accepted method of hemoglobin measurement requires the conversion of hemoglobin to

A. carboxyhemoglobin
B. cyanmethemoglobin
C. oxyhemoglobin
D. sulfhemoglobin

The answer is B. Hemoglobin in the circulation is normally found in several forms, including oxyhemoglobin, deoxyhemoglobin, carboxyhemoglobin, and methemoglobin. Each of these compounds has a separate peak absorbance and is therefore measured spectrophotometrically at different wavelengths. Conversion of these forms of hemoglobin to methemoglobin (oxidation of the $Fe^{+2} \rightarrow Fe^{+3}$) and reaction of the methemoglobin with NaCN to form cyanmethemoglobin (hemiglobincyanide) results in a stable compound that can be measured spectrophotometrically at 540nm. The only form of hemoglobin found in the circulation that will not form cyanmethemoglobin is sulfhemoglobin which, except in rare cases, is present only in very small amounts. (Lotspeich-Steininger et al., p. 108)

2. The "rule of three" means that the

A. MCV is three times the MCH
B. RBC count is three times the Hb
C. HCT is three times the MCH
D. HCT is three times the Hb

The answer is D. In the healthy individual, the hematocrit in percent is roughly three times the hemoglobin value in g/dL, which is, in turn, roughly three times the RBC count (ignoring the power of 10). This "rule of three" can be used to evaluate the probable acceptance of CBC results quickly. If the rule of three does not apply to a given sample, it can indicate a patient abnormality or an error in sample collection or testing. (Lotspeich-Steininger et al., p. 108)

3. Which of the following will result in a falsely decreased erythrocyte sedimentation rate (ESR)?

A. Presence of codocytes
B. Inflammatory reaction

C. Marked anemia

D. Slight tilting of the sedimentation rate tube

The answer is A. The process of red-cell sedimentation in the Wintrobe or Westergren tube requires rouleaux formation as the first step. Any condition or event that interferes with rouleauxing of red blood cells will result in a falsely decreased ESR value. The presence of codocytes or target cells impairs rouleaux formation. Severe anemia and any tilting of the tube during the test will result in a falsely elevated sedimentation rate value. The presence of an inflammatory state will cause a true increase in the value. (Lotspeich-Steininger et al., pp. 118–119)

4. One hundred fifty three nucleated RBCs are reported on a 100 cell differential. The uncorrected WBC count is 11.9×10^9/L. The corrected WBC count $\times 10^9$/L is:

A. 3.6

B. 4.7

C. 5.2

D. 8.0

The answer is B. The methods used to count WBCs will include any nucleated cells in that total. The following formula is used to correct the WBC count for the presence of nucleated RBCs in the peripheral blood:

$$WBC_{corr} = \frac{WBC}{100 + No.\ NRBC/100\ WBC} \times 100$$

$$WBC_{corr} = \frac{11.9 \times 10^9/L \times 100}{253}$$

(Lotspeich-Steininger et al., p. 311)

5. After staining a peripheral blood smear with Wright's stain and a buffer with the correct pH, the RBCs appear pale pink and the WBCs stain very weakly with little-to-no nuclear detail. One possible explanation is

A. the patient is experiencing diabetic alkalosis

B. the smear was stained while still wet

C. there was excessive washing of the smear

D. the slide was not on a flat surface, causing pooling of stain

The answer is C. Excessive washing of the smear will cause the stain to fade. (Brown, 6th ed., p. 101)

6. Given the following data, calculate the manual WBC count for this patient.

Dilution:	1:20
Depth:	0.1 mm
Area counted:	4mm²
Total number of cells counted:	120

A. 600/μL
B. 6,000/μL
C. 60,000/μL
D. 600,000/μL

The answer is B. The formula for a manual cell count is

$$\text{cells}/\mu L = \frac{\text{no. of cells counted} \times \text{dilution reciprocal} \times \text{depth conversion}}{\text{area counted}}$$

$$\text{cells}/\mu L = \frac{120 \times 20 \times 10}{4}$$

(Brown, 6th ed., p. 94)

7. Which of the following conditions would introduce a source of error into a manual WBC count?

A. Uneven distribution of leukocytes in the counting chamber
B. Immediate counting of cells
C. A sample with an extremely low WBC count
D. Using a 2% (vol/vol) solution of acetic acid as the diluting fluid

The answer is A. Erroneous results can be due to contaminated diluting fluid, incorrect diluting or loading of the hemocytometer, and an uneven distribution of leukocytes in the counting chamber. (Turgeon, pp. 354–355)

8. False-positive results may occur in the screening solubility test for hemo-globin S due to

A. decreased plasma proteins
B. hypolipidemia
C. adding more blood to the reagent than called for by test procedure
D. a hemoglobin value of less than 9 g/dL

The answer is C. Positive results in a screening solubility test for hemoglobin S are dependent on the relative insolubility of hemoglobin S, which creates a turbid solution. False-positive results in the screening solubility test for hemoglobin S may be caused by anything that increases that turbidity. Too much whole blood increases the potential for turbidity, as does the presence of excess plasma proteins or lipids. (Lotspeich-Steininger et al., p. 190)

9. After a gentle inversion of tube no. 1 of a freshly collected cerebrospinal fluid specimen, the specimen appeared slightly turbid (1+) and pale yellow. After centrifugation, the supernatant was clear and yellow. Which of the following statements is correct?

A. Methemoglobin is present
B. A traumatic tap has occurred
C. Free hemoglobin is present
D. Pathologic bleeding has occurred

The answer is D. If methemoglobin is present, the supernatant is brown. The supernatant is colorless after a traumatic tap, and a recent hemorrhage into the subarachnoid space will result in hemolysis and the release of free hemoglobin; as a result, the supernatant will be pinkish. Xanthochromia, or a yellow color, results from the breakdown of hemoglobin into bilirubin. It suggests bleeding into the subarachnoid space within the last two to three weeks. (Lotspeich-Steininger et al., p. 396)

10. The traditional diluent of choice for quantifying spermatozoa in seminal fluid contains

    A. sodium bicarbonate and formalin
    B. methylene blue
    C. dilute acetic acid
    D. normal saline

The answer is A. Formalin preserves and immobilizes spermatozoa so counting is more accurate. Stain is necessary when evaluating morphology. It is not recommended to evaluate morphology in a hemocytometer chamber. Dilute acetic acid is used to lyse red blood cells, which are not normally found in seminal fluid. Normal saline will simply dilute the fluid and will not immobilize spermatozoa, thus decreasing the accuracy of the count. (Strasinger, p. 163)

11. The following erythrocyte indices are obtained for a specimen:

MCV: 88 fL
MCH: 30 pg
MCHC: 34 g/dL

These erythrocytes on a Wright-stained smear should appear

    A. hypochromic, microcytic
    B. normochromic, microcytic
    C. normochromic, normocytic
    D. hypochromic, normocytic

The answer is C. The MCV, MCH, and MCHC are all within reference ranges; therefore, the erythrocytes are normal-sized with normal concentrations of hemoglobin. (Harmening, p. 57)

12. An increase in metamyelocytes, myelocytes, and promyelocytes in the peripheral blood can be referred to as

    A. Pelger-Huët anomaly
    B. a shift to the left
    C. agranulocytosis
    D. leukocytosis

The answer is B. A shift to the left means there is an increase in immature granulocytes (metamyelocytes, myelocyte, promyelocytes, and blasts). Pelger-Huët anomaly is an inherited condition in which hyposegmentation of the polymorphonuclear granulocyte's nucleus occurs. Agranulocytosis is the decrease or absence of granulocytes in either the bone marrow or peripheral blood. Leukocytosis is a general term referring to an increase of WBCs in the peripheral blood. (Harmening, p. 73)

13. Only 2.0 mL of blood is collected in a vacuum tube containing powdered EDTA that is designed for a 7.0 mL draw. Which of the following test results can be expected if this sample is used?

    A. Falsely lowered RBC count
    B. Falsely elevated hemoglobin
    C. Erroneously decreased hematocrit
    D. ESR of expected value

The answer is C. Since excessive anticoagulant causes shrinkage of red cells, the ESR and microhematocrit are affected. The number of red cells is not altered, nor is the amount of hemoglobin. Note that the calculated hematocrit as determined by electrical impedance instruments does not reflect this morphologic change. (Brown, 6th ed., p. 8)

14. The following values were plotted during the first six days of a new lot of control for leukocyte determination using an electronic particle counter:

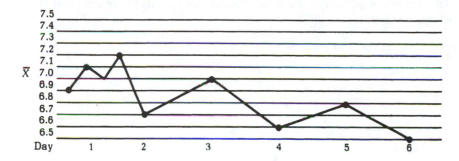

The coefficient of variation (CV) is 3.5%. Assume that these results are representative of the laboratory's usual performance of leukocyte count in the normal and low ranges. Evaluation of the statistical pattern and the coefficient of variation indicates that

    A. corrective action is unnecessary since the CV and plotted data are acceptable
    B. a dilutor check is necessary
    C. the control may be deteriorating
    D. calculation of a new mean and standard deviation is necessary

The answer is C. Continuously increasing variance in one direction points to a segment, control-sample, or instrument problem. If the drift were upward, one would suspect a dilutor error. In this instance, the drift is downward; therefore, the more likely factor is a deterioration of the control. Other possibilities are reagent deterioration and an electronic problem with the counting instrument. (Brown, 6th ed., p. 26)

15. While performing a WBC differential count on a capillary blood smear no platelets were observed. What action should be taken?

    A. Report the finding to your supervisor immediately
    B. Request a venous sample for an absolute platelet count
    C. Look at the edge of the smear for platelet clumping
    D. Report out the absence of platelets

The answer is C. Because of the nature of platelets, slides not prepared immediately after a capillary puncture may have excessive platelet clumping along the tail and margins of the stained slide. Slides with excessive clumping cannot be properly evaluated for platelet numbers and should be remade. (Henry, p. 597)

16. A patient's hemoglobin level is 12.3 g/dL. The erythrocytes appear normochromic on the Wright-stained smear. The hematocrit value that correlates with these data is

   A. 0.34 L/L
   B. 0.37 L/L
   C. 0.40 L/L
   D. 0.43 L/L

The answer is B. When RBCs are normochromic, an "average" MCHC of 33.3% can be inserted in the formula, which then can be solved for the Hct. This relation holds only if the RBCs are normochromic (have a normal MCHC of approximately 33–34%).

$$MCHC = \frac{Hb \times 100}{Hct}$$

$$MCHC = \frac{12.3 \times 100}{x}$$

$$33.3x = 12.3 \times 100$$
$$x = 0.369 \text{ or } 0.37$$

(Brown, p. 106)

17. A falsely elevated hematocrit is obtained on a defective centrifuge. Which of the following values will *not* be affected?

   A. MCH
   B. MCV
   C. MCHC
   D. All of the above

The answer is A. The MCV and MCHC use the hematocrit in their calculation. Therefore, only the MCH that uses Hb and RBC count would be unaffected by a falsely elevated hematocrit. (Brown, 6th ed., p. 106)

18. A patient's hematologic results from an electrical impedance instrument are

   WBC: 2.0×10^9/L
   RBC: 3.83×10^{12}/L
   Hb: 11.5g/dL
   Hct: 0.34 L/L
   PLT: 60.0×10^9/L

Blood-smear evaluation for quality-control purposes reveals acceptable cell distribution; normochromic, normocytic RBCs; 2 leukocytes per 40X field; and 10 platelets per oil-immersion field. The next step would be

A. report the results as obtained
B. repeat the leukocyte count
C. repeat the platelet count
D. repeat the RBC count

The answer is C. In general, one platelet per oil-immersion field is equal to 10,000–40,000/microliter (10–40 × 10^9/L). Therefore, this patient's platelet count would be expected to be greater than 100 × 10^9/L and should be repeated. All other data are compatible. (Brown, 6th ed., p. 104)

19. What effect would the use of a buffer with a pH of 6.0 have on a Wright-stained smear?

A. RBCs would be too pink
B. WBCs would be well differentiated
C. RBCs would be too blue
D. RBCs would lyse

The answer is A. The pH of the buffer is critical in a Romanowsky (Wright) stain. When the pH is too low (usual range is 6.4–6.7), the red cells take up more acid dye (eosin) and become too pink. Also, the white cells do not differentiate well, giving poor nuclear detail. (Brown, 6th ed., p. 101)

20. Which of the following red-cell inclusions can be detected with a supravital preparation that uses new methylene-blue N as the dye reagent but are not visible with Romanowsky stain?

A. Howell-Jolly bodies
B. Heinz bodies
C. Malarial trophozoites
D. Siderotic granules (Pappenheimer bodies)

The answer is B. There are only a few red-cell inclusions that cannot be seen on a Romanowsky stain. Heinz bodies, since they are composed of precipitated globin, have the same net charges as nonprecipitated globin and therefore are not visible with a stain based on acid-base principles. (Brown, 6th ed., p. 115)

21. Which of the following contain RNA and are usually identified by staining with brilliant cresyl blue or new methylene blue?

A. Heinz bodies
B. Reticulocytes
C. Siderotic granules
D. Howell-Jolly bodies

The answer is B. Brilliant cresyl blue and new methylene blue precipitate erythrocyte ribosomes into a network so that reticulocytes can be distinguished from cells containing Heinz bodies, Pappenheimer bodies, or Howell-Jolly bodies. (Brown, 6th ed., p. 113)

22. A manual hemoglobin determination using the cyanmethemoglobin reagent is performed on a known sickle-cell patient's whole blood. The blood/reagent mixture appears cloudy. The correct procedure is to

A. report the result as greater than 20 g/dL
B. allow the mixture to stand for at least 10 more minutes
C. recollect the specimen, making sure that there is a proper ratio of anticoagulant to whole blood
D. redilute the blood/reagent mixture using a 1 : 1 dilution with distilled water, determine the new value, and multiply the result by two

The answer is D. The blood/reagent mixture must be crystal clear prior to reading in the spectrophotometer. In situations of suspected hemoglobinopathies such as S or C, dilution with distilled water clarifies the solution and allows for accurate readings. Since the mixture has experienced an additional dilution, the value must be multiplied by 2. (Brown, 6th ed., p. 84)

23. The leukocyte count for a patient is 28.0×10^9/L. The differential shows 58 orthochromatic normoblasts and 10 polychromatophilic normoblasts per 100 WBCs. The leukocyte count is closest to

A. 2.8×10^9/L
B. 16.7×10^9/L
C. 17.7×10^9/L
D. 28.0×10^9/L

The answer is B.

$$\frac{\text{Uncorrected WBC} \times 100}{100 + \text{nucleated RBC}} = \text{corrected WBC}$$

$$\frac{28.0 \times 10^9 \times 100}{100 + 58 + 10} = \frac{2800 \times 10^9}{168} = 16.7 \times 10^9/\text{L}$$

(Lotspeich-Steininger et al., p. 311)

24. Using the estimated mean and standard deviation from the previous month, the following results were obtained the first two days new controls were used.

Instrument: particle counter
Dilutor: automatic

Assay values (published)

Normal WBC: 8.2 ± 0.6
Abnormal WBC: 15.5 ± 0.9
Normal RBC: 4.58 ± 0.09
Abnormal RBC: 1.54 ± 0.12

Laboratory Values

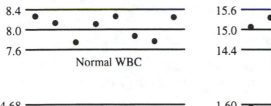

Normal WBC

Abnormal WBC

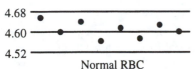

Normal RBC

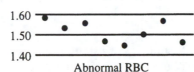

Abnormal RBC

A possible source of error is

A. poor mixing of controls
B. no obvious errors indicated
C. lysing agent expired
D. diluent contaminated with bacteria

The answer is B. Standard quality-control limits are $\pm$ 2 SDs. Since all the results fall within the accepted published range, no obvious error is present. No trends are represented in the data. Poor mixing would produce data that had a trend, and expired lysing reagent would tend to increase the WBC determinations. Diluent contamination would affect both WBC and RBC determinations, with an upward trend as bacterial growth increased. (Henry, p. 91)

25. The leukocyte count for an adult patient is 18.0×10^9/L. The differential shows

polymorphonuclear neutrophils:	56%
band neutrophils:	5%
lymphocytes:	25%
monocytes:	10%
eosinophils:	3%
basophils:	1%

The above data reveal an absolute increase in

A. polymorphonuclear and band neutrophils
B. lymphocytes and monocytes
C. monocytes and polymorphonuclear neutrophils
D. eosinophils and basophils

The answer is C. Absolute cell count = number of cells in percent $\times$ total WBC count. Although the percentages for polymorphonuclear neutrophils and monocytes fall within the normal range, these forms are increased in absolute numbers because the total count is increased. (Lotspeich-Steininger et al., p. 328)

26. Below are hematologic anticoagulants and corresponding characteristics of each. Select the one anticoagulant that does *not* match its characteristic.

A. Dipotassium EDTA—prevents platelet clumping
B. Sodium citrate—used for routine coagulation studies
C. Heparin—suitable for blood smears
D. Double oxalate—produces morphologic artifacts

The answer is C. Heparin is not suitable for blood smears because it gives a bluish background on Romanowsky-stained smears. (Lotspeich-Steininger et al., p. 18)

27. A student consistently makes peripheral blood smears that are too thin. You instruct the student to try

A. using a smaller drop of blood
B. using only capillary blood
C. increasing the angle of the spreader slide
D. applying more pressure on the spreader slide

The answer is C. Increasing the angle of the spreader slide results in a thicker smear. Using a smaller drop of blood or applying pressure can result in a thinner smear. Both capillary and anticoagulated blood should render equally satisfactory smears if other factors are correct, such as the angle of the spreader slide and the size of the drop of blood. (Lotspeich-Steininger et al., p. 23)

28. The most reliable criterion used to determine the maturity of a Wright-stained blood cell is the

A. size of the nucleus
B. color of the nucleus
C. nucleus-to-cytoplasm ratio
D. structure of the nuclear chromatin

The answer is D. The maturation stage of blood cells can best be determined by evaluation of the nuclear chromatin structure or pattern. The chromatin-pattern changes are more consistent. Size or color variables can be affected by slide preparation, quality of stain, and staining techniques. (Brown, 6th ed., p. 59)

29. Which characteristic differentiates the myelocyte from other myelocytic cells?

A. A kidney-bean–shaped nucleus
B. Presence of coarse nuclear chromatin
C. Presence of nucleoli
D. Appearance of specific granules

The answer is D. Identification of the myelocyte depends on noting the first appearance of specific granules. Other morphologic features that are helpful include the fine texture of the nuclear chromatin, absence of nucleoli, and lack of indentation in the nucleus. (Brown, 6th ed., p. 59)

30. Hematologic testing on an adult patient provides the following data.

Hb: 7.5 g/dL
Hct: 0.26 L/L

WBC: 14.6 × 10⁹/L
  neutrophils   80%
  lymphocytes   17%
  monocytes   3%

These results would best correlate with

A. normochromic RBCs, relative lymphocytopenia
B. hypochromic RBCs, absolute lymphocytopenia
C. normochromic RBCs, absolute lymphocytopenia
D. hypochromic RBCs, relative lymphocytopenia

The answer is D. The MCHC is 28.9%, which is below normal (32–25%). To determine whether the lymphocytopenia is absolute or relative, one must determine the actual number of lymphocytes per liter: 17% of 14.6×10^9/L is 2.5×10^9/L. The reference range for lymphocytes in the adult patient is $1.5 - 4.5 \times 10^9$/L. (Brown, 6th ed., p. 104)

31. Vigorous mixing of a whole-blood specimen collected with powdered EDTA as the anticoagulant results in

A. an acceptable specimen for routine hematologic tests
B. an acceptable specimen for special tests, such as leukocyte alkaline phosphatase
C. a falsely elevated WBC count
D. a falsely decreased hematocrit

The answer is D. If anticoagulated blood is mixed too vigorously, red cells will be lysed by the force of the mixing and hemolysis will result. The degree of hemolysis is directly proportional to the number of red cells lysed, and a falsely lowered hematocrit will result. (Lotspeich-Steininger et al., p. 112)

32. A clinical laboratory technician is reviewing a smear for quality-control purposes. The smear is wedge-shaped with smooth edges and extends over approximately 60% of the surface of the slide. On low-power (10×) examination, it is noted that granulocytes are clustered at the tail of the smear. On high (40×) magnification, the RBCs appear a buff pink. White cell nuclei appear dark blue to purple. This evaluation indicates that the smear is

A. acceptable
B. unacceptable because the smear is too long
C. unacceptable because the white cells are clustered at the tail
D. acceptable even though the RBCs are stained lightly

The answer is C. The smear should cover at least half the slide, and the edges should be smooth without any scratches or erratic areas. The quality of stain at the levels of magnification noted is acceptable. White blood cells should be evenly distributed throughout the body of the smear and not clustered at the edge. (Brown, p. 13)

33. A patient is admitted to the hospital with a tentative diagnosis of chronic lymphocytic leukemia. The WBC count is 250×10^9/L. One parameter that may be falsely elevated by this WBC count is the

A. hemoglobin
B. MCV
C. platelet count
D. reticulocyte count

The answer is A. Elevated WBC counts cause turbidity in the solution when whole blood is diluted with HiCN reagent whether this occurs in the manual procedure or in an automated instrument. This turbidity will effect the absorbance reading, and the dilution must be centrifuged prior to reading. (Brown, 6th ed., p. 84)

34. A positive sickle-cell screening using the protein-solubility method means that

A. the patient has a genotype of hemoglobin SS
B. the patient has a genotype of hemoglobin AS
C. hemoglobins D, Barts, or S may be present
D. hemoglobin S or C is definitely present

The answer is C. A protein-solubility screening test indicates the presence of any sickling hemoglobin or hemoglobin that is not soluble in dithionite. These hemoglobins include, but are not limited to, S, D, Barts, and some C. (Brown, 6th ed., p. 123)

35. During the examination of a cerebrospinal-fluid specimen from a 45-year-old man, the clinical laboratory technician noted the presence of rare choroid plexus cells in a total WBC count of 6/μL. These results are indicative of

A. malignant disease
B. inflammatory disease
C. degenerative disease
D. normal state

The answer is D. The total number of WBCs counted is within the standard reference ranges. Choroid plexus cells make up part of the lining of the cerebrospinal space. They will be found in both normal and abnormal cerebrospinal fluids and, since they were seen in a patient with a normal WBC count, can be presumed to be part of the normal shedding of these cells into the CSF. (Lotspeich-Steininger et al., pp. 397–399)

CLT Review Questions—Hemostasis

1. Oral anticoagulants such as coumarins

A. prolong the prothrombin time
B. act in the peripheral blood to decrease factor activity
C. prolong the APTT
D. are neutralized by protamine sulfate

The answer is A. The administration of coumarin interferes with the synthesis of factors II, VII, IX, and X in the liver by interfering with the utilization of vitamin K. The prothrombin time is prolonged since it is sensitive to the presence of three out of four Vitamin-K–dependent factors (II, VII, and X). (Brown, 6th ed., p. 216)

2. The following results were obtained for a patient:

Test	Results (sec)	Control (sec)
PT	25	12
APTT	80	32.5
thrombin time	10	12

The APTT and PT are both corrected with normal serum but not with adsorbed plasma. Select the factor deficiency that most likely is responsible for these results.

A. I
B. II
C. V
D. X

The answer is D. Normal serum contains factors IX, X, XI, and XII. Adsorbed plasma contains factors I, V, VII, XI, and XII. Correction of both tests by serum but not by adsorbed plasma suggests a deficiency in factor X. (Brown, 6th ed., pp. 225, 278)

3. All of the following conditions cause an increased (prolonged) thrombin time *except*

A. hypofibrinogenemia
B. increased fibrin-degradation products
C. heparin therapy
D. decreased prothrombin

The answer is D. Fibrin-degradation products interfere with the polymerization of fibrin, heparin acts along with antithrombin III to neutralize thrombin, and decreased fibrinogen levels result in prolonged thrombin times. (Brown, 6th ed., p. 222)

4. Plasma is diluted in a fibrinogen-activity determination to decrease the

A. amount of thrombin necessary
B. influence of inhibitors
C. amount of calcium needed
D. effect of deficiencies in other coagulation factors

The answer is B. Dilution of the plasma in this procedure produces an excess of thrombin, thus nullifying the effect of inhibitors and making fibrinogen the rate-limiting factor. (Brown, 6th ed., p. 229)

5. The quality-control data for normal and abnormal platelet controls have been acceptable for the last six days. A new lot number of normal control is run in parallel to the old lot number. What should be done with the following data?

	Results	Package insert acceptable range
Old lot number	$150 \times 10^9/L$	$140 \times 10^9/L \pm 30 \times 10^9/L$
New lot number	$160 \times 10^9/L$	$200 \times 10^9/L \pm 30 \times 10^9/L$

A. Use the acceptable range of the old lot number
B. Adjust the acceptable range to include the reading of $160.0 \times 10^9/L$
C. Rerun the new lot number; then run a new vial of control, if necessary
D. Recalibrate the instrument

The answer is C. The instrument should not be recalibrated nor the acceptable range adjusted until the new lot number of control has been thoroughly evaluated by rerunning the new control on a new vial. If the results are still out of range, check with the manufacturer for possible mislabeling of the control value. (Brown, 6th ed., p. 22)

6. A blood specimen for coagulation studies must be centrifuged

A. for no more than 5 minutes
B. with the cap on
C. after having been checked for any clotting
D. twice: once at 10,000 rpm for 10 minutes, then at 15,000 rpm for 5 additional minutes

The answer is B. The sample should be centrifuged with the cap on to prevent loss of CO_2 and alteration of pH. After centrifugation and drawing off the plasma, the remaining material should be checked for clots. Centrifugation requires only 15 minutes at $2,500 \times g$. (Brown, 6th ed., pp. 212–214)

7. Thawing of platelet-poor plasma that has been stored at $-40°C$ for coagulation studies should be performed at

A. 0–4°C
B. 4–8°C
C. 10–20°C
D. 35–38°C

The answer is D. Thawing of freshly frozen plasma for use in coagulation studies should be performed as rapidly as possible without damage to the proteins. 37°C is the preferred temperature. (Brown, 6th ed., p. 214)

8. A sample of whole blood drawn into a sodium citrate tube is evaluated for appropriateness of content. Approximately 90% of the expected amount of blood is seen. The specimen should be deemed

A. unacceptable
B. acceptable for platelet studies but not for some coagulation studies
C. acceptable for coagulation studies but not for platelet studies
D. acceptable for both coagulation studies and some platelet studies

The answer is D. Coagulation specimens are deemed acceptable if the blood drawn into the tube is at least 90% of the potential volume. The use of citrate as an anticoagulant is appropriate for both coagulation studies and for certain platelet studies such as platelet counts (with dilutional correction) and platelet aggregation. (Brown, 6th ed., pp. 212–214)

9. A clinical laboratory technician notes that a specimen for an APTT has been stored at room temperature for three hours prior to testing. The CLT should

    A. perform the APTT and report the results
    B. perform the APTT and report the results, noting the delay in processing
    C. dilute the sample 1:1 with buffered saline to correct the pH and perform the APTT
    D. request a new sample

The answer is D. Samples for APTT should be held at room temperature for no more than two hours. If longer delays are anticipated, the sample should be stored on ice. (Brown, 6th ed., pp. 212–214)

10. A patient with severe disseminated intravascular coagulation has an FDP result of greater than 200 μg/dL and a clottable fibrinogen value of 50 mg/dL. The fibrinogen level may have been affected by

    A. the presence of excess thrombin in the system
    B. the use of fibrinogen in the DIC process
    C. interference in the test caused by elevated fibrin-degradation products
    D. the semiquantitative nature of the test procedure

The answer is C. The presence of significantly high levels of fibrin-degradation products (>100μg/dL) will interfere with the test and cause a falsely decreased result. (Brown, 6th ed., p. 229)

11. A new lot of controls for prothrombin time has a mean of 12.2 sec with an SD of 0.4 sec. Which of the following control results would *not* be acceptable?

    A. 11.1 sec
    B. 11.5 sec
    C. 12.3 sec
    D. 12.6 sec

The answer is A. Controls ranges are generally given as ± 2 SD values or, in this case, from 11.4 to 13.0 sec. (Brown, 6th ed., p. 23)

12. An upward trend was observed over a six day period in a quality control plot for a prothrombin time procedure performed on an photo-optical instrument. This observation indicates

    A. a decrease in standard deviation values and thus a change in the reference range for the procedure
    B. a loss of precision
    C. a decreased coefficient of variation
    D. a loss of accuracy but not precision

The answer is B. Shifts, trends and increased scatter on a quality control plot all indicate a loss of precision with an increase in standard deviation and coefficient of variation. Reference values should not be altered unless there is a change in test method or principle.

13. A specimen is being tested from a patient with severe jaundice. The prothrombin time performed on an electro-optical instrument is 7.4 sec (control 12.0 sec). The clinical laboratory technician should

   A. request a new sample, drawn preferably as a microsample
   B. dilute the sample 1 : 1 and rerun the sample multiplying the result by 2
   C. perform the test on an electromechanical instrument
   D. put a patient blank prior to the patient's sample in the electro-optical instrument

The answer is C. The patient's jaundice may be causing the electro-optical instrument to report a false value. Repeating the procedure using a mechanical instrument will allow for an accurate result. (Lotspeich-Steininger et al., pp. 696–698)

14. A patient with an increased concentration of cryoglobulin is to be evaluated for a bleeding disorder. Which of the following instruments would be most likely to produce an accurate test result?

   A. Photo-optical instruments
   B. Electromechanical instruments
   C. Instruments that use chromogenic substrates
   D. Platelet aggregometry

The answer is B. Photo-optical instruments are more sensitive to the increased presence of certain substances than the electromechanical instruments. These include cryoglobulin, bilirubin, and hyperlipidemia. Instrument using chromogenic substrates are photo-optical as are platelet aggregometers. (Lotspeich-Steininger et al., pp. 696–698)

15. When operating an electromechanical-coagulation instrument for prothrombin-time tests, it is important to allow the patient samples to incubate at 37°C for

   A. at least 3 minutes but not longer than 10 minutes
   B. at least 5 minutes but not longer than 15 minutes
   C. at least 10 minutes but not longer than 20 minutes
   D. at least 15 minutes but not longer than 30 minutes

The answer is A. Samples must be incubated from 3 to 5 minutes for optimal results but not longer than 10 minutes. (Harmening, p. 595)

CLS Review Questions—Hematology

1. As the supervisory clinical laboratory scientist, you are asked to review a Wright-stained peripheral blood smear that shows clumping of leukocytes and platelets. Which of the following is the most probable cause for these morphologic changes?

   A. Smear was made from 1h-old heparinized blood
   B. Smear was made from 1h-old EDTA blood
   C. Excessive pressure was applied when making the smear from blood in the tip of a venipuncture needle
   D. Smear was made using fresh capillary blood

The answer is A. The effect of heparin on RBC morphology is negligible, but clumping of both leukocytes and platelets is seen. Nonanticoagulated blood will show no visible leukocyte artifacts, although platelet clumping is seen. (Brown, 6th ed., p. 13)

2. An EDTA-anticoagulated tube is received in the laboratory only partially filled, causing excessive concentration of EDTA. Since the patient was undergoing an MRI and would not be available to provide another specimen for an hour, the physician requested that the laboratory perform any test that would be reliable. Which of the following procedures would be accurate on this sample?

   A. Platelet count
   B. Hemoglobin
   C. Peripheral blood smear
   D. Spun hematocrit

The answer is B. Excessive EDTA causes RBCs to shrink, resulting in a decreased spun hematocrit, MCHC, and ESR. It also causes platelets to break up, falsely increasing the platelet count. Degenerative changes will occur in the WBCs, causing difficulty in interpreting a peripheral blood smear. The hemoglobin, however, is unaffected, since cells are hemolyzed in the reaction process. (Brown, 6th ed., p. 12)

3. Which of the following is appropriate in preparing an EDTA-anticoagulated specimen for analysis when it has been standing in a rack and not on a mechanical rotator?

   A. Shake vigorously by hand
   B. Invert gently at least 60 times
   C. Mix for a minimum of two minutes using a vortex mixer
   D. Invert 4–6 times

The answer is B. Inverting gently a minimum of 60 times by hand will ensure adequate mixing. An alternative is to place the specimen on a mechanical rotator for two minutes. Vigorous mixing or use of a vortex will hemolyze the cells and invalidate the results. (Henry, p. 555)

4. A patient has a hematocrit of 0.15 L/L. In order to obtain an acceptable wedge peripheral-blood smear, the clinical laboratory scientist should make the following adjustment:

   A. Use a hemocytometer cover glass as the spreader slide
   B. Push the spreader slide 50% slower than usual
   C. Permit some of the blood to get in front of the spreader slide
   D. Increase the angle of the spreader slide greater than 45°

The answer is D. When a specimen has a very low hematocrit, increasing the angle of the spreader slide higher than the normally recommended 30–45° results in a thicker smear. (Brown, 6th ed., p. 99)

5. When performing a manual differential on a Wright-stained blood smear, the clinical laboratory scientist noted a purplish black precipitate over the slide. One cause of this precipitate is

A. precipitation of paraproteins from the patient's blood
B. insufficient rinsing of the stain and buffer mixture
C. insufficient aging of the Wright's stain before use
D. failure to remove stain from the back of the slide

The answer is B. When the stain and buffer mixture is not completely rinsed from the slide, the stain may precipitate on the dried smear. One way to redissolve the precipitate is to cover the slide with Wright's stain for 5–10 seconds and flush with deionized or distilled water. (Lotspeich-Steininger, p. 35)

6. An automated platelet count performed on a venous blood specimen collected in EDTA is $40 \times 10^9/L$. The clinical laboratory scientist notes platelet clumps on the Wright-stained blood smear. The CLS should

A. perform a manual platelet count using the same specimen
B. redraw the specimen in sodium oxalate and repeat the count
C. redraw the specimen in sodium citrate and repeat the count
D. inform the physician that an accurate platelet count cannot be obtained on the patient

The answer is C. In-vitro platelet aggregation in EDTA-anticoagulated blood is the most common cause of a spuriously low platelet count. The large platelet aggregates may be counted as leukocytes by the instrument, resulting in a low platelet count. It is thought that platelet-specific antibodies that react only in EDTA and react best at room temperature cause the agglutination. When platelet clumping is suspected, the specimen should be redrawn and the count repeated using sodium citrate as the anticoagulant. (McKenzie, pp. 431–432)

7. A patient who underwent a bone-marrow transplant had daily leukocyte counts performed. Laboratory policy required that counts below $2.0 \times 10^9/L$ be performed manually. Since transplant patients usually have decreased counts, the laboratory scientist prepared a standard WBC Unopette (self-contained diluting device) resulting in a 1 : 20 dilution. Eighty-four leukocytes were counted in the entire area on both sides of the Neubauer hemocytometer. How should the leukocyte count be reported?

A. $0.4 \times 10^9/L$
B. $0.8 \times 10^9/L$
C. $0.9 \times 10^9/L$
D. $1.9 \times 10^9/L$

The answer is C. The entire area on both sides of the hemocytometer is $9mm^2 \times 2 = 18mm^2$. The depth of the hemocytometer is 0.1mm. The formula for cell counts using the Neubauer hemocytometer is

$$\frac{\text{no. of cells counted}}{\text{area} \times \text{depth}} \times \text{dilution factor} = \text{cells/mm}^3 \text{ or cells} \times 10^9/L$$

$$\frac{84}{18 \times 0.1} \times 20 = 933 \text{ cells/mm}^3 \text{ or } 0.9 \times 10^9/L$$

(Lotspeich-Steininger, 1st ed., p. 322)

8. A new clinical laboratory scientist in a hematology/oncology clinic consistently reads microhematocrit-control and patient values higher than co-workers do. Which of the following actions of the CLS could explain this discrepancy?

   A. Buffy coat is not being included
   B. Time of centrifugation is too long
   C. Speed of centrifugation is too high
   D. Microhematocrit tubes are allowed to sit and are not read within a few minutes of centrifugation

The answer is D. Allowing microhematocrit tubes to sit in the horizontal position longer than a few minutes after centrifugation may yield falsely elevated results. Answers A, B, and C would not result in elevated results. (Brown, 6th ed., p. 87)

9. An EDTA specimen from a known sickle-cell anemia patient is received for a microhematocrit and a hemoglobin determination using the cyan-methemoglobin principle. Values obtained are a hemoglobin of 10.7 g/dL and a hematocrit of 0.22 L/L. The CLS should

   A. centrifuge the hemoglobin and read the supernatant as the test sample
   B. mix the hemoglobin dilution 1 : 1 with distilled water, then read and multiply the results by 2
   C. repeat the hematocrit using heparinized hematocrit tubes
   D. repeat the procedure and, if similar results are obtained, report them immediately

The answer is B. Hemoglobins S and C can cause turbidity in the hemoglobin solution, causing falsely elevated results. The test sample can be cleared by diluting 1 : 1 with distilled water and multiplying the resultant value by 2. (Harmening, p. 535)

10. A hemoglobin value of 12.5 g/dL best correlates with a hematocrit value of

   A. 0.253 L/L
   B. 0.335 L/L
   C. 0.375 L/L
   D. 0.428 L/L

The answer is C. The mean corpuscular hemoglobin concentration in a normochromic cell is approximately one-third of the cell volume. Therefore, the hemoglobin will be approximately one-third of the packed-cell volume. (Lotspeich-Steininger et al., pp. 112–113)

11. A patient has an RBC count of $2.70 \times 10^{12}/L$, a hemoglobin of 5.5 g/dL, and a hematocrit of 0.19 L/L. What erythrocyte morphology would you expect to see on the peripheral blood smear?

   A. Microcytic, hypochromic cells
   B. Macrocytic, hypochromic cells
   C. Normocytic, hyperchromic cells
   D. Normocytic, normochromic cells

The answer is A. The formula for calculating the mean corpuscular volume (MCV) is

$$\frac{\text{Hct} \times 10}{\text{RBC}}$$

$$\text{MCV} = \frac{19 \times 10}{2.70} = 70.3 \text{ fL}$$

The normal range of the MCV is approximately 80–100 fL. An MCV of 70 fL indicates that the erythrocytes are smaller than normal, i.e., microcytic. The formula for calculating the mean cell hemoglobin concentration (MCHC) is

$$\frac{\text{Hgb}}{\text{Hct}} \times 100$$

$$\text{MCHC} = \frac{5.5}{19} \times 100 = 28.9 \text{ g/dL}$$

The normal range of the MCHC is approximately 32–36 g/dL. Values below 32.0 g/dL indicate hypochromia. (Harmening, p. 57)

12. When reviewing a peripheral blood smear, the clinical laboratory scientist notes many macrocytes. The MCV has been reported as 85 fL. This apparent discrepancy may indicate that

A. the smear was made from the wrong sample
B. the smear should be closely checked for spherocytes
C. the patient may have a hemolytic anemia
D. cold agglutinins may be present

The answer is A. When many macrocytes are seen on a blood smear, one would expect to see an MCV close to or above 100 fL. Although an MCV of 85 fL would be possible with spherocytes, the smear would not demonstrate macrocytes. A hemolytic anemia with many reticulocytes could cause a blood smear to appear macrocytic, but the MCV would not be as low as 85 fL. Cold agglutinins cause a falsely increased MCV. When there is lack of correlation between a hemogram and the blood smear, the identification on both the blood smear and the hemogram should be verified. If no laboratory error is discovered, the automated count should be repeated, and the blood smear should be prepared and evaluated again. (Lotspeich-Steininger, p. 559)

13. In the performance of a modified Westergren ESR, what is the recommended dilution?

A. 1 : 2 (1 volume diluent + 1 volume blood)
B. 1 : 3 (1 volume diluent + 2 volumes blood)
C. 1 : 4 (1 volume diluent + 3 volumes blood)
D. 1 : 5 (1 volume diluent + 4 volumes blood)

The answer is D. The modified Westergren ESR uses 4 volumes of whole blood diluted with 1 volume of either 0.109 m trisodium citrate or 0.85% sodium chloride prior to testing (1 : 5 dilution). (Brown, 6th ed., p. 109)

14. A Miller disc is used to perform reticulocyte counts. After counting 500 RBCs in square B, a total of 40 reticulocytes are seen in square A. How should the reticulocyte count be reported?

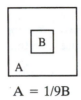

$$A = 1/9B$$

   A. 0.1%
   B. 0.9%
   C. 4.4%
   D. 8.0%

The answer is B. In the calibrated Miller disc, square B is one-ninth of square A. When 500 RBCs are counted in square B, theoretically the number of reticulocytes in 4,500 RBCs have been counted. The percent of reticulocytes is calculated as

$$\text{Reticulocytes (\%)} = \frac{\text{Total reticulocytes in square A}}{\text{Total RBCs in square B} \times 9} \times 100$$

$$\frac{40}{500 \times 9} \times 100 = 0.88 \cong 0.9\%$$

(Lotspeich-Steininger, p. 115)

15. Given the following results on a male patient, what is the reticulocyte-production index?

RBC count:	2.80×10^9/L
Hemoglobin:	9.0 g/dL
Hematocrit:	0.29 L/L
Uncorrected reticulocyte count:	3.0%

   A. 0.1
   B. 1.0
   C. 1.9
   D. 3.0

The answer is B. Reticulocytes normally remain in the peripheral blood approximately one day. When the bone marrow is under stress, as in anemia, reticulocytes may be released into the peripheral blood earlier than normal and thus may spend 2–3 days in the peripheral circulation. The reticulocyte-production index takes this increased circulation time into consideration and is a general indicator of the rate of effective erythropoietic response. Calculation:

$$\text{RPI} = \text{Reticulocytes (\%)}$$

$$\times \frac{\text{patient hematocrit (L/L)/normal hematocrit (0.45)}}{\text{maturation time in peripheral blood}}$$

With a hematocrit of 0.29 the maturation time is 2.0

$$3.0 \times \frac{0.29/0.45}{2.0} = 0.96 \cong 1.0$$

(Lotspeich-Steininger, p. 117)

16. Many schizocytes (schistocytes) are seen on a peripheral blood smear. One of the most common causes for these cells is

A. presence of an abnormal hemoglobin
B. high-titer cold agglutinins
C. deficiency of spectrin
D. microangiopathic anemia

The answer is D. Schizocytes are fragmented RBCs resulting from intravascular fragmentation caused by fibrin in small vessels or small-vessel disease. They may be seen in severe burns, megaloblastic anemia, and microangiopathic hemolytic anemia. (Henry, p. 588)

17. What erythrocyte morphology would be expected on the peripheral blood smear of a 50-year-old alcoholic with advanced cirrhosis?

A. pseudomacrocytosis, acanthocytes, codocytes
B. anisocytosis, microspherocytes, schizocytes
C. macrocytosis, schizocytes, dacryocytes
D. microcytosis, polychromasia, echinocytes

The answer is A. Pseudomacrocytosis is common in cirrhosis. The RBCs appear larger than normal due to an increase in surface area-to-volume ratio, but there is no increase in MCV or MCH. Both acanthocytes and codocytes may be seen in alcoholic cirrhosis as a result of abnormalities in plasma lipids that may alter the lipid composition of the cell membrane. (McKenzie, p. 183)

18. Which of the following procedures is unnecessary to confirm the majority of iron-related anemias?

A. Bone-marrow evaluation
B. Ferritin
C. Red-cell indices including RDW
D. Serum iron and total iron-binding capacity

The answer is A. Iron-related anemias may have numerous causes and can be confused with other diseases such as the thalassemias. It is important to determine the diagnosis and cause with as little trauma and cost to the patient as possible. The above tests can usually provide the necessary information without the need for a bone-marrow aspiration. (Lotspeich-Steininger, pp. 172–177)

19. A patient has a WBC count of 70.0×10^9/L, immature granulocytes, and dacryocytes on the peripheral blood smear. On the differential, 10 cells are seen that have a single nucleus, marked cytoplasmic granularity, and cytoplasmic blebs. What is the most likely identification of these cells?

A. Myelocytes
B. Lymphoblasts

C. Micromegakaryocytes
D. Plasma cells

The answer is C. The cells described are most likely micromegakaryocytes, which may be seen in myeloproliferative disorders (CML, AMM, etc.). (Brown, 6th ed., p. 79)

20. The background of a peripheral blood smear stained with Romanowsky-type stain appears very blue. The RBCs are stacked like coins. Fifteen percent of the WBCs are the size of a small lymphocyte with very blue cytoplasm. The nucleus is eccentric and there is a clear area next to it. These cells should be reported as

    A. nucleated RBCs
    B. blasts
    C. plasma cells
    D. micromegakaryocytes

The answer is C. Plasma cells have an eccentrically placed nucleus and a perinuclear hof. The cytoplasm stains deep blue due to the numerous ribosomes present. Plasma-cell dyscrasias are usually accompanied by increased immunoglobulins, which may cause the entire Romanowsky-stained smear to have a blue background. (Lotspeich-Steininger, p. 311; Brown, p. 325)

21. A hemoglobin electrophoresis pattern on cellulose acetate at pH 8.6 demonstrates a band in the S region. What other laboratory test could be performed to confirm the identity of this hemoglobin?

    A. Alkali denaturation
    B. Hemoglobin electrophoresis on citrate agar, pH 6.0
    C. Hemoglobin solubility
    D. Heat stability

The answer is B. Alkali denaturation is used for the differentiation of Hb F and Hb A, which do not migrate in the Hb S region. Acid electrophoresis is a useful procedure for fractionation of various hemoglobins. At pH 6.0–6.2, it distinguishes Hb S from Hb D. Hemoglobin solubility is a screening procedure for sickling hemoglobins. Heat stability is a nonspecific test for unstable, abnormal hemoglobins. (Lotspeich-Steininger, pp. 192–194)

22. A falsely elevated G-6-PD assay using the fluorescent spot test may be seen in persons with

    A. an increased RBC count
    B. a change in drug dosage
    C. the presence of many reticulocytes
    D. a deficiency of pyruvate kinase

The answer is C. Young RBCs (reticulocytes) produced in response to hemolysis have nearly normal G-6-PD levels. Accurate results may be obtained on patients with increased reticulocytes by centrifuging the specimen and removing the top layer before testing (contains reticulocytes), or by delaying testing for 2–4 months. (Lotspeich-Steininger, pp. 252–253)

23. A sucrose hemolysis screening test was set up as follows:

	Tube 1 (patient)	Tube 2 (control)
10% sucrose solution (mL)	0.85	0
50% suspension of patient RBCs (mL)	0.1	0.1
fresh serum (mL)	0.05	0.05
0.85% NaCl	0	0.85

The percent hemolysis calculated on the supernatant of tube 1 was 20%, and the percent hemolysis calculated on the supernatant of tube 2 was 18%. How should the test be interpreted?

A. A positive result suggests paroxysmal nocturnal hemoglobinuria
B. A negative result eliminates paroxysmal nocturnal hemoglobinuria
C. An invalid result suggests an incompatible serum may have been used. Test should be repeated with compatible serum
D. An invalid result suggests that the complement had been inactivated. Test should be repeated on a fresh serum specimen.

The answer is C. Fresh serum that is ABO blood-group compatible with the patient's RBCs should be used. Red cells in paroxysmal nocturnal hemoglobinuria lyse when suspended in a solution of low ionic strength (sucrose) containing complement. Since the control is positive, this makes the results invalid and suggests that the serum may have been ABO incompatible. (Turgeon, p. 388)

24. A peripheral blood smear contains 80% blast cells, which stain positively with Sudan black B and peroxidase. This result is consistent with a diagnosis of

A. acute lymphoblastic leukemia
B. acute undifferentiated leukemia
C. chronic myelocytic leukemia
D. acute myeloblastic leukemia

The answer is D. Lymphoid cells characteristically do not stain with Sudan black B and peroxidase. Undifferentiated cells have not matured enough to stain positively with either Sudan black B or peroxidase. Chronic myelocytic leukemia does not show 80% blast cells (unless the patient is in myeloblastic crisis). Therefore, this pattern is most consistent with acute myeloblastic leukemia in which blasts stain positively for Sudan black B and peroxidase. (Harmening, pp. 273–274)

25. Which of the following is the best specimen for the leukocyte alkaline-phosphatase (LAP) stain?

A. Smears made from blood anticoagulated with EDTA
B. Smears made from blood anticoagulated with 3.2% sodium citrate
C. Smears made from a finger stick and stored at room temperature for 24h
D. Smears made from capillary blood and stained immediately

The answer is D. EDTA has an inhibitory effect on LAP stain. Fresh capillary blood stained immediately is the preferred specimen, since delay in staining the blood smear causes loss of LAP activity. (Brown, 6th ed., pp. 132–133)

26. The presence of microorganisms, increased protein, and a high leukocyte count in cerebrospinal fluid (CSF) will cause the CSF to appear

A. bloody
B. oily
C. cloudy or turbid
D. clear and colorless

The answer is C. An increased WBC, increased protein, and presence of microorganisms can cause cloudiness or turbidity in CSF. Red blood cells from subarachnoid or intracerebral hemorrhage cause blood to be present in CSF. A traumatic tap may also cause blood to be present in the CSF and must be ruled out as a source. An oily appearance can result from injection of radiographic contrast media. (Brunzel, pp. 368–369)

27. A cytospin smear of CSF from an adult contains a few lymphocytes, monocytes, and ependymal cells. These findings indicate that the patient has

A. meningeal melanoma
B. bacterial meningitis
C. normal cytology in CSF
D. a traumatic brain injury

The answer is C. Normal CSF contains lymphocytes and monocytes. A few ependymal cells (cells that line the ventricles) may also be seen without indicating pathology. In meningeal melanoma, tumor cells would be seen. Increased neutrophils would indicate bacterial meningitis. Traumatic brain injury would likely be accompanied by RBCs. (Brunzel, p. 370–374)

28. Using an undiluted CSF specimen, 150 WBCs are counted in the four large corner squares on one side of the hemocytometer. What is the total WBC count per mm³?

A. 38
B. 375
C. 750
D. 3,750

The answer is B. Use the following formula.

$$\text{Cells/mm}^3 = \frac{\text{no. of cells counted} \times \text{dilution factor}}{\text{area} \times \text{depth}}$$

Since the fluid was undiluted, the dilution factor is 1. The area is 4 mm² and depth is 0.1 mm.

$$\text{Cells/mm}^3 = \frac{150 \times 1}{4 \times 0.1} = \frac{150}{0.4} = 375/\text{mm}^3$$

(Brown, 6th ed., p. 94)

Hematology and Hemostasis

29. In selecting material for smears of bone-marrow cell morphology, the clinical laboratory scientist should select

A. gray particles floating in blood and fat droplets
B. the last material aspirated
C. material free of fat
D. clotted specimens

The answer is A. Gray particles of marrow are visible with the naked eye floating in blood and fat droplets. These serve as landmarks for the microscopic review of stained bone-marrow smears. (Harmening, pp. 46–47; Henry, p. 622)

30. The type of bone-marrow specimen that is most valuable in estimating marrow cellularity and histologic structure is a

A. thin smear of aspirated marrow
B. thick smear of aspirated marrow
C. touch preparation of biopsied marrow
D. sectioned preparation of biopsied marrow

The answer is D. The histologic architecture and cellularity of bone marrow are best evaluated in a sectioned biopsy preparation because the relation of cells to each other is preserved. Individual cell morphology is best evaluated by thick or thin smears or touch preparations. (Harmening, p. 48; Henry, p. 622)

31. The following results are obtained on a bone-marrow differential:

Myeloblasts	1
Promyelocytes	5
Myelocytes	10
Neutrophilic bands	9
Segmented neutrophils	4
Eosinophils	1
Basophils	0
Lymphocytes	7
Monocytes	2
Plasmacytes	1
Normoblasts	60

What is the myeloid : erythroid ratio (M : E)?

A. 0.5 : 1
B. 0.7 : 1
C. 2.0 : 1
D. 3.0 : 1

The answer is A. The total percentage of myeloid cells (neutrophils, eosinophils, and basophils) observed in relation to the total percentage of erythroid precursors gives the M : E ratio. In the example given, the total of myeloid cells is 30% and the total of normoblasts is 60%; therefore, the M : E ratio is 30 : 60, or 0.5 : 1. (Lotspeich-Steininger, pp. 376–377)

32. A properly calibrated and controlled instrument that uses the principle of electronic impedance produces repeated (×3) values on a blood sample:

RBC: 4.01×10^{12}/L
HCT: 0.32 L/L
HB: 12.0 g/dL
MCV: 80 fL
MCH: 32 pg
MCHC: 37.5 g/dL

The most likely explanation for these results is

A. iron-deficiency anemia
B. hereditary spherocytosis
C. high titer of cold agglutinins
D. high reticulocyte count

The answer is B. In hereditary spherocytosis, the MCHC is often increased (greater than 36%) because of a decrease in cell surface area. The MCV is often in the low-normal range. In iron-deficiency anemia, one would expect a decreased MCHC. Cold agglutinins would cause a falsely decreased RBC and elevated MCV, along with an elevated MCHC. A high reticulocyte count might influence the MCV but would not affect the MCHC. (Brown, 6th ed., p. 294)

33. The following information is obtained from an electronic cell counter:

MCV   75 fL (N = 80–100 fL)
RDW   20% (N = 11–14)

Based on the above parameters, what RBC morphology would be expected on the peripheral blood smear?

A. normocytic cells that vary little in size
B. microcytic cells that vary little in size
C. microcytic cells with significant variation in size
D. macrocytic cells with significant variation in size

The answer is C. The MCV of 75 fL is decreased, suggesting microcytosis. An RDW of 20% is increased, and a variation in the size of the RBCs would be expected. Such a peripheral-blood morphology may be seen in iron deficiency or sideroblastic anemia. (Lotspeich-Steininger, p. 130)

CLS Review Questions—Hemostasis

1. Coagulation studies are ordered on a patient with a hematocrit of 0.18 L/L. What volume of 3.8% sodium citrate should be used in the collection?

A. 0.15 mL
B. 0.50 mL
C. 0.68 mL
D. 1.00 mL

The answer is C. The amount of 3.8% sodium citrate in evacuated tubes will provide a 1 : 9 ratio when the hematocrit is between 0.20 L/L and 0.55 L/L. A patient with an hematocrit of <0.20 L/L will have a relative increase in plasma volume, and the usual amount of anticoagulant will not be sufficient to maintain a 1 : 9 ratio. The ratio may be adjusted according to the following formula:

$$C = 1.85 \times 10^{-3} (100 - H) \times V$$

where C = volume of 3.8% sodium citrate in mL, V = volume of whole blood in mL, and H = hematocrit (%). Using 4.5 mL as the volume of blood, the amount of sodium citrate to be used when the patient hematocrit is 0.18 L/L will be:

$$1.85 \times 10^{-3} (100 - 18) \times 4.5 = 0.68 \text{ mL}$$

(Corriveau and Fritsma, p. 69)

2. Samples for laboratory studies involving hematology, chemistry, and hemostasis require the collection of a red-top tube, a tube containing sodium citrate, and an EDTA tube. What should the order of draw be to preserve the integrity of the specimen for coagulation studies?

   A. Red-top, sodium citrate, EDTA
   B. Sodium citrate, EDTA, red-top
   C. Red-top, EDTA, sodium citrate
   D. Sodium citrate, red-top, EDTA

The answer is A. If the tube for coagulation is drawn as part of a series, it should be drawn as the second or third tube in a series. It should never be the first tube drawn because of the possible contamination with tissue thromboplastin as the needle enters the skin. It should not follow a tube anticoagulated with EDTA (or heparin), because these anticoagulants may contaminate the specimen and invalidate results. (Corriveau and Fritsma, p. 71; Rodak, p. 12)

3. A specimen for determination of activated partial thromboplastin time is collected in sodium citrate at 9:30 AM and allowed to remain at room temperature in the collection center until delivery to the laboratory at 3:00 PM. What effect will this have on the results?

   A. Shortened due to increased glass activation
   B. Prolonged due to deterioration of factor VIII
   C. Prolonged due to deterioration of factor VII
   D. No effect

The answer is B. Factors VIII and V, which are measured by the APTT, are labile. Specimens should be tested within two hours of collection if they are maintained at room temperature. Specimens maintained at 2–8°C may be held up to four hours. Collection tubes are siliconized to prevent surface activation of procoagulants by glass. Factor VII is not labile and it is not measured by the APTT. (Corriveau and Fritsma, pp. 72–73; Brown, 6th ed., p. 214)

4. In the latex-agglutination method for determining serum fibrin/fibrinogen degradation products, which of the following can be a cause of false positive results?

Hematology and Hemostasis

A. The sample clots too rapidly
B. The specimen contains an enzyme inhibitor
C. Reptilase has been added to the patient specimen
D. The specimen is collected in a regular red-top tube instead of special FDP tubes

The answer is D. Special collecting tubes containing thrombin (to ensure complete removal of fibrinogen) and an inhibitor (to prevent further lysis) must be used. Otherwise, cross-reaction with fibrinogen, fibrin monomers, or polymers not completely clotted during sample preparation can cause false positives. (Brown, 6th ed., pp. 241–242)

5. In the performance of a bleeding-time test, the blood pressure cuff should be inflated to

A. 20 mm Hg
B. 40 mm Hg
C. 60 mm Hg
D. 100 mm Hg

The answer is B. In both the original Ivy bleeding-time test and its modifications, pressure is maintained at 40 mm Hg throughout the procedure. (Corriveau and Fritsma, p. 293; Brown, 6th ed., p. 268)

6. Enzymes measured in chromogenic substrate assays are of what class?

A. Serine proteases
B. Lysine arginases
C. Carboxyl anhydrases
D. Lyases

The answer is A. The blood-coagulation cascade depends on a series of reactions that are dependent on the enzymatic activity of serine proteases. (Lotspeich-Steininger, p. 704)

7. A patient has a normal prothrombin time (PT) and a prolonged activated partial thromboplastin time (APTT). To determine if the prolongation of the APTT is caused by a factor deficiency or a circulating anticoagulant, the clinical laboratory scientist should first

A. mix 1 part patient plasma and 1 part reagent plasma and repeat both the PT and APTT
B. mix 1 part patient plasma and 1 part reagent plasma and repeat the APTT only
C. perform a factor X assay. If prolonged, a factor X deficiency is indicated
D. perform a test for a lupus anticoagulant

The answer is B. To determine whether a factor deficiency or a circulating anticoagulant is responsible for a prolonged PT, APTT or thrombin time (TT), a mixture of equal parts of patient and normal reagent plasma should be prepared and tested following the protocol for the procedure that showed the prolongation. Only the system that showed the abnormal result is tested. If the result on the mixture is corrected into the normal range, a factor deficiency is suspected and the mixing test is repeated following a 60 minute incubation at 37°C. If the original prolonged test is corrected by the mixing procedure at both stages (with and without 60 minute incubation), a factor deficiency is likely. If either mixing test yields prolonged results, a circulating anticoagulant is suspected. If only the second mixing test does not correct, a factor VIII inhibitor is likely, as it reacts more slowly than the other circulating inhibitors. (Corriveau and Fritsma, pp. 111–112)

8. The mean of a normal prothrombin-time control is 12.2 sec. One standard deviation is 0.2 sec. According to Gaussian distribution, 95% of the control values should fall within what range?

   A. 11.6–12.8 sec
   B. 11.8–12.6 sec
   C. 12.0–12.4 sec
   D. 12.1–12.3 sec

The answer is B. According to Gaussian distribution, 95% of the values should fall within ± 2SD, or 0.4 sec. Therefore, the 2-SD range for this control is 11.8–12.6 sec. (Brown, 6th ed., pp. 23–24)

9. A decreased anticoagulant response to heparin therapy may be caused by decreased levels of

   A. antithrombin III
   B. platelet factor 4
   C. factor XIII
   D. thromboxane

The answer is A. Antithrombin III complexes with and inhibits thrombin and other activated serine proteases, e.g., factors XIIa, XIa, Xa, IXa, plasmin, and protein C. Heparin serves as a cofactor for this reaction. Low levels of antithrombin III result in decreased neutralization of these factors in the face of high levels of heparin since both AT-III and heparin are required. (Lotspeich-Steininger, pp. 640–641)

10. An abnormal APTT is not corrected into the normal range when the patient plasma is mixed in equal parts with normal plasma. This indicates

   A. a circulating inhibitor
   B. a factor deficiency
   C. dysfibrinogenemia
   D. von Willebrand's disease

The answer is A. When plasma from a patient with a prolonged APTT is mixed with an equal amount of normal plasma and another APTT is done, a normal result indicates that a plasma-factor deficiency exists. Only 50% of a plasma factor is needed for the APTT to be normal. If the APTT remains long, an inhibitor is suggested. (Brown, 6th ed., p. 251)

11. In the performance of coagulation tests, the abnormal control yields unacceptable results for both the PT and APTT. The normal control is within

acceptable limits for both procedures. What is the appropriate action for the clinical laboratory scientist?

A. Perform preventive maintenance on the instrument before retesting the controls
B. Repeat the abnormal control on a new bottle of control material before proceeding with the analysis
C. Continue with the procedure and report out only those patient results that are in the normal range
D. Continue with the procedure and report out only those patient results that are in the abnormal range

The answer is B. Since two test procedures are out of control, the integrity of the abnormal control should be questioned. A new bottle of abnormal control should be tested before any other action is taken. (Corriveau and Fritsma, pp. 79–80)

12. A patient with a history of frequent mild bleeding episodes has a normal PT and a moderately prolonged APTT, which is corrected by the addition of each of the following: normal plasma, factor VIII-deficient plasma, factor IX-deficient plasma. Which factor assay(s) should be run?

A. VIII
B. IX
C. XI and XII
D. None; a circulating inhibitor is present

The answer is C. Correction with normal plasma rules out the presence of a circulating inhibitor. Correction with factor VIII-deficient and factor IX-deficient plasmas rules out factor VIII and IX deficiencies. Therefore, the factors left as possibilities are XI and XII. (Corriveau and Fritsma, pp. 116–117)

13. An 18-year-old female was scheduled to have her wisdom teeth removed. Because the patient had a history of frequent nosebleeds, heavy menstrual periods, and easy bruisability, the surgeon ordered a full coagulation screen. The following results were obtained:

prothrombin time: 11.8 sec (N = 10–12 sec)
APTT: 40 sec (N = 25–35 sec)
platelet count: $300 \times 10^9/L$ (N = $150 - 450 \times 10^9/L$)
bleeding time: 13.0 minutes (N = 2–8 min)

Based on these results, what additional procedure should be performed?

A. Factor VII assay
B. Vitamin K level
C. Platelet-aggregation studies
D. Thrombin clotting time

The answer is C. The history and laboratory findings suggest von Willebrand's disease. Platelet-aggregation studies should be performed using epinephrine, ADP, collagen, and ristocetin. If von Willebrand's disease is present, aggregation with ristocetin may be decreased. Although a factor-VIII assay might be helpful, there is no indication for a factor-VII assay or a Vitamin-K level (PTT is normal). (Lotspeich-Steininger, p. 630)

14. On a patient's platelet-rich plasma (PRP) sample used to set the 0% baseline for platelet-aggregation studies, what should the platelet count be?

A. 100×10^9/L
B. 300×10^9/L
C. 400×10^9/L
D. 500×10^9/L

The answer is B. Aggregometry is performed on an aggregation meter, which is a special photometer with a stirring device that maintains platelet-rich plasma in an even suspension in a sample cuvette. PRP is adjusted to a count of 300×10^9/L and is used to set the 0% transmission-of-light baseline for the test. A suspension of platelet-poor plasma (PPP) is used to set the 100% baseline. (Corriveau and Fritsma, p. 294)

15. When operating an electrofibrometer system, care must be taken to ensure that the automatic pipet is turned off after each use. What will happen if the pipet is left in the "on" position?

A. The probe will fall down into the reactor well when you pick up the next sample
B. The timer will zero itself
C. The heating block will shut off
D. The electrodes will bend and no longer be parallel

The answer is A. To operate the fibrometer with an automatic pipet, the pipet switch must be in the "off" position and set to 0.1. The sample is then aspirated by depressing the plunger and releasing it with the fibrotip submersed in the sample plasma. The test-reagent cup is placed in the heated reactor well. The automatic pipet switch is set to "on" and the sample is delivered to the reaction cup by depressing the plunger. This causes the probe to fall down so that the electrodes are submersed. A cam causes the moving electrode to move in and out of the mixture until a clot forms and causes a current to flow between the two electrodes, stopping the timer. If the automatic pipet is not turned off after this function, the instrument will drop the probe when the next pipetting maneuver is made. (Brown, 6th ed., p. 393)

16. What reagent is added to conventional aggregometry to test platelets for release of dense granules as well as aggregation?

A. ATP
B. Firefly luciferase
C. Ristocetin
D. ADP

The answer is B. With the addition of firefly extract, luciferase, to conventional platelet aggregometry, two results can be monitored at the same time. This is called lumiaggregometry. The firefly extract illuminates when in contact with energized ATP. Platelet-dense granules contain both ADP and ATP. When platelets are activated, they release their granules and aggregate with each other. ADP causes the platelets to aggregate and ATP causes the luciferase to glow. Two photodetector systems in lumiaggregometry monitor both aggregation and granule release. This test can detect faulty release of granules and storage pool diseases. (Corriveau and Fritsma, p. 297)

17. What platelet-aggregation pattern would be expected for a sample from a patient with Bernard-Soulier syndrome if ristocetin is used as the agonist?

   A. Monophasic curve
   B. Biphasic curve
   C. Flatline
   D. Partially diminished curve

The answer is C. Persons with Bernard-Soulier syndrome have defective or missing glycoprotein receptors (GPIb) for von Willebrand Factor (vWF). Ristocetin gives a monophasic curve with normal platelets in the presence of vWF by agglutinating the platelets with vWF via the receptor. Bernard-Soulier syndrome platelets cannot connect to vWF. No aggregation occurs; therefore a flatline pattern results. Patients with all forms of von Willebrand disease, except type IIb, present a diminished curve corrected by the addition of exogenous vWF. (Harmening, p. 443)

18. In the performance of platelet aggregometry on patient samples, the instrument should be set to 100% transmittance using

   A. patient platelet-poor plasma
   B. patient platelet-rich plasma
   C. control platelet-poor plasma
   D. control platelet-rich plasma

The answer is A. The instrument should be adjusted to 100% transmittance using patient PPP. (Lotspeich-Steininger, p. 676)

References

Brown BA. *Hematology: Principles and Procedures* (5th ed). Philadelphia: Lea & Febiger, 1988.

Brown BA. *Hematology: Principles and Procedures* (6th ed). Philadelphia: Lea & Febiger, 1993.

Brunzel NA. *Fundamentals of Urine and Body Fluid Analysis.* Philadelphia: Saunders, 1994.

Corriveau DM, Fritsma GA. *Hemostasis and Thrombosis in the Clinical Laboratory.* Philadelphia: Lippincott, 1988.

Harmening DM. *Clinical Hematology and Fundamentals of Hemostasis* (2nd ed). Philadelphia: FA Davis, 1992.

Henry JB (ed). *Clinical Diagnosis and Management by Laboratory Methods* (18th ed). Philadelphia: Saunders, 1991.

Lotspeich-Steininger CA, Stiene-Martin EA, Koepke JA (eds). *Clinical Hematology: Principles, Procedures, Correlations.* Philadelphia: Lippincott, 1992.

McKenzie SB. *Textbook of Hematology.* Philadelphia: Lea & Febiger, 1988.

Rodak BF (ed). *Diagnostic Hematology.* Philadelphia: Saunders, 1995.

Strasinger SK. *Urinalysis and Body Fluids* (3rd ed). Philadelphia: FA Davis, 1994.

Turgeon ML. *Clinical Hematology: Theory and Procedures* (2nd ed). Boston: Little, Brown, 1988.

3

Immunohematology

Section Editors   Kathryn Doig and Michelle S. Wright

CLT Review Questions

Contributors

Suzanne H. Butch
M. Kathleen Huck
Marcia A. Kilsby
Betty Lynn Theriot

1. Whole blood collected in citrate-phosphate-dextrose with adenine (CPDA-1) may be stored for up to

   A. 48 hours
   B. 21 days
   C. 35 days
   D. 42 days

The answer is C. Blood collected in CPDA-1 is "good" for 35 days, mainly because the additive adenine provides a substrate from which erythrocytes can synthesize ATP. (Walker, p. 53)

2. The temperature of a refrigerator that contains stored blood or blood products should not exceed

   A. 4°C
   B. 6°C
   C. 8°C
   D. 10°C

The answer is B. According to American Association of Blood Banks (AABB) standards, the temperature in a refrigerator used to store blood or blood products must be maintained between 1–6°C. The refrigerator must also have a recording thermometer and an alarm system; often the alarm is set to trigger at 7°C. (Walker, p. 51)

3. The results of a physical examination performed on a female blood donor are as follows:

Last donation:	3 months ago
Age:	65 years
Hemoglobin:	12.8 g/dL
Pulse:	95 beats/min
Blood pressure:	170/90 mmHg
Weight:	112 lb
Temperature:	38°C

How many of the given values fall outside the acceptable limits set by the AABB and would result in the deferral of the donor?

A. None
B. One
C. Two
D. Three

The answer is B. Although several values are close to the limits, only one falls outside the acceptable range and would result in the donor being deferred. The oral temperature may not exceed 37.5°C. Other limits are as follows:

Last donation:	minimum interval is 8 weeks between donations
Age:	blood donors must be at least 17 years of age
Hemoglobin:	≥12.5 g/dL
Pulse:	50–100 beats/min with no pathologic irregularity
Blood pressure:	no higher than 180 mmHg systolic and 100 mmHg diastolic
Weight:	110 lb or more may donate 450 mL +/− 45 mL, plus 30 mL for processing tubes (Walker, pp. 1, 11–12)

4. What is the proper label for a blood product prepared as follows: About 12h after collection, a unit of whole blood collected in CPDA-1 is centrifuged at 4°C using a "heavy" spin. The plasma is expressed into a satellite bag and stored at 1–6°C for 24h. The plasma is then frozen at −18°C.

A. Fresh frozen plasma
B. Liquid plasma
C. Plasma
D. Recovered plasma

The answer is C. To be labeled as fresh frozen, plasma must be separated from cells within 6h of collection of the whole blood and frozen immediately to preserve the labile clotting factors. As the plasma in this unit is frozen and not liquid, it cannot be labeled liquid plasma. Recovered plasma is the name given to outdated plasma that is usually fractionated to produce products such as albumin. Therefore, since this plasma is not outdated, it must be labeled plasma. (Walker, p. 61)

5. A male donor appears generally healthy and has no history of recent surgery or travel outside the United States. He reports no risk factors for hepatitis or HIV. He takes blood-pressure medication twice daily. Physical examination reveals weight 155 lb, hemoglobin 15.5 g/dL, blood pressure 140/75 mmHg, oral temperature 37°C, and pulse 55 beats/min and regular. Based on the data provided, the clinical laboratory technician should

A. consult the physician regarding the donor's medication
B. accept the donor for plasma donation only
C. defer the donor based on the blood-pressure measurement
D. defer the donor based on the hemoglobin measurement

The answer is A. Taking medication is not automatically a cause for donor deferral, as most medications will not affect the recipient. However, the collection facility must be concerned about the ability of a donor taking medication for an underlying medical condition to tolerate the donation process. Therefore, the blood-bank physician should be consulted to assess the safety of the donation for the donor. (Walker, p. 5)

6. Both direct and indirect antiglobulin techniques require thorough washing. The following considerations are important for all procedures that use antiglobulin serum *except*

   A. antiglobulin serum can be added any time up to 40 min after completion of washing
   B. the cell button should be fully resuspended in the residual saline after decanting and before addition of wash saline
   C. the volume of wash saline should fill the tube at least three-quarters full
   D. washing is performed in as short a period of time as possible

The answer is A. The antiglobulin serum must be added immediately following the completion of washing. If this is not done, cell-bound IgG may detach from the red cells and remain free in the fluid medium. These unbound immunoglobulin molecules can inhibit the antiglobulin serum when it is added and, therefore, give a false-negative reaction. (Walker, p. 180)

7. A test tube containing known antibody and unknown cells has been incubated and spun. After dislodging the cell button completely, several large agglutinates are apparent with no small clumps or free cells visible. The background solution is clear. This reaction should be graded as

   A. 4+
   B. 3+
   C. 2+
   D. 1+

The answer is B. Using a semiquantitative method of grading reaction strength provides additional information that can be useful in solving problems such as ABO discrepancies or identifying atypical antibodies. A 4+ reaction appears as a single large agglutinate. The description above is 3+. A 2+ reaction may include several large agglutinates in a background of smaller clumps, but no free red cells. A 1+ reaction is characterized by multiple small clumps and a background of numerous free red cells. (Walker, p. 612)

8. The results of an agglutination test using successive dilutions of patient serum are shown below.

Tube no.	1	2	3	4	5	6	7	8	9	10
dilution	1:2	1:4	1:8	1:16	1:32	1:64	1:128	1:256	1:512	antigen control
patient	0	0	0	0	0	+	+	+	+	0

+ = agglutination; 0 = no agglutination

What do the results in tubes 1 to 5 represent?

   A. Activation of the complement sequence
   B. Prozone effect due to antibody excess
   C. Postzone effect due to antigen excess
   D. Technical error; these results cannot occur when the agglutination procedure is performed correctly

The answer is B. These results represent the classic prozone phenomenon due to antibody excess. It is thought that excess of antibody in relation to antigen prevents the formation of a lattice. (Walker, pp. 165, 652)

9. When performing ABO typing by the microplate method in U-bottom plates, the cell button appears round with a smooth perimeter after 30 min of settling. What is the interpretation of this appearance?

   A. The test is negative
   B. The test is weakly positive
   C. The test is strongly positive
   D. The test cannot be interpreted until the cells are resuspended

The answer is A. In a settling assay, a negative test appears as a smooth cell button in the bottom of a U-shaped microtiter plate. Positive tests, even those that are weakly positive, will have buttons with uneven or jagged edges. (Walker, p. 617)

10. The symbol cDE of the Fisher-Race system corresponds to the Wiener symbol

    A. R^o
    B. R^1
    C. R^2
    D. R^z

The answer is C. R^o corresponds to cDe, R^1 corresponds to CDe, and R^z corresponds to CDE. (Walker, p. 232)

11. Immune A and B alloantibodies differ from innate A and B alloantibodies in that the immune antibodies

    A. are generally IgG
    B. are unable to cross the placenta
    C. can be enhanced in reactivity by incubation at 4°C
    D. cause direct agglutination at room temperature

The answer is A. The major differences between innate and immune A and B alloantibodies are outlined below:

Class	Innate IgM	Immune IgG
ability to cross placenta	no	yes
optimal temperature of reactivity	<22°C	37°C
serologic characteristics	usually cause direct agglutination	usually require AHG for agglutination

(Walker, pp. 153, 210)

12. The presence of anti-A_1 is usually detected by the

    A. antibody screening procedure (indirect Coombs' test)
    B. reverse ABO grouping procedure
    C. red-cell typing antisera
    D. use of A_2 cells

The answer is B. Anti-A$_1$ will react with the A$_1$ cells used in reverse ABO grouping. Anti-A$_1$ will not react with group O cells used for antibody screening. Other antibodies will not react with anti-A$_1$ since no antigen is present. Anti-A$_1$ is not expected to react with A$_2$ cells. The pattern of reaction with A$_1$ cells but not O cells or A$_2$ cells confirms the identity of the antibody as anti-A$_1$. (Walker, p. 218)

13. The ABO typing of a patient's sample yields the following results:

Patient cells +		Patient serum	
Anti A	**Anti B**	**A$_1$ Cells**	**B Cells**
0	0	4+	3+

The patient's ABO blood group is

A. O
B. A
C. B
D. AB

The answer is A. In ABO typing, reagent antisera of known specificity are tested against the patient's red cells to detect the antigens on the cells. This is known as forward grouping, or front typing. A negative reaction with anti-A indicates that the A antigen is not present on the cells. Similarly, failure to react with anti-B indicates the lack of the B antigen on the cells. Lack of both antigens defines the individual as group O. In the ABO system, individuals typically possess in their serum the antibodies against the antigens that they lack on their cells. The presence of these antibodies is detected by testing the patient's serum against cells known to possess the A antigen and other cells known to possess the B antigen. This is known as reverse grouping, or back typing, and can be used to confirm the forward grouping. This patient's serum reacted with both the A cells and the B cells, indicating the presence of both anti-A and anti-B in the serum. This is the expected reaction of a group O individual. (Walker, pp. 204, 211)

14. The results of D typing on a patient using a high-protein anti-D reagent are

	Room temperature	AHG	Check cells
patient cells + anti-D	0	2+	Not Performed
patient cells + Rh control	0	2+	Not Performed

Which of the following is the correct interpretation of these results?

A. Rh negative, weak D (D^u) positive
B. Rh positive, weak D (D^u) positive
C. Rh negative, weak D (D^u) negative
D. Invalid Rh typing

The answer is D. When Rh or D typing is performed using a high-protein reagent, a high-protein control reagent is also reacted with the cells. This control lacks anti-D and is expected to give a negative reaction. Reaction of the Rh control serum with the cells is not due to anti-D reacting with the D antigen on the cells. Therefore, a positive reaction with the Rh control serum prevents interpretation of the presence or absence of D antigen on the tested cells, yielding an invalid Rh or D typing. (Walker, pp. 247–248)

15. An ABO grouping yielded the following results:

Patient cells +	Anti-A$_1$	Anti-A	Anti-B	Anti-A, B
	0	1+	0	1+

Patient serum +	A$_1$ cells	A$_2$ cells	B cells	O cells
	4+	0	3+	0

This patient's results are consistent with

A. group O
B. group AB
C. subgroup of A
D. group-O patient with unexpected alloantibody

The answer is C. Interpreting the results of the usual forward and reverse grouping (anti-A, anti-B, A$_1$ cells, and B cells) would suggest that the patient forward groups as an A, albeit weakly. The reverse grouping is that of a group O. When an ABO grouping reaction is weaker than 3+, it typically suggests that the reaction points to a problem. In this case, the weak reaction with anti-A indicates that the antigen may be present in a weakened form on the patient's cells. The failure of the cells to react with anti-A$_1$ confirms that the A$_1$ antigen, although found on most group-A cells, is not present. This pattern is consistent with the forward grouping reactions in patients with certain subgroups of the A antigen. The reverse grouping demonstrates a strong reaction against the A$_1$ cells. This is to be expected since the A$_1$ antigen is not present on the patient's red cells and is, therefore, foreign to the A-subgroup individual. No reaction is observed with the A$_2$ cells. As would be expected of a group-A individual, anti-B is present in the serum. The failure to react with group O cells suggests, but does not confirm, that the unexpected antibody is directed at an antigen in the ABO system. (Walker, pp. 208–209)

16. Below are the results of an ABO grouping:

Patient cells +	Anti-A	Anti-B	Patient serum +	A cells	B cells
	3+	0		0	0

The most likely interpretation of these results is that the patient

A. is a subgroup of A
B. is a group A newborn
C. is group A and has been multiply transfused with group O cells
D. has rouleaux due to multiple myeloma

The answer is B. These results demonstrate a discrepancy because the patient forward groups as group A but reverse groups as group AB. Since the forward grouping result is strong, it is likely that the patient is group A and the discrepancy is due to a "missing" anti-B. The reverse-grouping antibodies develop as a result of exposure to environmental antigens, probably in foods. As a result, infants up to six months of age may not demonstrate these antibodies. Elderly or immunocompromised individuals whose antibody production has declined may demonstrate a similar pattern of results. In these cases, forward-grouping results should be relied on to select blood for transfusion. (Walker, pp. 209–210, 215)

17. Antibodies in the Rh system typically

    A. bind complement and cause in-vitro hemolysis
    B. do not react with enzyme-treated cells
    C. react better at 37°C than at room temperature
    D. tend to be saline agglutinins

The answer is C. Most antibodies in the Rh system result from immunization due to either pregnancy or transfusion. They tend to be IgG, reacting best at 37°C in potentiating media or with antiglobulin or enzyme procedures. They rarely bind complement. (Walker, p. 246)

18. Which of the following lists four antibodies that all generally react strongly at 4°C?

    A. Anti-A, anti-P_1, anti-Le^a, anti-M
    B. Anti-B, anti-K, anti-I, anti-Fy^a
    C. Anti-H, anti-S, anti-Jk^a, anti-Le^b
    D. Anti-B, anti-N, anti-E, anti-Jk^b

The answer is A. The antibodies that usually react strongly at 4°C are anti-A, anti-B, anti-H, anti-P_1, anti-Le^a, anti-Le^b, anti-I, anti-M, and anti-N. (Walker, pp. 210, 220–221, 223, 260)

19. Group O, Rh-positive cells are used for antibody-screening tests because

    A. anti-A and anti-B do not react with O cells
    B. anti-A_1 is detected using O cells
    C. most recipients are O and Rh-positive
    D. weak A or B subgroups react with O cells

The answer is A. Group O cells are selected to avoid interference from ABO system antibodies. The cells are also selected to have as many red-cell antigens corresponding to common antibodies as possible on their surfaces. This is to allow detection of unexpected, clinically significant antibodies. Rh-positive cells are used to increase the likelihood of detecting unexpected anti-D. Anti-A_1 is not detected with O cells, but with A_1 cells. (Walker, p. 312)

20. From the abbreviated-cell panel depicted below, determine the most probable antibody or antibodies in the patient's serum.

Panel cell no.	Known antigens									Test results		
	C	D	E	c	e	K	k	M	N	37°C	AHG	Check cells
1	+	+	+	+	0	0	+	0	+	2+	3+	NP
2	0	+	0	+	+	0	+	+	0	0	0	2+
3	0	+	+	+	0	0	+	+	0	2+	4+	NP
4	+	+	0	0	+	+	+	+	+	0	0	2+
5	0	0	0	+	+	0	+	+	0	0	0	2+

AHG = antihuman globulin; NP = not performed

A. Anti-k

B. Anti-e

C. Anti-E

D. Anti-C and anti-e

The answer is C. From the panel antigens shown, possible antibodies are anti-C, -D, -E, -c, -e, -K, -k, -M, and -N. One first looks for negative test results to rule out antibodies against antigens present on nonreactive cells. For example, there are no reactions of patient serum with cell 2 at any phase of testing. Since these cells are positive for the D, c, e, k, and M antigens, corresponding antibodies must be absent or a positive reaction would have occurred. Thus, anti-D, -c, -e, -k, and -M have been eliminated from consideration. The only remaining possibilities are anti-C, -E, -K, and -N. Since cell 4 also does not react with the patient serum and has C, K, and N antigens on its surface, anti-C, -K, and -N are eliminated. This leaves anti-E as the only possible antibody in the patient's serum. Cell 5 is also negative when tested against the patient's serum, but this does not rule out any additional antibodies. The identification of anti-E is supported since E antigen is present on both cells 1 and 3, which were reactive with the patient's serum. The pattern of reactivity at 37°C, strengthening at AHG, is also consistent with anti-E. Antibodies in the Rh system are usually IgG and react best at 37°C and at the antiglobulin phase of testing. (Walker, pp. 335–336)

21. Below are the results of an antibody screen:

	LISS 37°C	AHG	Check cells
patient serum + screen cell I	0	0	2+
patient serum + screen cell II	0	0	2+

The correct interpretation of these results is that the

A. check cells did not react as expected; the results of the antibody screen cannot be interpreted

B. patient serum demonstrates an unexpected antibody reacting against antigens on both screening cells

C. patient serum demonstrates an unexpected antibody reacting against an antigen present on only one screening cell

D. patient serum demonstrates no unexpected antibodies

The answer is D. The antibody screening test is one example of an indirect antihuman-globulin test (AHG). The first step in interpretation is to evaluate the reaction of the check (Coombs' control) cells. If AHG has been added to the test and remains active, the addition of antibody-coated check cells will result in agglutination, as is the case in both tubes above. Since the check cells reacted, the results of the other phases of testing can be interpreted. No reaction occurred in either phase of testing or with either screening cell; therefore, the patient serum does not demonstrate any unexpected antibodies. The presence of most unexpected antibodies would be detected by a reaction of one or both of the screening cells at any phase of testing. (Walker, p. 312)

22. An antibody identification panel was performed on serum from a patient with a positive antibody screen. The panel tentatively identified the antibody as anti-c. Antigen typing on the patient's cells to aid in confirmation of the antibody identification gave the following results:

	Anti-c at 37°C
patient cells	0
Cc control cells	1+
CC control cells	0

Which of the following is the correct interpretation of the results?

A. Antigen typing is an inhibition test; the results indicate that the patient is c positive
B. The c typing on the patient cannot be interpreted because the positive control reacted only weakly
C. The patient is c negative and could have produced anti-c
D. The patient could not develop anti-c, so the antibody identification is in error

The answer is C. For antisera that are used infrequently, positive and negative control cells should be tested along with the patient's cells. Heterozygous control cells that are weakly positive should be selected to ensure that the antiserum will react with the patient cells if they too are heterozygous and carry a low dose of the antigen. Since the control cells reacted as expected, the results of the patient's typing can be interpreted. In this case, the results demonstrate that the patient's cells lack the c antigen. Individuals can develop antibodies to antigens that are considered by their immune systems to be foreign; i.e., to antigens they do not possess. Since this patient lacks the c antigen, the patient could develop anti-c, so the results of the antigen typing support the tentative identification of the serum antibody as anti-c. (Walker, pp. 343, 544)

23. An antibody-identification panel demonstrates possible anti-E and anti-K in a patient's serum. Which of the following group O cells could be used to absorb the patient serum and separate these antibodies so that anti-K remains in the absorbed serum?

Immunohematology

	Reactions of cells with:	
	Anti-E	**Anti-K**
A. Cell 1	0	0
B. Cell 2	+	0
C. Cell 3	0	+
D. Cell 4	+	+

The answer is B. To separate the two antibodies, a cell is selected that carries only one of the corresponding antigens on its surface. The serum is allowed to react with these cells so that one antibody will attach to its corresponding antigen present on the cells while the other antibody remains in the serum. In this case, cell 2 possesses the E antigen and lacks the K antigen. Allowing the serum to react with cell 2 would permit the anti-E to adsorb to the cells while the anti-K remains in the serum. The absorbed serum can then be tested to help confirm the presence of the anti-K. The anti-E can be eluted from the cells and the eluate tested like a serum sample to confirm the presence and identity of that antibody. (Walker, pp. 349–350)

24. The fundamental purpose of the crossmatch is to

A. detect recipient antibodies that are directed against donor red-cell antigens
B. prevent immunization of the recipient
C. prove that a recipient does or does not have an unexpected antibody in the serum
D. verify that the donor and recipient are Rh-identical

The answer is A. The crossmatch provides considerable safety in transfusion services. It can demonstrate that the ABO groups of recipient and donor are compatible, as in giving A blood to an A recipient or O blood to an A recipient. It can also be used to determine whether a recipient has detectable, unexpected antibodies directed against donor cells. However, the crossmatch cannot prove that a recipient has no unexpected antibodies, nor can it guarantee that immunizations will not occur. In the latter instance, for example, an Rh-positive donor can give a compatible crossmatch with an Rh-negative recipient; however, the Rh-positive cells, when transfused, may immunize the recipient to produce anti-D. The crossmatch does not verify that the donor and recipient are Rh-identical. (Walker, p. 312)

25. Choose the preferred criteria for donor units when issuing uncrossmatched blood for a patient for whom no pretransfusion testing can be completed.

A. ABO- and Rh-specific
B. ABO-specific, Rh-negative
C. ABO- and Rh-compatible
D. Group O, Rh-negative

The answer is D. In emergency situations, blood may be issued even though the recipient is neither typed nor crossmatched. If there is time for typing, blood that is type-specific (e.g., A positive donor to A positive recipient) should be issued. If blood that is type-specific is not available in sufficient quantity, type-compatible blood (e.g., O negative donor to A positive recipient) may be given. ABO-specific blood that is Rh-negative may be given when the recipient's ABO group has been determined but the Rh status has not. In dire emergencies, when no pretransfusion testing (e.g., ABO grouping and Rh typing) can be completed prior to transfusion, group O, Rh-negative blood should be issued. (Walker, p. 329)

26. The crossmatch can be limited to the immediate spin phase if

A. the recipient has been transfused within the last 72 hours without reaction
B. the recipient currently has a negative antibody screen and no previous history of an unexpected antibody
C. the blood selected for the recipient is ABO-group and Rh-type specific
D. the recipient is a newborn who has not yet developed unexpected antibodies

The answer is B. If a recipient has a negative antibody screen that includes an AHG phase, there is approximately 95% confidence that he/she does not have a demonstrable unexpected antibody. If the history is also negative, then concern about the transfusion stimulating a secondary immune response is minimal. Taken together, a negative history and negative screen indicate that there is negligible concern for a hemolytic transfusion reaction due to unexpected antibodies. However, the crossmatch must still detect the expected antibodies of the ABO system. Hence, the purpose of the crossmatch is narrowed to confirming that the donor and recipient are ABO-compatible; this can be determined in the immediate spin phase since ABO antibodies react best at 22°C or below. (Walker, p. 314)

27. Which of the following would be an acceptable alternative for a packed red-cell transfusion if ABO group-specific blood were not available?

A. Group A recipient with group B donor
B. Group B recipient with group AB donor
C. Group O recipient with a group A donor
D. Group AB recipient with a group B donor

The answer is D. The major crossmatch consists of recipient serum and donor cells. In option A, the A recipient has anti-B in the serum, which would react with the B cells of the donor. In option B, the B recipient has anti-A, which would react with the A antigenic sites of the AB donor. In option C, the group O recipient has anti-A and anti-B; the anti-A would react with the donor's group-A cells. In option D, the group AB recipient has neither anti-A nor anti-B in the serum; therefore, there are no ABO system antibodies to react with the B cells of the donor. Group A, B, or O blood can be given to an AB recipient, but only one blood group should be given to a single recipient if possible. (Walker, p. 315)

28. A patient has the phenotype O, CDEe. If transfused with blood from six group O, Rh-positive donors, the patient could theoretically produce the antibody

A. anti-D
B. anti-C
C. anti-c
D. none; the patient is Rh-positive

Immunohematology

The answer is C. Persons may produce alloantibodies to antigens they lack on their red cells. This patient, who has C, D, E, and e antigens on his/her red cells, could produce anti-c if transfused with blood possessing the c antigen. The chance of such a transfusion is high, since 31% of the white population and 9% of the African-American population are CDe/cde. (Walker, p. 236)

29. If the antiglobulin phase of the crossmatch is omitted, which of the following antibodies would probably not be detected?

   A. anti-K
   B. anti-A
   C. anti-P_1
   D. anti-N

The answer is A. Anti-K reacts best in the antiglobulin phase of testing, as do most of the antibodies in the Kell system. The same is true of antibodies in the Kidd and Duffy systems. Therefore, these antibodies may not be detected if the antiglobulin phase were omitted. Anti-A, anti-P_1, and anti-N react best at cold temperatures and would be detected on immediate spin. (Walker, p. 267)

30. Below are the results of pretransfusion testing on a recipient with no history of unexpected antibodies. The donor is group- and type-specific for the recipient.

	IS	LISS (37°C)	AHG	Check cells
patient serum + screen cell I	NP	0	0	2+
patient serum + screen cell II	NP	0	0	2+
patient serum + donor cells	0	NP	NP	NP

NP = not performed

Which of the following is a correct interpretation of these results?

   A. The compatibility of the donor cannot be determined without continuing the crossmatch through the antiglobulin phase
   B. The compatibility tests indicate compatibility, and the donor unit may be transfused into the recipient
   C. The antibody screen cannot be interpreted because an immediate spin phase was not performed
   D. The antibody screen cannot be interpreted because the check cells reacted

The answer is B. For a patient without a history of unexpected antibodies and a currently negative antibody screen through AHG, the crossmatch need only proceed through the immediate spin phase to assure ABO compatibility. In this case, the antibody screen is negative in both phases and the check cells reacted, indicating the presence of active AHG in the test system. The antibody screen can therefore be interpreted as negative. As the immediate spin crossmatch was also negative, the donor is considered compatible, and the unit may be transfused. (Walker, p. 314)

31. Direct antiglobulin testing was performed on a patient suspected of having autoimmune hemolytic anemia. The following results were obtained:

	Polyspecific AHG	Anti-IgG	Anti-C3d
patient cells	2+	2+	0
check cells	NA	NA	2+

NA = not applicable

What is the best interpretation of these results?

A. The test cannot be interpreted because the check cells did not react as expected
B. The patient's cells are coated with IgG
C. The patient's cells are coated with complement
D. The patient's cells are coated with IgG and complement

The answer is B. Since direct antiglobulin testing uses antihuman-globulin reagent, check cells must be added to negative tubes to ensure that the AHG reagent was added and is active. The test for the presence of the complement component C3d on the patient's cells is therefore interpreted as negative. For anti-C3d testing, the check cells must be coated with complement instead of, or in addition to, antibody. Since the check cells reacted, the anti-C3d added to the test was active. Direct addition of polyspecific and monospecific IgG antihuman sera to washed patient cells resulted in reactions, indicating that the AHG was added and active and detecting the presence of IgG on the patient's cells. The polyspecific reagent can detect the presence of both IgG and complement components. The monospecific reagents are then used to determine which specific molecule(s) are attached to the patient's cells. (Walker, pp. 176–178)

32. Which of the following tests can be used to determine the dosage of Rh-immune globulin needed for a postpartum woman to prevent Rh sensitization?

A. D-antigen typing by microplate
B. Donath-Landsteiner test
C. Kleihauer-Betke acid elution
D. Microscopic weak D (D^u)

The answer is C. The Kleihauer-Betke acid-elution test detects fetal cells in the maternal blood sample. A smear of the mother's peripheral blood is treated with citric acid. Fetal hemoglobin resists the acid and remains in the cells while the adult hemoglobins in the maternal cells are eluted. When the smear is subsequently stained with eosin, the fetal cells appear bright pink and the maternal cells appear as "ghosts." The proportion of fetal cells to maternal cells is counted and used to calculate the number of doses of Rh-immune globulin needed to clear the fetal cells from the maternal circulation. (Walker, p. 682)

33. All of the women described below are Rh-negative, weak D (D^u)-negative, and delivered Rh-positive infants and should receive Rh-immune globulin

except one. Identify the woman who would not benefit from the administration of Rh-immune globulin (RhIg).

A. Group O; positive antibody screen; anti-D identified; received antepartum RhIg
B. Group B; positive antibody screen; anti-D identified; did not receive antepartum RhIg
C. Group A; positive antibody screen; anti-K identified; did not receive antepartum RhIg
D. Group O; negative antibody screen; did not receive antepartum RhIg

The answer is B. Women are candidates for RhIg if they are Rh-negative, weak D (D^u)-negative, deliver Rh-positive infants, and have not developed endogenous anti-D. This woman fulfills the first two criteria; however, she appears to have endogenous anti-D in her serum. This differs from the woman described in option A. In her case, the anti-D detected and identified is most likely due to antepartum RhIg administration. She remains a candidate for postpartum RhIg to clear from her bloodstream the fetal cells that entered at delivery. (Walker, pp. 462–463)

34. Below are the preliminary results of the investigation of a reported transfusion reaction. The transfusion was stopped after infusion of approximately 1/2 of a unit of packed cells because the patient developed a fever. The posttransfusion sample was collected within 30 minutes of the time the transfusion was stopped. A review of records revealed that the patient was group A, Rh positive, while the donor was group O, Rh negative.

	DAT	**Serum hemolysis**
pretransfusion patient sample	neg	absent
posttransfusion patient sample	neg	absent

These results suggest that the patient

A. is having an acute hemolytic-transfusion reaction
B. is having a delayed hemolytic-transfusion reaction
C. may be having a transfusion reaction, but it is not hemolytic
D. is not having a transfusion reaction

The answer is C. Whenever a patient receiving blood develops a fever, a transfusion reaction is likely. The preliminary laboratory tests will detect acute hemolytic-transfusion reactions, as when ABO-incompatible blood is transfused, and a posttransfusion sample demonstrates a positive DAT or serum hemolysis while the pretransfusion sample is negative. Delayed hemolytic reactions do not develop until several days after the transfusion is complete and, thus, would not be the cause of the reaction described here. Febrile reactions are the most common and are due to recipient antibodies directed against WBCs that are present in residual amounts in most component preparations. Further investigation is required to confirm this cause. Until ruled out by further testing, the possibility of a nonhemolytic transfusion reaction must be maintained. (Walker, pp. 471–472, 477, 479–480, 483)

35. Laboratory studies of maternal and cord blood yield the following results:

Maternal blood	Cord blood
group O, Rh-positive; anti-c identified in serum	group A, Rh-positive; direct anti-globulin test 2+; anti-c identified in eluate

If exchange transfusion is required, the best choice of blood is

A. A, Rh-negative, c-positive
B. O, Rh-positive, c-negative
C. A, Rh-positive, c-positive
D. O, Rh-negative, c-negative

The answer is B. Donor blood of the baby's ABO group should be selected when known—*if* it is compatible with the mother's serum. In this instance, the group O mother, with anti-A in her serum, would react with A cells if these were used. Thus, O red cells should be selected. Since the mother has anti-c in her serum, blood lacking the c antigen should be used. Therefore, group O, c-negative cells, such as CDe/CDe, should be selected. Since both mother and baby are Rh-positive, Rh-positive blood should be used to increase the likelihood of obtaining c-negative blood (D-negative, c-negative blood is rare). (Walker, p. 453)

36. Fresh frozen plasma should be thawed by

A. allowing it to come slowly to room temperature
B. slow thawing in the refrigerator to prevent bacterial growth
C. rapid thawing in a water bath at 56°C
D. rapid thawing in a microwave not to exceed 37°C

The answer is D. Thawing fresh frozen plasma must occur rapidly enough that bacteria cannot grow; thus, room-temperature thawing is too slow. Allowing plasma to thaw in the refrigerator prevents this problem due to the inability of most bacteria to multiply at 4°C; however, this is impractical because it greatly increases the time required to thaw the plasma for transfusion. Warming is required to thaw the plasma in a timely manner. The temperature cannot exceed 37°C because coagulation factors and other plasma proteins will be denatured. Both microwaves and waterbaths are acceptable as long as the temperature remains at or below 37°C. (Walker, p. 70)

37. Which of the following methods is acceptable for disposal of units of blood that must be discarded?

A. Chemical decontamination by mixing with bleach
B. Freezing with subsequent quick thawing, resulting in hemolysis
C. Incineration
D. Irradiation

The answer is C. Incineration and autoclaving are the only acceptable methods for ensuring that blood-borne pathogens are destroyed. (Walker, p. 523)

Immunohematology

38. The date is February 15th. The expiration dates of four units of packed red cells in the blood-bank refrigerator are given below. Which of these must be removed from inventory today?

    A. February 14
    B. February 15
    C. March 1
    D. March 14

The answer is A. Unit A has passed expiration and must be removed from inventory. Unit B is usable today but, if not transfused, must be removed from inventory tomorrow. Under exceedingly urgent conditions, if no other options are available, a unit just past outdate may be transfused. The benefit to the patient will be reduced as red-cell viability has probably fallen below 70%. However, this may be preferable to no transfusion or transfusion of incompatible units in an emergency situation. (Walker, p. 58)

39. A unit of blood is returned to the blood-transfusion facility. It had been issued 20 minutes previously. A patient emergency prevented the transfusion from being attempted. The nurse had taken the precaution of placing it in the refrigerator on the nursing floor where drugs are kept. The unit has not been entered and still has two segments attached. Assuming that visual inspection reveals no hemolysis or other abnormalities, can the unit be reissued?

    A. Yes; all requirements for reissue have been met
    B. No; the unit was not maintained at the appropriate temperature
    C. No; at least three segments are required for investigation of a possible transfusion reaction
    D. No; once a unit has left the transfusion facility, it cannot be reentered into inventory

The answer is A. Most blood banks will accept for reissue a unit of blood that has been out of their monitored refrigerator for less than 30 minutes. The fact that this unit was refrigerated during this time provides even greater assurance that the temperature of the blood did not exceed 10°C. However, well-meaning hospital staff may place the unit too near the freezer compartment of the nursing-floor refrigerator; therefore, inspection of the unit for hemolysis is essential prior to reissue. Additionally, the unit had not been entered, eliminating concerns of possible contamination and at least one segment was still attached to allow for any further pretransfusion testing. (Walker, p. 68)

CLS Review Questions

1. A donor unit contains a warm-reacting (37°C) unexpected antibody. That unit should be

    A. treated as any other unit for transfusion
    B. used only for purposes other than red-cell transfusion (e.g., plasma components)
    C. used only as frozen, deglycerolized red cells
    D. used as red-blood cells, or the equivalent, with the plasma removed

The answer is D. Donor units containing antibody that is reactive at 37°C should be processed into components that contain only minimal amounts of plasma. The antibody contained in the unit will be reduced in quantity, and when transfused will become diluted within the recipient's body. (Walker, p. 20)

2. All of the following tests on donor units are required *except*

    A. HBsAg
    B. anti-HTLV I
    C. anti–Epstein-Barr
    D. anti-HCV

The answer is C. Epstein-Barr virus, the causative agent for infectious mononucleosis, can be transmitted by transfusion. However, this occurrence is rare. Since the disease is usually mild and the transmission rate by transfusion is low, testing for this virus is not required. Hepatitis B and C viruses and HTLV I cause serious diseases that are the more common causes of transfusion-transmitted infections. All units transfused must be tested for exposure to these viruses. (Walker, p. 84)

3. A donor history reveals the following information:

Traveled to an area endemic for malaria 18 months ago; has had no antimalarial drugs or malarial symptoms
Has seasonal hay fever; presently asymptomatic
Has not eaten for the past 12 hours
Takes an occasional sleeping pill

    How many of these results exclude the person from giving blood for routine transfusion?

    A. None
    B. One
    C. Two
    D. Three

The answer is A. Although none of the conditions listed should exclude the donor, items concerning hay fever, fasting, and sleeping pills do warrant additional consideration. If the donor is taking aspirin-containing medications, the blood should not be the only source of platelets for a patient. Because lack of eating often causes more donor reactions than usual, a light snack before donation is advisable. The occasional use of hypnotics often is acceptable, but it is advised in such instances that the donor's verbal approval to donate be documented in the donor record. (Walker, pp. 5, 6, 8)

4. The clinical laboratory scientist is determining hemoglobin values on donors using the copper-sulfate method. When a drop of one donor's blood was added to the 1.053 specific-gravity copper-sulfate solution, the drop sank into the solution about 1/2 inch, hesitated there, and then rose. This indicates that

    A. the donor has sufficient hemoglobin to be accepted for donation
    B. the copper-sulfate solution is contaminated and should be replaced

C. the donor is anemic and should not be accepted for donation

D. the donor is acceptable only if female

The answer is C. In the copper-sulfate method of hemoglobin determination, a drop of blood with a hemoglobin concentration of 12.5 g/dL or greater will sink in a solution of specific-gravity 1.053. The failure of the blood to sink indicates that the donor's hemoglobin level is less than 12.5 g/dL, and, therefore, the donor is anemic. Since donation may be risky for this donor, the donor should be deferred. In past years, different minimum hemoglobin concentrations were specified for male and female donors. Recently, a single value has been established for all donors, regardless of gender. (Walker, p. 12)

5. A unit of whole blood is spun using a heavy spin, and the plasma is removed into a transfer pack 24 hours after collection. The plasma unit is then frozen solid and later thawed at 4°C, at which time the liquid portion is removed. The remainder of the unit should be

A. labeled as cryoprecipitated AHF and frozen at −30°C

B. labeled as fresh frozen plasma and frozen at −18°C

C. placed in the refrigerator and labeled liquid plasma

D. discarded due to incorrect preparation

The answer is D. The described procedure would result in the preparation of cryoprecipitated AHF; however, it is necessary to begin such preparation within eight hours of whole-blood collection to preserve the labile clotting factor. Therefore, the cryoprecipitated AHF cannot be transfused. The remainder of the whole-blood unit may be used as RBCs and plasma. (Walker, p. 728)

6. Below is the label for a patient sample submitted to the blood bank for type and crossmatch. Assuming that the date is today, is the sample acceptable for testing?

Thomas, Marilyn
ID 76-15405
7-15-96   15:05   CB

A. The sample is acceptable

B. The sample is not acceptable because it lacks the patient's room number or location

C. The sample is not acceptable because it lacks the name of the patient's physician

D. The sample is not acceptable because the patient's middle name or initial is missing

The answer is A. The label must contain the patient's first and last names, identification number, and the date the specimen was collected. Some institutions may require additional information, such as physician, time of collection, or the initials of the phlebotomist. (AABB Standards, 16th ed. page 25)

7. A serum has been tentatively determined to contain anti-c and anti-Fy^a. Which of the cells below would best adsorb the serum and separate the antibodies so that anti-Fy^a would be recovered from the eluate of the adsorbing cells?

  A. CcDEe, Fy(a+b−), Kk
  B. ce, Fy(a−b+), Kk
  C. CDe, (Fya+b+), kk
  D. CDe, Fy(a+b−), kk

The answer is D. When using adsorption to separate antibodies, the cells selected must possess the antigen corresponding to only one of the antibodies. Since the anti-Fy^a was to be recovered from the eluate of the adsorbing cells, the cells must have the Fy^a antigen but must not have the c antigen on their surfaces. Both cells C and D meet this requirement. However, cell D is homozygous for the Fy^a antigen; this would increase the sites available to adsorb anti-Fy^a and render it the better choice. (Walker, p. 349)

8. Which of the following cells would be the best choice to use in titration of only anti-Jk^a in a serum containing both anti-Jk^a and anti-Jk^b?

	Anti-Jk^a	Anti-Jk^b
A. Cell 1	0	0
B. Cell 2	+	0
C. Cell 3	+	+
D. Cell 4	0	+

The answer is B. The cell used for the titration must have on its surface the antigen corresponding to the antibody to be titered and lack the antigen(s) corresponding to antibody(ies) in the same serum that are not to be titered. (Walker, pp. 651–654)

9. Which of the following best reflects the discrepancy seen in a sample demonstrating the acquired-B–like phenomenon?

  A. Forward group appears to be B, but reverse group seems to be O
  B. Forward group appears to be AB, but reverse group seems to be A
  C. Forward group appears to be O, but reverse group seems to be B
  D. Forward group appears to be B, but reverse group seems to be AB

The answer is B. Some group A individuals, such as those with carcinoma of the colon, massive infection with gram-negative organisms, or intestinal obstruction, have been observed to acquire a B-like antigen. This may result from the action of bacterial deacetylase, which converts the primary A-antigen determinant, N-acetyl-galactosamine, to N-galactosamine; this is similar to the primary D-galactose determinant of B antigen. Interestingly, the natural anti-B in the patient's serum does not react with the B-like antigens on her own cells, whereas most other examples of anti-B, such as anti-B–typing serum, react with the patient's cells. (Walker, p. 216)

10. A patient whose blood is a subgroup of A gives the following red-cell reactions when tested against various antisera:

Antisera	Reactions of patient's RBCs
Dolichos biflorus:	negative
anti-A:	mixed-field agglutination
anti-A,B:	mixed-field agglutination

This patient has an anti-A_1 in the serum. The subgroup is most likely

A. A_1
B. A_2
C. A_3
D. A_m

The answer is C. The mixed-field reactions with anti-A and anti-A,B are characteristic of the A_3 subgroup. Occasionally, A_3 persons have anti-A_1 in their serum. Mixed-field agglutination is not seen in any other subgroup of A. (Walker, p. 208)

11. Select the most likely cause for the ABO forward and reverse reactions given below:

Cell grouping			Serum grouping			
anti-A	anti-B	anti-A,B	A cells	B cells	O cells	Auto control
4+	0	4+	0	0	0	0

A. polyagglutinable cells
B. immunodeficiency
C. acquired A-like antigen
D. A subgroup

The answer is B. The strong reactions in the forward grouping indicate a group A individual. However, no agglutination is seen in the reverse grouping, in which the serum of a group A person possessing anti-B should react with B cells. One would not expect reactions with A cells or O cells. The autocontrol is negative, ruling out an autoantibody. The lack of agglutination in all of the serum groupings indicates that an immunodeficiency state should be suspected. Immunodeficient persons do not produce antibodies demonstrable at 22°C (room temperature). (Walker, p. 218)

12. The transfusion service receives an order for 4 units of packed red cells for a surgical patient. Blood grouping and typing results are as follows:

Cell grouping		Serum grouping	
anti-A:	0	A cells: +	
anti-B:	+	B cells: +	
anti-A,B:	+		
anti-D:	0 (IS and AHG)		
Rh control:	0 (IS and AHG)		

The next step required to solve this problem is to

A. draw a new blood sample from the patient and repeat all test procedures
B. set up a cell panel to identify the antibody causing the typing problem

C. test the patient's serum with A_2 cells and the patient's red cells with anti-A_1 lectin

D. repeat the ABO-antigen grouping using 3×-washed, saline-suspended cells

The answer is B. There is a discrepancy in the ABO grouping. The patient's forward grouping indicates a group B; however, the serum gives reactions with both A and B cells. Since the weak-D testing results at AHG give no reaction, the cells are known to be free of coating antibody, so the forward typing results are probably reliable. The problem is most likely due to the presence of an unexpected antibody in the patient's serum that is reacting with the reagent B cells. In this instance, performing a panel to identify the antibody is the most appropriate course of action. (Walker, p. 219)

13. Below are the results of a type and screen on a patient with lymphoma who is scheduled for surgery the following day. In this laboratory, cells are not washed for routine typing.

Cell grouping	Serum grouping
anti-A: 4+	A cells: 2+
anti-B: 1+	B cells: 4+

	37°C LISS	AHG	Check cells
patient serum + screening cell I	2+	0	2+
patient serum + screening cell II	2+	0	2+

Which of the following techniques would be most useful in resolving the ABO discrepancy and obtaining reliable antibody screening results?

A. Autologous absorption
B. Saline-replacement technique
C. Antibody-identification panel
D. Use of polyspecific AHG rather than monospecific AHG

The answer is B. If the weaker grouping results are ignored, the patient forward and reverse groups as an A. The weak cell reaction with anti-B and the serum reaction with A cells suggest that these results are unreliable. Since patient cells are not washed prior to grouping tests in this laboratory, patient serum is present in all of the tubes; however, patient cells are present only in the cell-grouping tubes. Therefore, the problem is most likely to be with the patient's serum. The antibody-screening results also indicate a serum problem. An antibody detected at 37°C in LISS would most often react with even greater strength in the AHG phase of testing. In this case, the reactions disappear at AHG. Before AHG is added to the test system, the cells are thoroughly washed, removing all patient serum. Since this seems to have eliminated the reactions, rouleaux is suspected. Rouleaux is typically seen in patients with multiple myeloma but may also be observed in association with lymphocytic leukemias or lymphomas. Saline-replacement technique is used when rouleaux is present. In this technique, patient serum is allowed to react with the reagent cells. The tubes are then centrifuged but are not resuspended for reading. The serum is removed, an equal amount of saline is added, and the tubes are recentrifuged and read for agglutination. True agglutination will not be dispersed, but rouleaux will. (Walker, p. 643)

14. The ABO-grouping and Rh-typing results on a donor are given below. High-protein anti-D reagent was used.

Cell grouping		Serum grouping
anti-A:	0	A cells: 4+
anti-B:	0	B cells: 3+
anti-D (IS):	0	
Rh control (IS):	0	
anti-D (AHG):	2+	
Rh control (AHG):	2+	

The most appropriate next step is

A. label the unit O, Rh negative, D^u positive
B. label the unit O, Rh positive
C. perform a DAT on the donor cells
D. wash the donor cells to remove rouleaux and retype

The answer is C. The patient's ABO grouping is unremarkable. In the test for weak D at AHG, however, the Rh control is reacting. The Rh control should be negative. The Rh control for a high-protein reagent contains the protein and additives that are included in the anti-D reagent but lacks the exogenous antibody. High protein is added to reagents to reduce the zeta potential and allow cells to come closer together. This enables IgG antibodies to cause visible agglutination at room temperature, speeding the typing reaction. When cells coated with endogenous antibody are tested in this environment, the antibodies already present on the red cells may crosslink and cause agglutination without the addition of exogenous antibody in the anti-D reagent. When the test for weak D is performed by adding AHG after 37°C incubation, the AHG will react with the endogenous antibody on the cell in the Rh control tube. Since the presence of endogenous antibody coating the red cells is often the cause of a reaction with the Rh control, a DAT should be performed. The DAT will detect endogenous antibody coating red cells and either confirm this as the cause of the problem or suggest that further testing is necessary. (Walker, pp. 248–250)

15. All of the following are characteristic of cold agglutinins *except*

A. they react optimally at temperatures between 1–10°C
B. the reactions obtained are reversible after warming
C. they react strongly with cord cells
D. they will agglutinate most adult human red cells, regardless of blood group

The answer is C. Cold agglutinins are antibodies that react best at low temperatures and are, therefore, clinically unimportant in most cases. Most are anti-I and react with most adult human red cells because they carry the I antigen. Since cord cells have very little I antigen, they do not react with most cold agglutinins. The reactions are reversible on warming, since the antibodies tend to dissociate from antigen at higher temperatures. (Walker, p. 223)

16. A patient has incompatible crossmatches and a positive antibody screen in the antiglobulin phase. The patient's serum is tested against a panel of reagent red cells. Reactions are shown below:

Cell No.	D	C	E	c	e	M	N	S	s	Le^a	Le^b	P₁	K	k	Fy^a	Fy^b	Jk^a	Jk^b	Saline RT	LISS 37°	LISS AHG	Check Cells	Ficin 37°C	Ficin AHG	Check Cells
1	0	+	0	+	+	0	+	0	+	+	0	+	0	+	0	+	+	0	0	0	0	2+	0	0	2+
2	+	+	0	0	+	+	+	+	+	0	+	0	+	+	0	0	+	+	0	+	3+	NP	+	3+	NP
3	+	+	0	0	+	+	+	+	0	0	+	+	0	+	+	+	+	+	0	0	1+	NP	0	0	2+
4	+	0	+	+	0	0	+	0	+	+	0	+	0	+	0	+	0	+	0	0	0	2+	0	0	2+
5	+	0	+	+	+	0	+	0	+	+	0	+	0	+	+	0	0	+	0	0	2+	NP	0	0	2+
6	0	0	+	+	+	+	0	0	+	0	+	0	+	0	+	0	0	+	0	2+	4+	NP	2+	4+	NP
7	0	0	0	+	+	0	+	0	+	0	+	0	0	+	0	+	+	0	0	0	0	2+	0	0	2+
8	0	0	0	+	+	0	0	0	+	0	+	0	0	+	0	+	+	0	0	0	0	2+	0	0	2+
9	0	0	0	+	+	+	+	+	0	+	0	+	+	0	0	+	+	+	0	2+	4+	NP	2+	4+	NP
10	0	0	0	+	+	0	+	+	+	+	0	+	0	+	+	+	+	+	0	0	1+	NP	0	0	2+
11 Cord	/	/	/	/		/	/	/	/	0	0	/	/	/	/	/	/	/	0	±	2+	NP	±	2+	NP
Auto	+	+	0	+	+	+	0	+	+	0	+	+	0	+	0	+	+	0	0	0	0	2+	0	0	2+

RT = room temperature; LISS = low ionic strength salt solution;
AHG = antiglobulin test; NP = not performed.

What are the most probable antibodies?

A. Anti-S and anti-k
B. Anti-S and anti-Fy^a
C. Anti-K and anti-Fy^a
D. Anti-s, anti-K, and anti-Fy^a

The answer is C. The autocontrol is negative, indicating that these are alloanti-bodies. Cells 1, 4, 7, and 8 give negative reactions with the patient's serum. Antibodies that would have reacted with the antigens on these cells can then be eliminated. This leaves three possibilities: anti-S, anti-K, and anti-Fy^a. All of these antibodies react optimally in the antiglobulin phase of testing. The reactions seen in LISS at 37°C coincide with the pattern shown for anti-K. K antigen is present on cells 2, 6, and 9, and cells 6 and 9 are KK while cell 2 is Kk. The reactions correspond to the dose of the antigen, with stronger reactions seen when testing with the homozygous cells 6 and 9. The LISS-AHG phase of testing increases the reaction with cells 2, 6, and 9; additionally, reactions are seen with cells 3, 5, and 10. Cells 3, 5, 6, and 10 possess the Fy^a antigen. Ficin treatment destroys the Duffy antigens, and cells will no longer give reactions with anti-Fy^a. Following ficin treatment, only cells 2, 6, and 9 react (corresponding with anti-K); this indicates that the Fy^a has been removed from the cells by the ficin treatment. The antibodies identified by this panel are anti-K and anti-Fy^a. Anti-S cannot be ruled out, however, because the patient is S-antigen positive, it is unlikely that Anti-S is present in the patient's serum. (Walker, p. 341)

17. Anti-D and anti-Fy^a have been tentatively identified in a serum. To provide 95% confidence in the proper identification of the antibodies, which set of cells and serum results would be expected?

		Anti-D	Anti-Fy^a	Patient serum
A.	3 cells	+	0	+
	3 cells	0	+	+
	3 cells	+	+	+
B.	3 cells	+	0	+
	3 cells	0	0	+
	3 cells	0	+	+

		Anti-D	Anti-Fy^a	Patient serum
C.	3 cells	+	+	0
	3 cells	+	0	+
	3 cells	0	0	0
D.	3 cells	+	0	+
	3 cells	0	+	+
	3 cells	0	0	0

The answer is D. Whenever an antibody panel is used to identify antibodies, the possibility exists that the patient's serum is reacting against a low-incidence antigen present on a panel cell that is unidentified, or that an additional antibody is present but masked by reactions of other antibodies. The likelihood of the reaction being due to an unsuspected antigen is reduced when the serum containing the antibody reacts with three or more cells carrying the suspected antigen. Confidence is further increased when the serum is negative with three or more cells lacking the antigen. Therefore, to provide 95% confidence in the correct identification of the antibody, three cells carrying the antigen and three cells lacking the antigen corresponding to the antibody identified should be tested against the serum containing antibody. The cells carrying the antigen should all react with the serum, and the cells lacking the antigen should not react with the serum. When multiple antibodies are identified, three cells carrying antigen 1 but not antigen 2, three cells carrying antigen 2 but not antigen 1, and three cells lacking both antigens must be tested. All of the cells carrying either antigen 1 or antigen 2 should react, but the cells lacking both antigens should not react with the serum. (Walker, p. 649)

18. Given the panel of reagent red cells below tested against patient serum at IS, 37°C with LISS, and AHG, which cells would show agglutination at some phase of testing if the serum contained antibodies to M and Fy^a?

Cell no.	D	C	E	c	e	K	k	Fy^a	Fy^b	M	N
1	+	+	0	0	+	+	+	+	0	+	+
2	+	+	0	0	+	0	+	0	+	+	0
3	+	0	+	+	0	0	+	+	0	0	+
4	+	0	0	+	+	0	+	0	+	0	+
5	0	+	0	+	+	0	+	0	+	+	+

A. Cells 1, 2, 3, and 5
B. Cells 1 and 3
C. Cells 1, 2, and 5
D. Cell 4 only

The answer is A. The patient's serum should react with each cell that carries M antigen and each cell that carries Fy^a antigen. It is likely that reactions with M-positive cells would occur in the IS phase of testing and weaken or disappear on warming, and the reactions with Fy^a-positive cells would not appear until the AHG phase. Cells that are homozygous for either antigen may demonstrate stronger reactions. (Walker, pp. 259–260, 271)

19. The results of an antibody screen are

	37°C LISS	AHG	Check cells
patient serum + screening cell I	0	2+	NA
patient serum + screening cell II	1+	3+	NA

Assuming that the test has been performed correctly and the serum contains only a single antibody, how can the difference in reaction between the two cells be explained?

A. Dose
B. Larger drops of screening-cell II were used
C. Prozone reaction with screening cell I
D. Rouleaux is present

The answer is A. *Dose* refers to the number of antigen sites on the cell surface and is controlled by the number of genes coding for production of the antigen. Possessing a single gene (i.e., being heterozygous) for a given antigen produces fewer antigen sites on the cell, or one dose of antigen. Possessing two genes (i.e., being homozygous) for an antigen at one locus produces roughly twice the number of antigen sites on the cells, or a double dose. If the antibody concentration in the two tubes is the same, as when a single serum is tested against two different screening cells, a stronger reaction can occur with a cell carrying a double dose of the antigen. (Walker, p. 189)

20. The antibody panel below can be used to identify antibodies against all of the following antigens *except*

Cell no.	D	C	E	c	e	K	k	Fy^a	Fy^b	Jk^a	Jk^b	M	N
1	+	+	+	0	0	0	+	+	+	+	0	+	+
2	+	+	0	+	+	0	+	0	+	0	+	+	0
3	+	+	0	+	+	0	+	+	0	+	+	0	+
4	+	0	+	+	0	0	+	+	0	+	+	+	+
5	0	0	0	+	+	0	+	+	+	+	0	+	+

A. Fy^a
B. Jk^b
C. M
D. K

The answer is D. A given panel of cells can be used to identify antibodies to antigens that are known to be present on the panel cells. Antibodies to antigens that are *not* present on panel cells cannot be identified, since the serum tested will not react with any cells. In this case, K antigen is not present on any of the cells, so a reaction with anti-K cannot occur. Antibody present in a patient serum can react with antigen present but not identified on a panel cell, such as a low-incidence antigen. In that case, the antibody cannot be identified, and additional cells known to carry low-incidence antigens will need to be tested. (Walker, p. 164)

21. Which of the following is performed as routine pretransfusion testing on *all* patients?

    A. Antibody panel identification
    B. Antiglobulin-phase crossmatch
    C. Direct antiglobulin testing
    D. Examination of prior transfusion records

The answer is D. Whenever a transfusion is ordered, the patient's previous transfusion history should be checked. This can alert the clinical laboratory scientist to prior transfusion reactions that can be avoided or to the presence of unexpected antibodies in the patient's serum, which may now have fallen below detectable levels. In some cases, disease may cause changes in ABO-grouping results; previous records may help resolve discrepancies. (Walker, p. 309)

22. If a patient has anti-c in the serum, which of the following units of red cells may he or she receive without expecting a reaction due to this antibody?

    A. R^1R^1
    B. R^1R^2
    C. R^1r
    D. r'r

The answer is A. A person who has anti-c should receive blood that does not carry the corresponding c antigen to prevent a transfusion reaction. R^1R^1 = CDe/CDe; R^1R^2 = CDe/cDE; R^1r = CDE/cde, and r'r = Cde/cde. Therefore, the only unit that does not carry the c antigen is R^1R^1. (Walker, p. 316)

23. A donor's cells give incompatible major crossmatches in the antiglobulin phase of testing with seven different recipients of the same ABO group and Rh type as the donor. Based on these results, the donor might be expected to be positive on

    A. anti-I testing
    B. direct antiglobulin testing
    C. indirect antiglobulin testing
    D. k-antigen typing

The answer is B. The major crossmatch tests recipient serum against donor red cells. Therefore, something on this donor's cells must be reacting with all recipient sera. The indirect antiglobulin test is eliminated, since donor serum (not cells) is tested in that procedure. Similarly, since anti-I is present in serum, it would not be the cause of the problem. Because most individuals are k positive, anti-k is very rare. For the k antigen on the donor cells to be a problem, all seven recipients would have to have anti-k in their serum, an extremely unlikely event. The most likely cause of the problem is an unexpected antibody coating the donor cells, which would give a positive direct-antiglobulin test. Coated donor cells, since antibody is already present before addition of recipient serum, will react in the antiglobulin phase of all major crossmatches performed regardless of the recipient serum added to the test system. (Walker, p. 327)

24. A patient requiring a transfusion has a positive autologous control at immediate spin. All serum tests done at 37°C and with AHG are negative. The antibody is identified as anti-I. The patient's history reveals transfusion of several units of blood at another institution within the past month. What is the procedure of choice to obtain compatible blood at this time?

A. Absorb the patient's serum with the donor cells at 4°C
B. Absorb the patient's serum with the patient's cells at 4°C
C. Perform all tests at 37°C and convert to the antiglobulin phase
D. Perform warm autoabsorptions with the patient's cells and the patient's serum

The answer is C. The patient's serum must not be absorbed with the donor cells, as any alloantibodies present may also be absorbed out. Since the patient history includes recent transfusion, autoabsorption at any temperature is inappropriate, because donor cells will still be present in the patient's blood, and alloantibodies may be adsorbed onto the transfused cells in the patient sample. The procedure of choice is testing while avoiding the temperature at which the anti-I reacts. (Walker, pp. 370–371)

25. Which of the following differences between donors and recipients will the major crossmatch performed at the IS, 37°C LISS, and AHG phases of testing usually detect? In each situation, no unexpected antibodies are present except those indicated.

A. Group O patient mistyped as A; donor is A
B. Rh-negative patient mistyped as Rh-positive but with no unexpected antibodies; donor is Rh-positive
C. Patient with AHG-reacting anti-Jk^a; donor is Jk(a−b+)
D. Rh-positive patient; donor is Rh-negative

The answer is A. Group O individuals have anti-A and anti-A,B in their serum, which will react with the A antigen on the donor's cells. An Rh-negative patient having no anti-D in the serum, as in option B, will not react with the D antigen on the donor's Rh-positive cells. In option C, the patient has an antibody, but the donor lacks the corresponding antigen; therefore, no reaction will occur. In option D, the Rh-positive patient, having no unexpected antibodies in the serum, would be expected to have a compatible crossmatch with the Rh-negative donor cells. (Walker, pp. 326–327)

26. A patient is typed as group O, Rh-positive and crossmatched with five units of red cells. The patient's antibody screening test and one compatibility test show agglutination in the antiglobulin phase. All other test results are negative. Of those listed below, the most probable antibody is

A. anti-I
B. anti-K
C. anti-M
D. anti-k

The answer is B. Anti-I and anti-M, which react best at room temperature and below, are eliminated. Although anti-k is expected to react in the antiglobulin phase, it is directed against a high-incidence antigen. If anti-k were present in the patient's serum, all donor units and screening cells would be expected to be incompatible. The optimal phase for anti-K reactivity is the antiglobulin phase. Although anti-K would be expected to give an incompatible crossmatch in one of ten cases, the occurrence of one in five crossmatches in this instance is still possible. (Walker, p. 267)

27. A woman is diagnosed as having immune hemolytic anemia (IHA). Her direct antiglobulin test is positive, but an indirect antiglobulin test is negative. Absorption-elution techniques are employed to help identify the causative antibody. The eluate gives the following agglutination patterns with these group-O cells:

    cDE/cDE: ±
    cdE/cDE: ±
      cde/cde: 4+
    cDE/cde: 2+
    CDe/cDE: 2+

From these results, the specificity of the antibody appears to be

    A. anti-C
    B. anti-E
    C. anti-c
    D. anti-e

The answer is D. In this situation, the antibodies that could cause IHA are assumed to be anti-C, -D, -E, -c, or -e. A spectrum of reactivities from ± to 4+ is observed, indicating multiple antibodies or a dosing antibody. If we consider only the 2+ and 4+ reactions for a moment, the possibility of the antibody being anti-c, anti-D, or anti-E is unlikely, since only ± results were obtained with cells cDE/cDE and cdE/cDE. Anti-C is eliminated because a 2+ reaction is seen with cell cDE/cde, which lacks the C antigen. In contrast, cell cde/cde carries the e antigen in the homozygous form, and a 4+ reaction is seen. In addition, 2+ reactions are seen in cells cDE/cde and CDe/cDE, on which e is carried in the heterozygous form. These results indicate a dosage effect. Therefore, anti-e is the most logical antibody. Additional resolution of the ± reactions may be indicated depending on the policies of the individual blood bank regarding the possible clinical importance of such reactions. (Walker, p. 367)

28. A blood sample from a neonate was received for typing and DAT. The test results on the mother and neonate are given below:

	Mother's results	Baby's results
anti-A	0	0
anti-B	0	4+
A cells	4+	NP
B cells	4+	NP
anti-D	0	4+
DAT	0	0
Rh control	NP	2+
anti-M	0	4+
anti-K	0	1+

The mother has anti-M and anti-K in her serum. No other unexpected antibodies were detected. The baby is being given penicillin for a streptococcal infection. The most likely cause for the baby's positive DAT is

A. maternal anti-D coating the baby's Rh-positive cells
B. maternal anti-M coating the baby's M-positive cells
C. maternal anti-K coating the baby's K-positive cells
D. drug-induced hemolytic anemia due to penicillin administration

The answer is C. Anti-K is most often IgG, which is able to cross the placenta into the fetal circulation where, in this case, it can attach to the baby's cells carrying the corresponding K antigen. Anti-M is also present in the maternal serum; however, it is most often an IgM antibody and IgM cannot cross the placenta. So no anti-M would be available to attach to the M antigen on the baby's cells. No anti-D has been detected in the maternal serum, so even though she is Rh-negative, the positive DAT is not due to anti-D. Although the baby is on penicillin, neonates are not likely to produce antibody in response to any antigen stimulus in the first four months of life. Since IgG antibodies to the drug-RBC complex cause the positive DAT associated with penicillin–induced hemolytic anemia, the penicillin is not the cause of the problem in this case. (Walker, pp. 260, 440, 449)

29. A Kleihauer-Betke acid-elution test is performed to determine the dosage of Rh-immune globulin (RhIg). Once the cells have been counted, the percentage of fetal cells in the maternal circulation is determined to be 2.2%. The procedure manual directs the use of the following formula to calculate the Rh-immune globulin dosage:

$$\frac{\% \text{ fetal cells} \times 50}{30} = \text{doses of RhIg}$$

How many doses of RhIg should this woman receive?

A. 2
B. 3
C. 4
D. 5

The answer is D. 2.2 × 50 divided by 30 equals 3.6. However, the method is imprecise, and undertreatment must clearly be avoided. Therefore, when the number to the right of the decimal point is less than 5, round down and add 1 dose. When the number to the right of the decimal point is greater than 5, round up and add 1 more vial. In this case, round up to 4 and then add 1 more dose; the correct dosage would be 5 vials. (Walker, p. 465)

30. In which of the following situations would the administration of Rh-immune globulin (RhIg) *not* be indicated? None of the women has received antenatal RhIg.

	Mother	Newborn
A.	r′r; no antibody detected	R⁰r; DAT positive
B.	rr; no antibody detected	R¹r; DAT negative

Immunohematology

	Mother	Newborn
C.	rr; anti-E in serum	R^1r; DAT positive
D.	r'r; anti-D in serum	R^2r; DAT positive

The answer is D. Administration of RhIg prevents the formation of anti-D by the mother. If the mother has already been immunized to the D antigen and has produced anti-D, RhIg would not be of benefit. If anti-D is detected in maternal serum, however, the clinical laboratory scientist must determine whether the woman received RhIg antenatally. If so, she should receive additional immunoprophylaxis after delivery, because the anti-D in her serum may be due to the RhIg and not represent immunization to the D antigen. (Walker, pp. 462–464)

31. A 44-year-old woman has a hemoglobin level of 6.1 g/dL. Leukocyte and platelet counts are within reference limits. The patient is group O, Rh-negative and has no unexpected blood-group antibodies in her serum. Crossmatches are compatible. However, 15 min after the first transfusion is started, she experiences a sudden anaphylactic reaction, including difficulty in breathing and hives. Subsequent units of transfused washed red cells are tolerated well. The most probable explanation for these findings is that the

    A. patient has antibodies against WBCs
    B. patient has antibodies against IgA
    C. donor has IgG antibodies
    D. patient has antiplatelet antibodies

The answer is B. These signs and symptoms are most characteristic of an allergic reaction, of which urticaria (hives) is the most common sign. IgA-deficient patients who have developed anti-IgA may experience anaphylactic reactions. Such reactions occur after the infusion of a small amount of blood or plasma and are characterized by coughing, nausea, respiratory distress, and shock. Antihistamines, such as diphenhydramine, are effective in reducing the incidence of allergic reactions. However, washed red cells, which have IgA removed, have proven even more effective in preventing an allergic reaction of this type. (Walker, p. 481)

32. The primary investigation of a transfusion reaction yields the following results. (The records show that the patient and donor are both group O, Rh-positive.)

	DAT	Serum/plasma hemolysis
pretransfusion patient sample	0	absent
posttransfusion patient sample	0	present
pretransfusion donor segment	0	absent
sample from the donor unit	0	present

These results are consistent with

    A. acute hemolytic transfusion reaction
    B. allergic reaction

C. transfusion of hemolyzed blood

D. delayed transfusion reaction

The answer is C. The presence of hemolysis in the posttransfusion patient sample when it was not present in the pretransfusion sample suggests that the transfusion caused the hemolysis. Immunologic causes such as ABO incompatibility must be considered, but nonimmunologic causes must also be considered. Generally, nonimmunologic causes create hemolysis within the donor unit prior to transfusion so that hemolyzed blood is being transfused into the recipient. The patient reacts to the free hemoglobin with fever and other symptoms as if the hemolysis were happening in vivo. Nonimmunologic causes of hemolysis of the unit include bacterial contamination, infusion of inappropriate fluids with the blood, use of inappropriate infusion sets, use of improper devices to increase the rate of infusion, improper warming of the unit, or improper storage of the unit. These occur after the pretransfusion testing has been performed on the segment, so it shows no hemolysis. However, a sample of blood taken directly from the bag implicated in the transfusion reaction shows the presence of hemolysis and, together with a negative DAT on the recipient's posttransfusion sample, confirms the nonimmunological cause. (Walker, pp. 474–475)

33. Which of the following matings has the potential to result in hemolytic disease of the newborn (HDN) due to antigens in any of the systems identified?

	Mother's phenotype	Father's phenotype
A.	O, DCcEe	O, DCe
B.	A, DCcEe, Kk	O, DcE, kk
C.	B, dce	O, DCce
D.	AB, Dce, Jk(a−b+)	A, dce, Jk(a−b+)

The answer is C. HDN can occur when the fetus has antigens, inherited from the father, that the mother lacks. In option A, the father has no antigens that the mother lacks. In option B, the Rh and Kell systems antigens are no problem, because the mother has all of the antigens carried by the father. The ABO system is also compatible, because the child of the mating would be either A or O. In option C, the mother lacks both D and C antigens, which are carried by the father and could be passed to the fetus. In option D, the father has no Rh or Kidd system antigens not carried by the mother, and since the mother is AB, no ABO incompatibility between mother and fetus is possible. (Walker, p. 440)

34. A mother is group O, Rh-negative and has anti-K in her serum. Her baby is group B, Rh-positive and requires an exchange transfusion. Assuming that the exchange crossmatch is performed using the maternal serum, which of the following units would be expected to be compatible?

A. O, Rh-negative, K-positive

B. B, Rh-positive, K-negative

C. O, Rh-positive, K-negative

D. B, Rh-negative, K-positive

The answer is C. The blood used for an exchange transfusion must lack the antigen against which the maternal antibody is directed. In this case, the mother has anti-K in her serum; hence, only K-negative units can be considered. Additionally, the unit must be compatible with the baby's blood group. In this case, group B or O, Rh-negative or Rh-positive blood would be compatible with the baby. However, since the maternal serum is being used for the crossmatch, type-B cells cannot be used. Therefore, only group O cells lacking the K antigen, either Rh-positive or Rh-negative, will be expected to be compatible. (Walker, p. 453)

35. What is the preferred hematocrit level in small-volume transfusions given to neonates?

A. 45%
B. 50%
C. 55%
D. 65%

The answer is D. Hematocrits can be adjusted to any required percentage by collecting the whole blood into a multipack system and expressing the plasma into a satellite bag. The cells and plasma are then mixed in a second satellite bag to the required level. When using 12-h settling, the resulting hematocrit is approximately 65%, which is the preferred concentration when transfusing small volumes to neonates. Since neonates do not compensate well for changes in blood volume, a unit with a relatively high hematocrit, comparable to that of a healthy neonate, is preferred. (Walker, p. 447)

36. A unit of packed red cells was issued to the floor nurse for a patient transfusion at 13:51 h. The patient was taken to radiology before the nurse could start the infusion; the blood bag and all ports were unentered. The unit was placed in the drug refrigerator on the floor. The temperature of this unmonitored refrigerator was reported as 10°C. At 15:12 h, the blood is returned to the transfusion service. Can this unit be returned to inventory and reissued?

A. Yes, because it has been returned to the transfusion service within 2 h of issue
B. Yes, because it has not been entered
C. No, because the unit was outside a monitored refrigerator for more than 30 min
D. No, because the temperature of the drug refrigerator was ≤10°C

The answer is C. Packed red-cell units returned to the transfusion service intact less than 30 min after issuance (i.e., outside a monitored refrigerator for less than 30 min) are reissuable. After 30 min, regardless of storage away from the transfusion service, units are considered to be warmed and cannot be reissued. The only exception to this rule is when the unit is stored in a refrigerator monitored by the transfusion service in an alternate location, such as the surgical area or the emergency room. (Walker, p. 69)

37. The clinical laboratory scientist has recently been promoted to a supervisory position in the transfusion service of a small rural hospital. He feels that the optimal blood inventory should be reviewed. The data for the previous 3 mo of group A, Rh-positive blood usage is given below. Assuming that it is representative of a 6-mo period, what should the optimal inventory of A-positive units be for this institution?

Week	Usage
1	3
2	12
3	4
4	2
5	0
6	5
7	3
8	2
9	4
10	3
11	3
12	4

A. 3
B. 4
C. 5
D. 8

The answer is A. In calculating the optimal inventory, any weeks with unusually high usage should not be included in the calculation, so week 2 is not included. The usage in each of the remaining weeks is averaged (33/11 = 3). This provides an average usage across several weeks, which is the optimal inventory. (Walker, p. 591)

38. While inspecting the donor units in the blood-bank refrigerator, the clinical laboratory scientist notes a greenish appearance in the plasma of one unit. What course of action should be taken?

    A. Ignore this appearance and leave the unit in the available inventory
    B. Remove the unit from the inventory pending completion of a bacterial culture on the unit
    C. Discard the unit following appropriate precautions
    D. Return the unit to the donor center

The answer is A. On exposure to light, the yellow of bilirubin pigments in the plasma can be converted to green. This is not a cause for concern. However, other colors, such as purple, brown, or red, can indicate contamination or other harmful changes in the unit, and it should be removed from inventory. Clots or cloudiness in the plasma are also causes for removing the unit from the inventory. (Walker, p. 67)

References

AABB Technical Standards (16th ed). Washington, DC: American Association of Blood Banks, 1995.

Walker RH (ed). *Technical Manual of the American Association of Blood Banks* (11th ed). Washington, DC: American Association of Blood Banks, 1993.

4

Microbiology

Section Editor   **Joyce A. Zook**

CLT Review Questions

Contributors

Rebecca Janine Fithen
Frances A. Morgenstern
Hal S. Larsen
Margaret J. H. Fuller
Donna L. Oblack
John P. Seabolt

1. Which of the following characteristics is *not* used to isolate or identify *Staphylococcus aureus?*

   A. "Pitting" on sheep-blood agar
   B. Fermentation of mannitol
   C. Positive catalase test
   D. Positive coagulase test

The answer is A. *S. aureus,* which is the most important pathogenic staphylococcus, generally ferments mannitol and produces catalase and coagulase enzymes. Mannitol salt agar is a selective and differential agar used for the primary isolation of staphylococci. Even though *S. aureus* ferments mannitol to produce acid in the medium surrounding the colonies, this ability is shared by other staphylococci. Definitive identification of *S. aureus* usually involves characterization of the isolate as a catalase-positive, gram-positive coccus that is coagulase-positive. Pitting on sheep-blood agar is a characteristic typical of organisms such as *Eikenella corrodens;* it is not observed in *Staphylococcus aureus.* (Ballows et al., pp. 228–229)

2. To differentiate between a coagulase-negative staphylococcus species and a micrococcus species, which of the following tests can be used?

   A. Furazolidone (100 µg/disk) susceptibility
   B. Catalase
   C. Novobiocin susceptibility
   D. Urease

The answer is A. Differentiation between staphylococci and micrococci can be made using the furazolidone-disk test. Staphylococci and *Stomatococcus* sp. are susceptible to furazolidone (100 µg disk) whereas *Micrococcus* sp. are resistant. A catalase positive reaction is expected from both staphylococci and micrococcus. Novobiocin and urease tests may be used to assist in differentiating *Staphylococcus* sp. (Baron, Peterson, and Finegold, p. 329) All members of the family *Micrococcaceae* are resistant to (show no-zone or up to 9-mm zone around) the 100 µg furazolidone disk; all other clinically significant cocci are susceptible (zones of 15–35 mm). (Ballows et al., pp. 222–223)

3. A pustule drainage submitted for culture is plated onto primary media. After an 18-h incubation, the sheep-blood agar plate reveals a predomi-

nance of beta-hemolytic, white, porcelain-like colonies. Gram stain shows gram-positive cocci. The colonies test catalase-positive. The most appropriate test for additional identification of the isolate is

A. bacitracin
B. bile esculin
C. bile solubility
D. coagulase

The answer is D. Facultatively anaerobic gram-positive cocci that are beta-hemolytic on sheep-blood agar can presumptively be considered to be of the *Micrococcaceae* or *Streptococcaceae* family. Most members of the *Micrococcaceae* family are strongly catalase-positive, whereas the *Streptococcaceae* are catalase-negative or weakly positive. The coagulase test will definitively identify *Staphylococcus aureus,* the most likely causative agent from this specimen source. Bacitracin, bile esculin, and bile solubility are tests used in the identification of streptococci that are ruled out by a positive catalase result. (Ballows et al., p. 227)

4. A 43-year-old female patient complains of a very sore throat. The throat swab that is submitted for routine culture grows a variety of diphtheroids: alpha- beta-, and nonhemolytic streptococci; staphylococci; and *Neisseriae.* The next step is to

A. report it as normal throat flora
B. ask for a repeat collection to get a better specimen
C. identify the beta-hemolytic streptococcus species
D. identify the *Neisseria* species

The answer is C. Routine throat cultures on persons over approximately 10 years of age are taken primarily to detect the presence of *Streptococcus pyogenes.* Any amount of group-A, beta-hemolytic streptococci is considered pathogenic and of concern because of the possibility of subsequent rheumatic fever or acute glomerular nephritis. In this patient, therefore, the beta-hemolytic streptococcus species should be identified. All the other organisms enumerated in this specimen may be encountered in the normal oropharyngeal flora, including nongroup-A, beta-hemolytic streptococci. (Ballows et al., p. 238)

5. A nasopharyngeal culture grows a predominance of a beta-hemolytic colony-type on sheep-blood agar at 18 h. The isolate is susceptible to a 0.04 unit of bacitracin. The most likely identification is beta-hemolytic streptococcus,

A. group A
B. group B
C. group D
D. not group A, B, or D

The answer is A. *Streptococcus pyogenes* is a probable etiologic agent of pharyngitis. This isolate is presumptively identified as beta-hemolytic streptococcus, group A, by demonstration of susceptibility to bacitracin. Group-A streptococci are also bile-esculin–negative and hippurate-hydrolysis–negative. Group-B streptococci hydrolyze hippurate. Group-D streptococci hydrolyze esculin in the presence of 40% bile. Other beta-hemolytic streptococci that are not in group A, B, or D are generally resistant to bacitracin and negative to the other reactions given in this problem. (Ballows et al., pp. 248, 1,221)

6. Which of the following characteristics is *not* consistent with *Streptococcus pneumoniae?*

A. Alpha hemolysis on sheep-blood agar
B. Bile-solubility–positive
C. Gram-positive, oval-shaped cocci in pairs
D. Positive catalase test

The answer is D. *S. pneumoniae* is a gram-positive, oval, or lancet-shaped coccus that is seen microscopically in pairs and chains. On sheep-blood agar, colonies produce alpha hemolysis. Definitive identification requires a negative catalase test to differentiate it from *Aerococcus viridans* and either a bile solubility test or susceptibility to ethylhydrocupreine hydrochloride (optochin) to differentiate it from viridans streptococci. (Ballows et al., p. 238)

7. Neisseria species can be identified and differentiated by

A. bile esculin hydrolysis
B. carbohydrate utilization
C. nitrate test
D. oxidase test

The answer is B. Members of the genus *Neisseria* are identified by demonstrating acid production from the degradation of carbohydrates. The standard basal medium is cystine trypticase agar (CTA) into which 1% filtered sterilized carbohydrate is added. Conventional carbohydrate testing includes the utilization of glucose, lactose, maltose, sucrose, and fructose. Nitrate reduction differentiates *Moraxella catarrhalis* from members of the genus *Neisseria*. Since all *Neisseria* are oxidase-positive, the oxidase test is not useful in their differentiation. Bile-esculin hydrolysis is not used for testing this group of bacteria. (Ballows et al., p. 263)

8. A small gram-positive rod that causes neonatal meningitis and septicemia is

A. *Escherichia coli*
B. *Corynebacterium diphtheriae*
C. *Listeria monocytogenes*
D. *Streptococcus agalactiae*

The answer is C. *L. monocytogenes* is a small gram-positive rod that causes meningitis and septicemia in neonates, the elderly, and immunocompromised patients. *E. coli* is a gram-negative rod. *C. diphtheriae* is a small gram-positive rod that can cause diphtheria in nonimmunized hosts. *S. agalactiae* is a gram-positive coccus. (Ballows et al., p. 287)

9. The X and V factors required for growth of *Haemophilus influenzae* are contained in

A. brain/heart infusion broth
B. chocolate agar

C. sheep-blood agar
D. thioglycollate broth

The answer is B. Chocolate agar is enriched with hemin (or X factor) and NAD coenzyme (or V factor). Among the more fastidious organisms, both *Haemophilus* and *Neisseria* species will grow on chocolate agar. (Ballows et al., p. 465)

10. On a sheep-blood agar plate, *Haemophilus influenzae* satellites around colonies of

A. diphtheroids
B. *Streptococcus pyogenes*
C. *Haemophilus parainfluenzae*
D. *Staphylococcus aureus*

The answer is D. *H. influenzae* has two growth requirements. The X factor, hemin, is a heat-stable substance associated with hemoglobin and directly available in sufficient quantity in routine sheep-blood agar. The V factor (NAD) is a heat-labile coenzyme that can be supplied by adding yeast or potato extract to routine media. Alternately, certain bacteria such as staphylococci, *Neisseriae,* pneumococci, and some other microorganisms synthesize the required NAD that enables *H. influenzae* satellitism. (Ballows et al., p. 466)

11. The specimen of choice for the isolation of *Bordetella pertussis* from a suspected case of whooping cough is

A. blood
B. cerebrospinal fluid
C. nasopharyngeal swab
D. throat swab

The answer is C. Whooping cough is an upper respiratory infection. Whereas a throat swab is sufficient for the recovery of some agents of upper respiratory infections, optimal recovery of *B. pertussis* is achieved by culture of a nasopharyngeal swab or aspirate. (Ballows et al., p. 472)

12. Family characteristics of the *Enterobacteriaceae* include

A. fermentation of glucose
B. fermentation of lactose
C. production of indophenol oxidase
D. failure to reduce nitrates

The answer is A. All species of the family *Enterobacteriaceae* are gram-negative rods that ferment glucose. Indophenol oxidase is not produced. Most species are capable of reducing nitrates to nitrites, but only some species ferment lactose. (Ballows et al., p. 360)

13. Twenty patients on a surgical ward develop urinary tract infections after catheterization. In each instance, the isolated organism grows on sheep-blood agar as a large, gray colony, and on MacConkey agar as a large, flat, pink colony. The oxidase-negative, gram-negative rod produces the

same biotype and is resistant only to tetracycline. Additional biochemical results are as follows:

Phenylalanine deaminase (PAD): negative
Urease: negative
Hydrogen sulfide (H_2S): negative
Lysine decarboxylase: negative
Ornithine decarboxylase: positive
Indole: positive
Citrate: negative

The most probable identity of this organism is

A. *Escherichia coli*
B. *Enterobacter cloacae*
C. *Enterobacter aerogenes*
D. *Proteus vulgaris*

The answer is A. *E. coli,* the cause of this nosocomial outbreak, is one of the most frequent causes of hospital-acquired bacteriuria. Definitive identification of *E. coli* is confirmed by the PAD-negative, H_2S-negative, citrate-negative, indole-positive, urease-negative results. Both *Enterobacter* species are indole-negative and citrate-positive. *Proteus* species are PAD-positive and H_2S-positive and would be non-pink colonies on MacConkey agar. (Ballows et al., p. 361)

14. A mucoid, lactose-positive colony type on MacConkey agar that is indole-negative and citrate-positive is

A. *Escherichia coli*
B. *Klebsiella pneumoniae*
C. *Proteus vulgaris*
D. *Serratia marcescens*

The answer is B. *K. pneumoniae* is a lactose-positive, gram-negative rod on MacConkey agar. The IMViC reaction is $\theta\theta++$. Typical strains produce copious amounts of capsular polysaccharide that render the colony macroscopically mucoid. None of the alternative organisms are mucoid. *E. coli* has a positive indole and a negative citrate. *P. vulgaris* is lactose-negative on MacConkey agar, generally swarms on sheep blood agar, and has positive indole and citrate reactions. *S. marcescens* is lactose-negative on MacConkey agar. (Ballows et al., p. 362)

15. *Escherichia, Klebsiella,* and *Proteus* species are frequently normal flora of the

A. gastrointestinal tract
B. respiratory tract
C. superficial skin surfaces
D. urinary tract

The answer is A. Many of the organisms of *Enterobacteriaceae* colonize the gastrointestinal tract, and as such, have been termed "coliforms." Among the commonly encountered *Enterobacteriaceae, Salmonella* and *Shigella* are notable in that they are never normal flora. The genera given in this question are all normal fecal flora. While they may be isolated from superficial skin surfaces, the respiratory or urinary tracts, they are not considered as normal microflora from these sites. (Ballows et al., p. 360)

16. A discharge from an infected ear grows a colorless colony type on Mac-Conkey agar that swarms on sheep blood agar. This oxidase-negative, gram-negative rod is resistant to tetracycline and colistin on a routine Kirby-Bauer antimicrobial susceptibility test and gives the following biochemical reactions:

Phenylalanine deaminase (PAD): positive Ornithine: positive
Hydrogen sulfide (H_2S): positive   Indole: negative
Urease: positive   Citrate: positive
Lysine: negative

The organism described is

A. *Citrobacter freundii*
B. *Morganella morganii*
C. *Proteus mirabilis*
D. *Proteus vulgaris*

The answer is C. Chronic otitis externa is usually associated with infection of pseudomonads or *Proteus* species. Here, the biochemical results confirm the presence of *P. mirabilis*. *C. freundii* is PAD-negative, *M. morganii* is H_2S-negative and indole-positive, and *P. vulgaris* is ornithine-negative and indole-positive. (Ballows et al., p. 360)

17. A gram-negative rod biochemically compatible with the genus *Salmonella* fails to agglutinate in the polyvalent somatic antisera for *Salmonella* serotyping. What is the next step in the definitive identification of this organism?

A. Report the organism as a *Salmonella* polyvalent O-positive species and send the isolate elsewhere for additional identification
B. Wash a suspension of the isolate in saline and retest it in the *Salmonella* polyvalent antiserum
C. Boil a saline suspension of the organism for 15 min, cool, and retype in *Salmonella* polyvalent antiserum
D. Retest the isolate using the individual somatic antisera from each serogroup, A through E

The answer is C. Occasional strains of *Salmonella* fail to agglutinate in polyvalent O antiserum. Some *Salmonella* species possess K antigens that render them nonagglutinable in the live, unheated form. These antigens can be inactivated by heating a saline suspension of the isolate at 100°C for at least 15 min. On retesting the cooled saline suspension in the *Salmonella* polyvalent antiserum, agglutination may occur. If agglutination occurs and group-specific antisera are available, individual grouping may be performed. Boiled suspensions that do not react in the polyvalent test may be *Salmonella* strains that belong to groups other than those represented in the typical polyvalent antiserum that includes groups A through E. (Baron et al., p. 383)

18. A gram-negative rod is isolated from a patient with second- and third-degree burns. The isolate produces a bluish green pigment and a characteristic fruity odor. Other characteristic observations are

Triple sugar iron: alk/alk
Motility: positive
Oxidase: positive
Oxidative/fermentation glucose:
  oxidative utilization only

The most probable genus of this isolate is

A. *Acinetobacter*
B. *Alcaligenes*
C. *Moraxella*
D. *Pseudomonas*

The answer is D. *Pseudomonas aeruginosa* is a probable infective agent in a burn patient. This organism is the only one that produces pyocyanin, a blue-green water-soluble pigment, and a fruity, grapelike odor. Although all pseudomonads are nonfermenters, most can utilize glucose oxidatively. Most pseudomonads produce indophenol oxidase, and are motile. *Alcaligenes* and *Moraxella* are nonsaccharolytic. *Acinetobacter* (*Herellea*) degrades glucose oxidatively but is oxidase-negative. *Acinetobacter* and *Moraxella* are nonmotile, and *Alcaligenes* is motile. (Ballows et al., p. 431)

19. After 48 h of incubation on anaerobic sheep-blood agar, *Clostridium perfringens* appears as a

A. large, flat, fringy colony with a double zone of hemolysis
B. white, butyrous, nonhemolytic colony with a glistening surface
C. gray, mucoid colony with a zone of alpha hemolysis
D. colony with a pearl-like surface and a single zone of beta hemolysis

The answer is A. A double zone of hemolysis is typical for *C. perfringens*. The inner zone of complete hemolysis is distinct and surrounded by an indistinct zone of partial hemolysis. (Ballows et al., p. 506)

20. A *Bacteroides* species grows as a

A. gram-negative rod on an anaerobic sheep-blood agar plate
B. gram-positive rod on an anaerobic sheep-blood agar plate
C. gram-negative rod on a capneic sheep-blood agar plate
D. gram-negative coccobacillus on a capneic sheep-blood agar plate

The answer is A. Anaerobic sheep-blood agar is used for the recovery of anaerobic bacteria. Therefore, an obligate anaerobic *Bacteroides* species will grow on the anaerobic sheep-blood agar plate as a gram-negative rod. Sheep-blood agar incubated in an increased CO_2 atmosphere is a nonselective, general-purpose plating medium for the isolation of facultative anaerobes. Capneic conditions do not support an anaerobe's growth. (Ballows et al., p. 538)

Microbiology

21. Isolation of *Campylobacter jejuni* from a patient with gastroenteritis is optimized by

A. incubation at 35–37°C
B. selective enrichment in selenite broth
C. a microaerophilic environment
D. an anaerobic environment without CO_2

The answer is C. *Campylobacter* species are oxidase-positive, curved gram-negative rods that can cause a wide spectrum of infections in humans. Gastrointestinal disease is associated with *C. jejuni.* This microbe is fastidious but grows on Skirrow's or supplemented Campy blood-agar medium. Broth enrichment of the specimen can be set up in Campy thio. Selenite enrichment, which is recommended especially for the recovery of *Salmonella,* will not enhance the recovery of this microbe. Incubation at 42°C is desirable since *C. jejuni* thrives better at 42°C than at 35°C. Since this organism is a strict microaerophile, it grows best in an environment of less than 6% O_2. It also requires 5–10% CO_2. This atmosphere can be achieved easily by using the CampyPak microaerophilic generator envelope (BBL Microbiology Systems, Cockeysville, Md.) in a GasPak jar without a catalyst. Alternatively, evacuation and replacement of a jar with 5% O_2, 5% CO_2, and 90% N_2 gas mixture will achieve the desired environment. (Ballows et al., p. 403)

22. In the *N*-acetyl-L-cysteine–alkali method of processing sputum specimens for mycobacterial culture, the *N*-acetyl-L-cysteine serves as a

A. buffer
B. decontaminant
C. digestant
D. pH stabilizer

The answer is C. *N*-acetyl-L-cysteine is a mucolytic agent that digests tenacious sputum specimens. Sodium hydroxide is a decontaminant. Phosphate buffer (pH 6.8) stabilizes the pH to stop the action of the *N*-acetyl-L-cysteine and sodium hydroxide solution. (Ballows et al., p. 307)

23. A sputum specimen is submitted to the laboratory accompanied by a request for an AFB culture. All of the following are standard protocol for processing this specimen *except*

A. use of a refrigerated centrifuge with bucket covers and safety domes for high-speed concentration
B. use of both liquid and solid media for setup of AFB culture
C. use of concentrated potassium hydroxide for decontamination procedure
D. use of a laminar-flow biological safety cabinet for processing the specimen

The answer is C. A refrigerated centrifuge is needed because of the high speed and length of time required to sediment the AFB organisms (which are more buoyant than non-AFB organisms). The covers and safety domes as well as the use of a laminar-flow biological safety cabinet are necessary during these steps to prevent aerosolization of the specimen, which potentially carries the infective AFB organisms. For optimal recovery of AFB organisms, both liquid media (BACTEC) and solid media are recommended. NALC (*N*-

acetyl-L-cysteine sodium hydroxide) is the most common method for liquefaction and decontamination of AFB specimens (nonsterile sites). The sodium hydroxide used in this reagent is a 4% solution, not a concentrated solution. (Baron et al., pp. 594–598)

24. Routine sterilization of artificial culture media by autoclaving is recommended at

    A. 15 psi at 121°C for 15 min
    B. 10 psi at 121°C for 10 min
    C. 15 psi at 200°F for 15 min
    D. 10 psi at 220°F for 10 min

The answer is A. Artificial culture media are routinely sterilized by moist heat under pressure of 15 psi at 121°C for 12 to 15 min. These conditions are sufficient to kill thermoresistant spore-forming bacilli commonly found in the laboratory environment. Overheating the medium can result in degradation of some of the basic nutrients in artificial media. Inadequate sterilization may result in contamination of the medium. (Ballows et al., p. 1,226)

25. When acetone-alcohol is inadvertently omitted from the gram-stain procedure, streptococci and *Neisseriae* will be stained, respectively,

    A. purple and red
    B. purple and purple
    C. red and red
    D. red and purple

The answer is B. Iodine is a mordant that complexes with crystal violet and the cytoplasmic contents of bacteria. This complex cannot be eluted from gram-positive organisms such as streptococci because of their cell wall structure. Because of high lipid cell-wall content in gram-negative organisms, acetone-alcohol treatment confers high permeability to the cell wall, which results in elution of the crystal violet complex. If the decolorizer is omitted, therefore, gram-negative bacteria such as *Neisseriae* will remain purple. (Ballows et al., p. 31)

26. The color of a nonacid-fast bacillus following the acid-alcohol step and before counterstaining in the acid-fast stain procedure is

    A. blue
    B. red
    C. colorless
    D. green

The answer is C. Due to their high lipid content, acid-fast bacilli resist staining with ordinary dyes. Alcoholic basic aniline dyes are usually used to penetrate the cell. Depending on the method used, penetration may be augmented by the addition of heat or a wetting agent. After the initial staining step with carbol-fuchsin, virtually all intact bacteria should appear red. Once stained, acid-fast bacilli resist decolorization with acid-alcohol and remain red. Most other bacteria are readily decolorized with acid-alcohol and appear colorless until a counterstain is applied. Methylene blue is commonly used to counterstain. (Koneman et al., p. 24)

Microbiology

27. MacConkey agar is used for the isolation of members of the family *Enterobacteriaceae* because the medium is

   A. inhibitory and differential
   B. differential and enriched
   C. enriched and selective
   D. selective and supplemented

The answer is A. MacConkey agar contains ingredients that select for *Enterobacteriaceae* and related gram-negative bacilli. That is, it contains bile salts and crystal violet, which inhibit the growth of gram-positive bacteria and some fastidious gram-negative bacilli. Additionally, this medium contains lactose and neutral red indicator, which make it differential for lactose fermentation, essential in the differentiation of enteric pathogens such as *Salmonella* and *Shigella.* (Koneman et al., p. 115)

28. Ethylhydrocupreine hydrochloride (optochin) is a chemical used to differentiate

   A. Catalase-positive *Streptococcus* species from catalase-negative *Staphylococcus* species
   B. *Streptococcus pneumoniae* from alpha-hemolytic streptococci
   C. *Enterobacteriaceae* from non-*Enterobacteriaceae*
   D. Group-D enterococci from group-D nonenterococci

The answer is B. Ethylhydrocupreine hydrochloride (optochin) is a quinine derivative that selectively inhibits the growth of *Str. pneumoniae*. Pneumococcal cells exposed to this chemical are lysed due to changes in surface tension, and a zone of inhibition greater than 14 mm results. Generally, the *viridans* streptococci are relatively resistant to optochin, resulting in no zone of inhibition. (Koneman et al., pp. 449–450)

29. A lysine-iron agar (LIA) slant shows a red slant over a yellow butt. This reaction indicates that the organism

   A. deaminates lysine
   B. decarboxylates lysine
   C. ferments lactose
   D. produces H_2S

The answer is A. LIA tests for fermentation of glucose, lysine decarboxylase (LDC), H_2S production, and lysine deaminase. Lysine deaminase is evidenced by a red-slant reaction and indicates the tribe *Proteeae*. A yellow butt reveals fermentation of glucose with a negative LDC. Decarboxylation of lysine is evidenced by a purple-butt reaction. H_2S formation results in the production of a black precipitate in the butt of the tube. (Koneman et al., plate 3–4D)

30. Which of the following statements regarding Simmon's citrate agar is *incorrect?*

   A. Blue color is an alkaline reaction
   B. Citrate is the only source of carbon in the medium
   C. Glucose is the carbohydrate in the medium
   D. Growth on the slant is interpreted as a positive reaction

The answer is C. Simmon's citrate agar tests for the ability of an organism to utilize citrate as a sole source of carbon. Growth on the slant indicates this ability. Most organisms that grow will produce sufficient alkaline products to turn the bromthymol blue indicator from green to blue. Since the principle of this test is to determine the ability to utilize citrate as the only source of carbon, no other carbon-containing compounds, such as glucose, are ingredients in this medium. (Koneman et al., pp. 121–123)

31. The reagent(s) used to detect a positive phenylalanine-deaminase reaction is(are)

A. sulfanilic acid and alpha-naphthylamine
B. *p*-aminodimethylbenzaldehyde
C. alpha-naphthol and potassium hydroxide
D. ferric chloride

The answer is D. Phenylalanine deaminase deaminates the amino acid phenylalanine to phenylpyruvic acid. This alpha-keto acid forms a visible green-colored complex with 10% ferric chloride. Within the family *Enterobacteriaceae,* only members of the tribe *Proteeae* possess the deaminase required to deaminate phenylalanine. (Koneman et al., p. 124)

32. To eliminate the antibacterial properties of blood and simultaneously introduce an adequate volume of blood for recovery of microorganisms from septicemia, the recommended blood-to-broth ratio in the blood-culture bottle is approximately

A. 1 : 2
B. 2 : 1
C. 1 : 10
D. 10 : 1

The answer is C. A minimal blood dilution of 1 : 10 in blood-culture broth virtually eliminates the inhibitory effect of previous antimicrobial chemotherapy on the recovery of microorganisms from the blood. Additionally, it dilutes the antibacterial properties of the serum. (Koneman et al., p. 97)

33. Which of the following specimens is acceptable for the evaluation of clinically important anaerobes?

A. Feces
B. Sputum
C. Peritoneal fluid
D. Superficial wound

The answer is C. Feces, sputa, and superficial wounds are frequently contaminated with normal microflora of the gastrointestinal tract, oropharyngeal area, and skin, respectively. Only those specimens that are likely to be devoid of contaminating organisms, such as peritoneal (or other aspirated body fluid) are acceptable for anaerobic evaluation. (Koneman et al., p. 15)

34. A urine is received in the laboratory for culture. If the specimen cannot be plated immediately, it should be held

Microbiology

A. in the freezer
B. in the refrigerator
C. at room temperature
D. in the 35°C incubator

The answer is B. Refrigeration is a practical and safe method to hold a urine specimen until it can be plated. In this manner, a urine may be held for up to 24 h without significant alteration in bacterial population. It is paramount to refrigerate urine specimens immediately to avoid bacterial growth and significant increase in numbers of organisms in the urine. (Koneman et al., p. 80)

35. Standardized testing conditions for the Kirby-Bauer agar-disk diffusion antimicrobial susceptibility test include all of the following *except*

A. use of Mueller-Hinton media
B. standard inoculum size
C. incubation at 35°C
D. incubation in 8–10% CO_2

The answer is D. Some testing variables that can affect the results of the Kirby-Bauer antimicrobial-susceptibility test include composition of the medium, inoculum size, incubation conditions, and drug stability. Mueller-Hinton medium should be tested to assure that the medium pH is 7.2 to 7.4 and the approximate depth is 4 mm. Inoculum turbidity should be standardized to equal that of a No. 0.5 McFarland barium-sulfate standard. Incubation of the plates at 35°C is recommended, since methicillin results are not reliable at 37°C. Because capneic incubation decreases the pH of the medium and affects the properties of some antimicrobials, aerobic incubation is required. (Koneman et al., pp. 623–624)

36. The pair of organisms that would provide a good positive and negative control for phenylethyl-alcohol (PEA) blood agar is

A. *Pseudomonas aeruginosa* and *Escherichia coli*
B. *Haemophilus influenzae* and *Streptococcus pyogenes*
C. *Enterococcus* and *E. coli*
D. *Staphylococcus aureus* and *Str. pyogenes*

The answer is C. Phenylethyl-alcohol agar is a selective medium for the isolation of gram-positive cocci including staphylococci and streptococci. This medium inhibits the growth of gram-negative bacteria. Since *E. coli* and *P. aeruginosa* are two gram-negative organisms, no positive growth control is included in option A. Similarly, no negative control is included in option D, since both organisms are gram-positive. Option B could be correct since it includes both a gram-negative and gram-positive organisms; however, because the sheep-blood enrichment of PEA does not support the growth of *H. influenzae*, it does not challenge the inhibitory characteristics of this medium. In option C, an enterococcus species tests the PEA for ability to support growth, and *E. coli* tests for the inhibition of growth. (Koneman et al., p. 58)

37. Which of the following organisms will give the appropriate positive and negative reactions for quality control of the test listed?

	Positive	Negative
A. Gram stain	*E. coli*	*Neisseria meningitidis*
B. Indole	*E. coli*	*Proteus vulgaris*
C. Catalase	*S. aureus*	*S. epidermidis*
D. Oxidase	*Pseudomonas aeruginosa*	*E. coli*

The answer is D. Quality control requires that the performance of stains, media, and reagents be tested for the desired positive and negative reactions using stock culture strains of known stability. The performance characteristics of the oxidase reagent are tested adequately using *P. aeruginosa* as the positive control and *E. coli* as the negative control. Both *E. coli* and *N. meningitidis* are gram-negative. Both *E. coli* and *P. vulgaris* are indole-positive. Both *S. aureus* and *S. epidermidis* are catalase-positive. (Baron et al., pp. 105–106)

38. A fungal colony grows rapidly on Sabouraud's dextrose agar as a white colony type with a dense production of aerial, blue-green spores. On lactophenol cotton blue preparation, swollen-tipped conidiophores bear sterigmata and conidia in chains. The most likely identification of this isolate is

A. *Aspergillus*
B. *Helminthosporium*
C. *Penicillium*
D. *Scopulariopsis*

The answer is A. *Aspergillus* species are rapid-growing fungi that produce densely colored surfaces. Microscopically, septate, hyaline hyphae are seen with swollen-tipped conidiophores. Sterigmata that radiate from the conidiophores bear chains of spherical conidia. *Penicillium* and *Scopulariopsis* produce freely branching, slender conidiophores of the penicillus type. *Helminthosporium* is a dematiaceous fungus. (Koneman et al., p. 815)

39. A saprobic yeast that inhabits airborne dust, skin, and mucosa grows rapidly and produces an orange-to-red color. This isolate most likely belongs to the genus

A. *Cryptococcus*
B. *Geotrichum*
C. *Rhodotorula*
D. *Saccharomyces*

The answer is C. *Rhodotorula* is a common yeast that is saprobic and found in airborne dust, skin, and mucosa. Cultures grow within 24 to 48 h on Sabouraud's dextrose agar with colonies that are small, shiny, rounded, and orange-to-red. The color is due to carotenoid pigments that are produced by the genus. (Koneman et al., p. 808)

40. The function of 10% potassium hydroxide in the direct examination of skin, hair, and nail scrapings is to

A. preserve fungal elements
B. kill contaminating bacteria
C. clear and dissolve debris
D. fix preparation for subsequent staining

Microbiology

The answer is C. Direct examination of specimens submitted for fungal analysis can be crucial to early initiation of antifungal therapy. Ten-percent potassium hydroxide mounting fluid is recommended for the examination of skin, hair, and nail scrapings to clear and dissolve keratinous material that would render the preparation difficult to evaluate for fungal elements. (Koneman et al., p. 801)

41. A potentially pathogenic yeast that is normal flora in the oropharyngeal cavity and may produce thrush is

A. *Aspergillus fumigatus*
B. *Candida albicans*
C. *Cryptococcus neoformans*
D. *Rhizopus oryzae*

The answer is B. Although *Candida albicans* may be part of the normal oropharyngeal flora, oral candidiasis is commonly called thrush. *Cryptococcus neoformans* is another yeast that may rarely be part of the oropharyngeal flora, but it does not cause thrush. *A. fumigatus* and *R. oryzae* are true molds that are opportunistic pathogens of man. (Koneman et al., p. 841)

42. In an iodine preparation of feces, an amebic cyst appears to have a basket nucleus and a large glycogen mass that stains reddish brown. The most probable identity of the cyst is

A. *Entamoeba histolytica*
B. *Iodamoeba bütschlii*
C. *Naegleria fowleri*
D. *Entamoeba hartmanni*

The answer is B. A cyst with the large, well-defined glycogen mass describes *I. bütschlii. Entamoeba* cysts have such masses only when very immature; however, these cysts have one to four nuclei and chromatoid bars, which are not present in *Iodamoeba* cysts. *N. fowleri* is found in tissues, not in stool contents. (Garcia et al., pp. 24–25)

43. The infective stage of this parasite consists of an egg with a thin hyaline shell, with one flattened side and, usually, a fully developed larva within. The parasite is

A. *Enterobius vermicularis*
B. Hookworm
C. *Ascaris lumbricoides*
D. *Giardia lamblia*

The answer is A. *Enterobius* fits the description given in this item. Hookworm eggs are thin-shelled with an internal four- to eight-cell stage, which pulls away from the shell, resulting in an empty peripheral space. *Ascaris* has a thick shell with an albuminous coat that may be mamillated. *Giardia* cysts are oval with four nuclei within. (Garcia et al., p. 192)

44. The direct iodine preparation is best used to detect protozoan

A. eggs
B. trophozoites
C. cysts
D. larvae

The answer is C. Protozoan cysts stained with a weak iodine solution are refractile and show yellow-gold cytoplasm and brown glycogen. Although trophozoites also may be visible in iodine preparations, they are more easily detected by permanent stained slide or by their motility in unstained direct wet preparations. (Garcia et al., p. 505)

45. Parasites that are detected by direct visualization in a peripheral blood smear are

A. *Ascaris*
B. *Entamoeba*
C. *Giardia*
D. *Plasmodium*

The answer is D. *Plasmodium* species are the causative agents of malaria. Laboratory diagnosis of those blood-borne parasites involves preparing thick- and thin-film blood smears. Wright's or Giemsa stain may be used. *Ascaris, Entamoeba,* and *Giardia* are generally intestinal tract parasites. (Garcia et al., p. 123)

46. Chlamydiae differ from viruses in that chlamydiae

A. are true bacteria
B. are obligate intracellular organisms
C. produce intracellular inclusions
D. are isolated in tissue-culture systems

The answer is A. Chlamydiae have some characteristics in common with bacteria and some characteristics of viruses. Chlamydiae are bacteria that possess bacterialike cell walls and are gram-negative, although they usually cannot be visualized by Gram's stain. Like viruses, chlamydiae are obligate intracellular organisms that can be visualized as intracellular inclusions using a Giemsa or Giménez stain. Similar to viruses, tissue-culture techniques are required for growth and isolation. Unlike viruses that possess either RNA or DNA, chlamydiae contain both. (Ballows et al., p. 1,045)

47. A specimen for viral culture is collected on a Friday and must be held for processing until the following Friday. In general, the optimal temperature for holding this specimen is

A. 35°C
B. 4°C
C. −20°C
D. −70°C

The answer is D. Specimens for viral isolation should be collected as soon as possible after the onset of the illness, preferably within 3 days, and refrigerated promptly. If processing will be performed within 5 days, the specimen may be held at 4°C or on ice. To hold for long periods, the specimen should be frozen at −70°C. Freezing at −20°C is not recommended since some viruses are labile at this temperature. (Baron et al., p. 648)

48. A procedure that directly determines beta-lactamase production by a microorganism is based on detection of a(n)

A. zone of susceptibility around an ampicillin disk
B. zone of inhibition around an oxacillin disk
C. increased acidity due to the release of penicilloic acid
D. increase in pH due to the reduction of iodine

The answer is C. The direct detection of beta-lactamase production is most commonly performed by demonstrating the ability of the microbe to convert penicillin to penicilloic acid. The rapid acidimetric method uses a pH indicator to detect the decrease in pH in response to cleavage of the beta-lactam ring to form penicilloic acid. The iodometric method centers on the ability of penicilloic acid to reduce iodine and, therein, decolorize a starch-iodine solution. Neither of the screening tests using ampicillin or oxacillin disks tests directly for beta-lactamase production. (Koneman et al., p. 639)

49. The antimicrobial testing protocol for gram-negative bacteria should routinely include

A. clindamycin
B. erythromycin
C. gentamicin
D. oxacillin

The answer is C. Standard testing protocols for gram-negative bacteria routinely include antimicrobials such as amikacin, ampicillin, cephalosporins, gentamicin, tetracycline, ciprofloxacin, and sulfamethoxazole-trimethroprim. Clindamycin, erythromycin, and vancomycin are used routinely in gram-positive batteries. (Ballows et al., p. 1,070)

50. In a broth-dilution method of antimicrobial-susceptibility testing, the tube with the lowest concentration of antimicrobial in which there is no visible growth is the minimal

A. antimicrobial concentration
B. bacteriocidal concentration
C. inhibitory concentration
D. lethal concentration

The answer is C. The minimal inhibitory concentration (MIC) of an antimicrobial is the lowest concentration of the drug that inhibits the growth of the organism as compared to a negative growth control. The minimal bacteriocidal concentration (MBC) is the lowest concentration of the drug that kills the organism. The MBC is also known as the minimal lethal concentration (MLC). The minimal antimicrobial concentration has no meaning per se. (Koneman et al., p. 630)

CLS Review Questions

1. An early morning clean-catch, midstream urine specimen yields these results on urinalysis:

Appearance: yellow, cloudy   Protein: 1+
Specific gravity: 1.025   Blood: negative
pH: 8.0   Ketones: negative
Glucose: negative   Bilirubin: negative
Nitrite: positive
Microscopic: no casts, 15 to 25 WBCs per high-power field; many bacteria present

The results of this urinalysis indicate that

A. the bacteria present are the result of collection into a nonsterile container and correlate to a probable original count of less than 10^4 CFU/ml
B. the bacteria present are the result of a delay of several hours in processing and correlate to probable original count of less than 10^4 CFU/ml
C. significant urinary-tract infection that correlates to a probable original count of greater than 10^5 CFU/ml should be suspected
D. nephrotic syndrome should be considered, and the bacteria are merely coincidental

The answer is C. The combination of a cloudy, concentrated (specific gravity ≥ 1.024), alkaline urine that is positive for nitrite and protein and in which WBCs are found on microscopic examination indicates probable urinary-tract infection. Urine specimens that are not examined while fresh may deteriorate, and small numbers of contaminating bacteria can multiply, splitting urea, producing nitrite, and increasing the pH. However, large numbers of WBCs would not be found in that instance. Large numbers of WBCs without an alkaline pH and positive nitrite reaction may indicate either an inflammation without infection or a short urine transit time during which significant bacterial growth has not occurred. (Ballows et al., pp. 23–24)

2. This adult disease is more appropriately considered an intoxication than an infection because the preformed neurotoxin that is ingested causes the symptoms of neuromuscular paralysis. The agent that produces the toxin is

A. *Bacillus cereus*
B. *Clostridium botulinum*
C. *Clostridium tetani*
D. *Staphylococcus aureus*

The answer is B. The spores of *C. botulinum* occur in the soil ubiquitously. Intoxication in adults results from consumption of inadequately preserved foods in which spores of *C. botulinum* germinate and produce the neurotoxin. In this country, the incriminated foods are usually canned vegetables. Infant botulism is a special case resulting from ingestion of the spores with subsequent colonization of the intestinal tract and production of the toxin in situ. *S. aureus* food poisoning results from ingestion of preformed enterotoxin and causes severe vomiting and diarrhea. Ingestion of *B. cereus*–contaminated food results in a profuse, watery diarrhea. *C. tetani* causes tetanus (lockjaw), which manifests with classical neuromuscular symptoms. However, the pathogenesis requires a deep-tissue wound, contaminated with soil-containing spores, that becomes necrotic and sufficiently deoxygenated to allow proliferation of the organism. Once the primary *C. tetani* infection is established, the neurotoxin tetanospasmin is produced and spreads to the central nervous system where neuromuscular symptoms result. (Ballows et al., p. 512)

3. Two siblings arrive at the emergency room. Both had antecedent sore throats about 2 to 3 weeks earlier that grew beta-hemolytic streptococci; now they present with different clinical symptoms. The brother displays edema and hypertension, and RBC casts are seen in the urine. The sister complains of fever and joint pains and has carditis. The diseases that these siblings have are most likely

   A. erysipelas and glomerulonephritis
   B. glomerulonephritis and rheumatic fever
   C. rheumatic fever and scarlet fever
   D. scarlet fever and erysipelas

The answer is B. Although beta-hemolytic streptococcus group A can cause several types of disease, it most commonly causes an infection of the pharynx and adjacent areas. Symptoms from *Streptococcus pyogenes* arise initially from an acute upper respiratory infection. If inadequately treated, delayed complications can result, such as the two cardinal sequelae described in these siblings. The sister exhibits rheumatic fever, in which carditis and arthritic joints are major features. The brother displays acute glomerulonephritis with typical kidney pathology. Erysipelas and scarlet fever are skin manifestations of *S. pyogenes*. Erysipelas is an inflammatory skin disease in which large numbers of streptococci are present in the periphery of the lesions. Scarlet fever is a superficial skin rash resulting from the production of the unique scarlatinal toxin. (Baron et al., pp. 334–336)

4. Purulent material is obtained from a carbuncle and submitted for bacterial culture. The direct smear reveals many gram-positive cocci and WBCs. The culture shows growth in the primary broth and on the sheep-blood agar plate and no growth on the MacConkey agar plate. The colonies on the blood-agar plate are butyrous, white, and beta-hemolytic. Both glucose and mannitol are fermented. Although the slide coagulase test is negative, the tube coagulase test is positive. The most probable identity of this isolate is

   A. *Micrococcus* sp.
   B. *Staphylococcus aureus*
   C. *Staphylococcus epidermidis*
   D. *Staphylococcus saprophyticus*

The answer is B. *S. aureus* is a gram-positive coccus frequently isolated from this site. The positive coagulase tube test, which demonstrates the presence of "free" coagulase, is the best test to identify *S. aureus* definitively. Not all strains of *S. aureus* possess "bound" coagulase, as evidenced in the data from the negative slide coagulase test. Most strains of *S. aureus* also ferment mannitol. Micrococci do not utilize glucose anaerobically. Staphylococci other than *S. aureus* are coagulase-negative. (Baron et al., pp. 334–336)

5. Which of the following is unique to *Pseudomonas aeruginosa?*

   A. Growth at 30°C
   B. Production of pyocyanin, a blue or blue-green pigment
   C. Beta-hemolysis on both sheep- and horse-blood agar
   D. Oxidation of O-F glucose medium

The answer is B. No other bacteria except *Pseudomonas aeruginosa* produces pyocyanin, a blue-green pigment; demonstration of this pigment is sufficient for the identification of this organism. All *Pseudomonas aeruginosa* strains are able to grow at 42°C; this ability is also shared by several other *Pseudomonas* species. *Pseudomonas aeruginosa* is beta-hemolytic on sheep-blood agar, and it oxidizes O-F glucose medium; however, these are not unique features of this organism. Other gram-negative bacilli in the nonfermenter group may also exhibit these characteristics. (Baron et al., p. 395)

6. On thiosulfate-citrate–bile-salts–sucrose (TCBS) agar, colonies of *Vibrio vulnificus* appear

   A. yellow
   B. colorless
   C. olive green
   D. black

The answer is C. Most clinically significant vibrios appear as olive-green colonies on TCBS, including most *Vibrio vulnificus* strains. Yellow colonies appear on TCBS when the organisms are sucrose-fermenters (including *V. cholerae*). None of the vibrios produce colorless or black colonies on TCBS. (Baron et al., p. 431)

7. A gram-negative coccobacillary organism that is isolated from synovial fluid on chocolate agar resembles either a *Moraxella* species or *Neisseria gonorrhoeae*. The single best test to distinguish between these organisms is

   A. beta hemolysis
   B. glucose degradation
   C. motility
   D. oxidase production

The answer is B. *Moraxella* species and *N. gonorrhoeae* can be isolated from similar specimen sources such as the genitourinary tract, blood, and synovial fluid. The micromorphology of *Moraxella* is coccobacillary, sometimes resembling a gonococcus. The single best test for distinguishing *N. gonorrhoeae* from a *Moraxella* species is carbohydrate degradation. *N. gonorrhoeae* forms acid from glucose, whereas *Moraxella* species are metabolically inactive in carbohydrate-utilization tests. Both *Neisseria* and *Moraxella* produce indophenol oxidase and are nonmotile. *Moraxella* species are nonhemolytic on sheep-blood agar. Because *N. gonorrhoeae* does not routinely grow on sheep-blood agar, beta hemolysis is irrelevant. (Baron et al., pp. 359–360)

8. A lumbar puncture is performed on an 82-year-old woman who is receiving immunosuppressive therapy. The direct Gram's stain of the CSF reveals small gram-positive rods and numerous WBCs. At 18 h, a small translucent colony type grows on sheep-blood agar with a narrow zone of beta hemolysis. Identification of this isolate could be made by demonstration of

A. tumbling motility
B. metachromatic granulation
C. hippurate hydrolysis
D. capsule formation

The answer is A. *Listeria monocytogenes* is a small gram-positive rod often associated with meningitis in infants and elderly adults. The organism is an opportunistic pathogen in patients with predisposing conditions such as malignancies and blood dyscrasias, and, as in this instance, in patients receiving immunosuppressive therapy. Growth on sheep-blood agar yields small, round translucent colonies with a faintly detectable narrow zone of beta hemolysis. Key characteristics for the identification of *L. monocytogenes* include blackening of routine bile-esculin agar, tumbling motility at 25°C, and development of an umbrella-like area of motility in a semisolid medium incubated at 25°C. Metachromatic granulation is a characteristic attribute of *Corynebacterium diphtheriae*. The ability to hydrolyze hippurate is a characteristic of *Streptococcus agalactiae*. The ability to form a capsule is not an attribute of *L. monocytogenes*. (Baron et al., pp. 458–460)

9. An acute infectious respiratory outbreak occurs in the overcrowded poverty-stricken central core of a United States–Mexico border town. A 5-year-old girl was admitted to the city hospital 48 h ago and has expired. Her 7-year-old brother was admitted as a prime candidate in the epidemic. Physical examination of this child reveals fever and pseudomembranous, white patchy spots in the pharynx, but no sore throat. The probable diagnosis is

A. diphtheria
B. epiglottitis
C. pertussis
D. trench mouth

The answer is A. The infectious outbreak described is consistent with diphtheria. Diphtheria is an acute infection in which the organisms localize in the oropharyngeal area multiplying in number to produce the notorious pseudomembrane and exotoxin. It is the diphtherial exotoxin that causes myocarditis and congestive heart failure. At risk are unimmunized children who in this country are likely to inhabit crowded border towns or central-city ghettos. Treatment for active cases involves the administration of specific antitoxin as soon as possible. (Baron et al., p. 462)

10. A dairy farmer who has an intermittent fever, progressive weakness, and night sweats is suspected of having undulant fever. A likely etiologic agent that requires an atmosphere of 10% CO_2 and is urease-positive in 1 to 2 h is

A. *Bacillus anthracis*
B. *Bacillus cereus*

C. *Brucella abortus*
D. *Brucella melitensis*

The answer is C. Brucellosis in cattle causes contagious abortion, or Bang's disease, and commonly results from infection with *Brucella abortus*. Undulant fever in humans is a generalized infection with several typical clinical manifestations, one of which is described above. *B. abortus* is the only *Brucella* species that requires up to 10% CO_2 for primary isolation. It also is urease-positive in 1 to 2 h. *Brucella melitensis* is most often found in sheep and goats, does not require CO_2 for growth, and varies in its ability to split urea. *Bacillus anthracis* is the etiologic agent of anthrax in cattle and, secondarily, in humans. *Bacillus cereus* causes food poisoning in humans. (Ballows et al., pp. 457–459)

11. A patient is admitted to the hospital with symptoms of appendicitis. A stool specimen for culture reveals a gram-negative bacillus that is oxidase-negative, catalase-positive, urease-positive, and weakly fermentative. The slant of Kligler's iron agar (KIA) is orange-yellow. These reactions suggest the possibility of

A. *Yersinia enterocolitica*
B. *Escherichia coli*
C. *Plesiomonas shigelloides*
D. *Pasteurella multocida*

The answer is A. *Y. enterocolitica* and *Yersinia pseudotuberculosis* are capable of causing a mesenteric lymphadenitis that clinically simulates appendicitis. The genus *Yersinia* differs from the genera *Pasteurella* and *Plesiomonas* in that *Yersinia* is cytochrome oxidase–negative, whereas *Pasteurella* and *Plesiomonas* are oxidase-positive. The positive urease reaction differentiates *Yersinia* from *E. coli*. Sucrose fermentation distinguishes the two species of *Yersinia*. *Y. enterocolitica* ferments sucrose and *Y. pseudotuberculosis* does not. (Baron et al., pp. 370–371)

12. A stool culture from an adult appears to have two lactose-negative colony types on Hektoen and xylose-lysine-deoxycholate agar. One colony type retains the original color of each medium and the other has black centers. Stool screen data are as follows:

Medium	Isolate 1	Isolate 2
triple-sugar iron (TSI)	alkaline/acid, no gas, H_2S-negative	acid/acid, gas, H_2S-positive
lysine-iron agar (LIA)	lysine-negative, H_2S-negative	red slant, lysine-negative, H_2S-positive
urease	negative	positive

Based on these data, an important step is to

A. set up confirmatory tests for campylobacter sp.
B. set up *Shigella* agglutinations
C. set up *Salmonella* agglutinations
D. report the culture as negative for enteropathogens

The answer is B. The stool-screen reactions for isolate 1 are typical of those expected for a *Shigella* species. However, they are also consistent with a possible lysine-negative *E. coli* or *Aeromonas hydrophila;* therefore, biochemical confirmation and *Shigella* agglutination should be performed for this isolate. *Campylobacter* sp. would be isolated on selective media incubated at 42°C. Testing on these isolated includes Gram stain, motility, catalase and oxidase; not TSI and LIA incubations. Since the stool screen on isolate 2 indicates reactions that are typical for a *Proteus* species, no additional workup is necessary for this isolate. (Baron et al., pp. 370–371)

13. Both blood and urine cultures are positive for an oxidase-negative, gram-negative rod that is colorless on MacConkey's agar. Biochemical reactions include the following:

Phenylalanine deaminase: negative   DNase: positive
H_2S: negative   Arabinose: alkaline
Indole: negative   Lysine decarboxylase: positive
Citrate: positive   Ornithine decarboxylase: positive
Rhamnose: alkaline

This organism, an opportunistic pathogen, should be susceptible to

A. ampicillin
B. cephalothin
C. colistin
D. gentamicin

The answer is D. This patient's blood and urine cultures are positive for the opportunist *Serratia marcescens*. The biochemical reactions are all typical and the positive DNase or alkaline rhamnose, coupled with the alkaline arabinose reaction, pinpoints the identification. The typical antibiogram for *Serratia marcescens* shows resistance to ampicillin, cephalothin, and colistin. (Ballows et al., p. 367)

14. The metabolism of glucose by the *Klebsiella-Enterobacter-Serratia* group is as follows:

Glucose → 2,3-butanediol + 2 CO_2 + H_2

The reaction is the basis for the

A. glucose oxidase reaction
B. methyl red test
C. oxidative/fermentation (O-F) glucose test
D. Voges-Proskauer test

The answer is D. All members of the family *Enterobacteriaceae* metabolize glucose to pyruvate via the Embden-Meyerhof pathway. The subsequent metabolism of pyruvate results in either mixed organic acid end products or the formation of neutral 2,3-butanediol end product. In the methyl-red test mixed acid end products decrease the acidity of the medium to approximately pH 4.4, where the methyl-red indicator in the medium is red. In the Voges-Proskauer test, the neutral 2,3-butanediol end product is detected by a colorimetric reaction. The Klebsielleae utilize the butylene-glycol pathway, which results in a negative methyl-red test and a positive Voges-Proskauer test. (Baron et al., pp. 376–377)

15. A stool specimen is submitted for culture from a patient with gastroenteritis, nausea, and vomiting. A gram-negative rod grows on TCBS agar as a large green colony type. Additional screening characteristics include

Triple-sugar iron (TSI): alk/acid   Catalase: positive
H_2S: negative   Nitrate: positive
Oxidase: positive   Lysine: positive

The most probable presumptive identification of this isolate is

A. *Aeromonas hydrophila*
B. *Shigella flexneri*
C. *Vibrio parahaemolyticus*
D. *Yersinia enterocolitica*

The answer is C. TCBS is an excellent selective and differential medium for the isolation of vibrios. Most fecal flora and gastrointestinal pathogens are inhibited on this medium. *V. parahaemolyticus* appears as a large, blue-green colony on TCBS agar at 24 h of incubation. Key characteristics include TSI-alk/acid, oxidase-positive, and lysine-positive reactions. *Shigella* and *Yersinia* are oxidase-negative and lysine-negative. Although *Aeromonas* is oxidase-positive, it is lysine-negative. (Ballows et al., p. 388)

16. A patient specimen from an endotracheal intubation reveals a nonmotile gram-negative coccobacillary rod that grows on MacConkey agar as a lactose-negative colony at 24 h. It is a nonfermentative organism. A large battery of conventional biochemicals yields the following reactions:

O-F glucose (aerobic): acid   Lactose: alkaline
O-F glucose (anaerobic): alkaline   Maltose: alkaline
Oxidase: negative   Mannitol: alkaline
TSI: alkaline/no change   Sucrose: alkaline
Orthonitrophenyl galactoside (ONPG): negative   Xylose: acid

This isolate also produces acid from a 10% lactose agar slant. The identification of this isolate is

A. *Acinetobacter*
B. *Alcaligenes faecalis*
C. *Moraxella osloensis*
D. *Pseudomonas cepacia*

The answer is A. This isolate is *Acinetobacter anitratus,* which is a nonmotile coccobacillary gram-negative nonfermentative microbe. Its key reactions using the King criteria are glucose oxidizer, MacConkey-positive, and oxidase-negative. Typical reactions include the production of acid from O-F xylose and a 10% lactose slant. *Alcaligenes faecalis* is nonsaccharolytic and motile with peritrichous flagellation. *M. osloensis* is nonsaccharolytic and nonmotile. Although *P. cepacia* is an oxidizer, it is motile with polar flagellation and ONPG-positive. (Ballows et al., p. 415)

17. Which result is *not* consistent with the identification of *Mycobacterium fortuitum?*

A. Arylsulfatase positive
B. Niacin positive

C. Growth on MacConkey agar
D. Growth in 5% NaCl

The answer is B. *M. fortuitum* may be differentiated from the other rapid-growing mycobacteria by its positive arylsulfatase reaction within 3 to 5 days and its growth on MacConkey agar within 5 days. This saprobe also grows in 5% NaCl in 3 to 5 days. Although niacin may aid in distinguishing between *M. fortuitum* and *M. chelonei*, niacin accumulation varies among strains of *M. chelonei.* (Baron et al., p. 613)

18. An acid-fast bacillus (AFB) has been isolated from the sputum of a patient suspected to have a mycobacterial pulmonary disease. The organism is a slow-growing isolate that produces cream- to tan-colored colonies when grown in the dark in the incubator and after exposure to light. This organism is most likely which of the following mycobacteria?

A. *Mycobacterium avium-intracellulare* complex
B. *Mycobacterium chelonei*
C. *Mycobacterium kansasii*
D. *Mycobacterium scrofulaceum*

The answer is A. Mycobacteria that are slow-growing nonphotochromogens include the TB complex, *M. ulcerans,* and the Runyon group-III species. The *M. avium-intracellulare* complex includes AFB in Runyon group III, capable of causing serious pulmonary disease similar to tuberculosis. *M. chelonei* is a Runyon group-IV rapid grower. *M. kansasii* and *M. scrofulaceum* are slow-growing AFB that are group-I photochromogens and group-II scotochromogens, respectively. (Baron et al., p. 612)

19. *Nocardia* species that cause nocardiosis often are

A. obligate anaerobes
B. gram-variable
C. partially acid-fast
D. spore-forming rods

The answer is C. *Nocardia* species are nonspore-forming, branching, gram-positive bacilli. They are characterized as being partially acid-fast; i.e., they retain the carbolfuchsin when decolorized with a diluted acid-alcohol solution. *Nocardia* species are generally aerobic, although they tend toward microaerophilic or capnophilic requirements. (Baron et al., p. 605)

20. A direct Gram's stain of a pelvic mass from a patient with an IUD shows numerous pus cells and branching, beaded gram-positive rods. Heaped, lobate colonies grow anaerobically and develop a molar-tooth appearance after several days of incubation. The most probable identity is

A. *Actinomyces israelii*
B. *Mycobacterium phlei*
C. *Nocardia asteroides*
D. *Trichosporon capitatum*

The answer is A. The description of the anaerobic, branched, gram-positive rods is typical of *Actinomyces. A israelii,* which develops mature molar-tooth–

type colonies, has been shown to be present in the cervix of approximately 5 to 25% of women using IUDs and has been implicated in pelvic infections complicated by IUDs. None of the other three alternatives are anaerobes. (Baron et al., p. 516)

21. A lung abscess is cultured. At 24 h of capneic incubation, no growth is detected on any of the primary agar plates. Gram-negative rods are seen in the thioglycollate broth. After 48 h, the growth includes

    Anaerobic sheep blood agar: 3+ gram-negative rods
    Anaerobic laked-blood agar with kanamycin-vancomycin (K-V): 3+ gram-negative rods

    The isolate fluoresces a brick-red color under long-wave ultraviolet exposure. If allowed to incubate several more days, the colonies would be visibly

    A. black-pigmented
    B. yellow-pigmented
    C. orange-pigmented
    D. blue-pigmented

The answer is A. Anaerobic gram-negative rods that are initially nonpigmented on laked-blood agar with K-V and fluoresce brick-red when exposed to ultraviolet light (365 nm) are of the *Prevotella melaninogenicus* group. With age, the fluorescence disappears and a brown-black pigment is produced. These bacteria are important pathogens in respiratory infections and are seen in other infections as well. (Baron et al., p. 529)

22. Two organisms that are thought to act synergistically to produce an ulcerative infection of the gums, commonly called trench mouth, are

    A. streptococci and staphylococci
    B. yeast and fusiforms
    C. fusiforms and treponemes
    D. spirochetes and treponemes

The answer is C. This ulcerative or pseudomembranous infection of the gums is thought to be a fusospirochetal disease related to *B. vincentii* and *F. necrophorum*. Demonstration of Vincent's infection can be made by staining smears with Gram's crystal violet for 1 min and examining them for the presence of numerous white cells, fusiform bacilli, and spirochete organisms. Culture of mouth lesions or pseudomembrane is of no value. (Baron et al., p. 224)

23. A physician inquires about repeated sputum specimens, negative on routine bacterial culture, that are reported to contain only normal oropharyngeal flora. The patient is a 67-year-old man who smokes 15 to 20 cigarettes a day and has persistent cough, malaise, and a fever of 102–105°F. Treatment with routine antimicrobials such as penicillin and cephalothin has not been effective; the cough and fever persist. The most recent direct Gram's stain of sputum shows 3+ PMNs, mucus present, and rare epithelial cells. A likely etiologic agent is

    A. *Haemophilis influenzae*
    B. *Legionella pneumophila*

C. *Pseudomonas aeruginosa*
D. *Streptococcus pneumoniae*

The answer is B. Repeatedly negative sputum cultures from an elderly patient who smokes, has pneumonia with persistent cough and high fever, and does not respond to routine drug therapy are suggestive of legionellosis. Definitive diagnosis requires isolation of the organism from the lung tissue on a special medium, such as buffered charcoal yeast extract agar, or a rapid immunodiagnostic approach. Erythromycin is the drug of choice. *H. influenzae* would be detected on Gram's stain and grow on chocolate agar on routine sputum culture. Both *P. aeruginosa* and *S. pneumoniae* can be recovered from routine sputum cultures. (Baron et al., p. 571)

24. Which of the following descriptions characterize *Pasteurella multocida?*

A. Gram-negative coccoid bacillus
B. Growth on MacConkey agar
C. Beta-hemolytic on sheep-blood agar
D. Obligate anaerobe

The answer is A. *P. multocida* is a small coccobacillary gram-negative rod that is a facultative anaerobe. It grows on sheep-blood agar as a small translucent colony type that is nonhemolytic and fails to grow on MacConkey agar. Among the pasteurellae, *P. haemolytica* is beta-hemolytic on blood agar and grows on MacConkey agar, and *P. aerogenes* grows on MacConkey agar. (Baron et al., pp. 420–422)

25. Which of the following media has a high protein content and requires sterilization by inspissation?

A. Löwenstein-Jensen egg
B. Sheep-blood agar
C. Thioglycollate
D. Christensen's urease

The answer is A. Inspissation is a moist-heat method of sterilization in which the medium thickens by coagulation and evaporation when exposed to a temperature of 75°C on 3 consecutive days for 2 h each day. This sterilization method is generally used to avoid altering the appearance of media that contain high amounts of protein, egg, or serum. Thioglycollate is autoclaved routinely; sterile sheep blood is added to basal agar after autoclaving; and urea must be filter-sterilized for incorporation into Christensen's urease. (Ballows et al., p. 1,259)

26. All of the following describe the orthonitrophenyl galactoside (ONPG) test *except*

A. it detects the presence or absence of the enzyme beta-galactosidase in an organism
B. it is positive for organisms that are pink or red on MacConkey agar and negative for those that are colorless on MacConkey agar at 24 h
C. it is positive for isolates that are capable of fermenting lactose but lack the permease
D. it detects the decarboxylation of ONPG to ornithine and galactose

The answer is D. Rapid lactose-fermenting bacteria possess two enzymes: lactose permease enhances transport of lactose across the cell wall, and beta-galactosidase cleaves the galactoside bond of lactose, producing glucose and galactose. The glucose is then degraded by the Embden-Meyerhof pathway, producing mixed-acid fermentation. In conventional lactose-fermentation tests, such as that using MacConkey agar, both enzymes must be present to evidence a rapid positive test. Some species appear to be nonlactose fermenters at 18 to 24 h because they lack the permease activity, even though they possess beta-galactosidase. Because ONPG readily permeates the cell and is structurally similar to lactose, the ONPG test detects only beta-galactosidase activity. By circumventing the need for permease, ONPG rapidly identifies these late lactose-fermenting bacteria. (Ballows et al., p. 1,267)

27. Bacteria that are glucose oxidizers in Hugh-Leifson (H-L) O-F medium produce an alkaline/no change reaction in Kligler iron agar (KIA) because

  A. these organisms produce insufficient amounts of acid to be detected on KIA
  B. the lactose component in KIA inhibits glucose oxidation in this medium
  C. the concentration of glucose in KIA is higher than in the O-F medium
  D. KIA detects only fermentation of lactose

The answer is A. Fermentation media such as KIA contain 2% peptone and 0.1% glucose. In contrast, Hugh-Leifson O-F medium contains 0.2% peptone and 1% glucose or other carbohydrate. The decrease in peptone reduces the formation of alkaline end products from oxidation of amino acids. The increase in carbohydrate enhances production of acids. Consequently, Hugh-Leifson O-F medium is a more sensitive medium for detecting weak-acid production. Nonfermentative bacteria, such as *Pseudomonas aeruginosa,* which utilize glucose oxidatively, produce small amounts of acid in Hugh-Leifson O-F medium exposed to air. Because KIA contains a low concentration of glucose, these organisms resort to oxidative utilization of peptone to form amines that result in an alkaline/no change reaction on KIA. (Baron et al., pp. 388–389)

28. Physical examination of a 20-year-old man seen in the emergency room reveals nuchal rigidity and a temperature of 102°F. Direct Gram's stain of the CSF reveals numerous WBCs and a few gram-negative diplococci. The isolate grows on sheep-blood agar and is oxidase-positive. Acid production occurs in the cystine trypticase agar (CTA) carbohydrates as follows:

Glucose: acid
Lactose: acid
Maltose: acid
Sucrose: acid

The most appropriate action to take is

  A. identify the organism as meningococcus and report it
  B. identify the organism as *Moraxella* and set up additional tests to determine the species
  C. Gram-stain and subculture the CTA sugars to check them for purity

D. perform an antimicrobial-susceptibility test as a confirmation of the identification

The answer is C. This situation represents a classic presentation of meningococcal meningitis, diagnosed on the basis of clinical symptoms and preliminary culture results. Because meningococci ferment glucose and maltose exclusively, and *Moraxella* species are unable to attack carbohydrates, it appears that the CTA sugars are contaminated. The possibility that the sugars contain more than the patient's isolate could be established by Gram's stain and subculture. Antimicrobial susceptibility testing does not aid identification when the carbohydrate reactions are discrepant. (Koneman et al., p. 377)

29. Special handling or methods are required when blood cultures are requested on a patient to rule-out any of the following diagnoses *except*

   A. brucellosis
   B. candidemia
   C. systemic tuberculosis
   D. typhoid fever

The answer is D. Routine blood cultures will become positive for *Salmonella* sp. organisms (agent of typhoid) within the first few days of incubation. Blood is the best specimen for recovery of *Brucella* during febrile illness. Biphasic media enhances growth of *Brucella* sp; the culture should be incubated at least 21 days and subcultured periodically before reported as negative. With candidemia and fungemia the organisms often do not grow rapidly in routine blood culture media and may require up to 2 weeks incubation. *M. tuberculosis* is optimally cultured in special media such as Middlebrook 7H9 broth, in special biphasic media; prolonged incubation (> 5 days) may be required for positive cultures. (Baron, Peterson, and Finegold, p. 205)

30. Safety precautions designed to minimize laboratory-acquired infections when working with *Mycobacterium tuberculosis* in a clinical laboratory would prevent spreading of these organisms by

   A. aerosol production
   B. ingestion
   C. superficial contact
   D. contact with fomites

The answer is A. Tuberculosis is initiated by inhalation of droplet nuclei of less than 5 μm. Inhalation of infectious aerosols is the major biohazard to microbiology laboratory personnel. To minimize laboratory-acquired infection, safety precautions are designed that prevent spread of aerosols and inhalation of droplet nuclei. (Koneman et al., p. 49)

31. To check for positive and negative reactions, select the appropriate set of quality-control microorganisms for the following tests:

   Bile esculin hydrolysis
   Bacitracin susceptibility
   6.5% NaCl tolerance
   Hippurate hydrolysis

A. *Streptococcus pyogenes,* viridans streptococcus, enterococcus
B. *Str. pyogenes, Str. agalactiae,* enterococcus
C. *Staphylococcus aureus, Str. pyogenes,* enterococcus
D. *Str. agalactiae,* viridans streptococcus, enterococcus

The answer is B. An appropriate quality-control set of microorganisms would be as follows:

Test	Positive reaction	Negative reaction
Bile esculin hydrolysis	Enterococcus	*Str. pyogenes*
Bacitracin susceptibility	*Str. pyogenes*	*Str. agalactiae*
6.5% NaCl tolerance	Enterococcus	*Str. pyogenes*
Hippurate hydrolysis	*Str. agalactiae*	*Str. pyogenes*

(Koneman et al., pp. 448–451)

32. From the dimorphic fungi and major identifying morphologic features listed, select the species whose major characteristics are *not* described correctly.

A. *Blastomyces dermatitidis:* thick-walled yeast cells with single, broad-based buds at 37°C
B. *Coccidioides immitis:* barrel-shaped arthrospores at 25°C
C. *Histoplasma capsulatum:* spherical, tuberculated macroaleuriospores at 25°C
D. *Sporothrix schenckii:* thick-walled yeast cells with multiple buds at 25°C

The answer is D. The morphologic features of the dimorphic molds that cause disease in humans are of major importance in determining the etiology of these sometimes life-threatening illnesses. Pertinent criteria of the thermally dimorphic species are as follows:

Blastomyces dermatitidis: at 37°C tan- to cream-colored colonies with wrinkled surfaces and waxy sheen; microscopically, large, thick-walled yeast cells that have single buds attached by a broad base
Coccidioides immitis: at room temperature, white-to-brown colonies with cottony aerial mycelia; microscopically, septate hyphae dissociate and fragment into barrel-shaped arthrospores
Histoplasma capsulatum: at room temperature, silky-smooth, white-to-tan colonies; microscopically, echinate, tuberculated, spherical macroaleuriospores (macroconidia)
Sporothrix schenckii: at room temperature, smooth cream-to-white colonies that turn brown with age; microscopically, branched slender conidiophores with small conidia arranged in flowerettes or in a sleeve arrangement

(Koneman et al., p. 836)

33. *Fusarium* species have on occasion been associated with corneal ulcers, ulcerated skin conditions, and mycetoma. Typical macromorphologic and micromorphologic features are

A. rapid growers that usually produce a lavender pigment and crescent-shaped, septate macroconidia
B. rapid growers that darken with age and produce aseptate hyphae with rhizoids

C. slow growers that are velvety and light tan with a salmon-colored reverse, and seldom produce macroconidia
D. slow growers that are gray-brown and produce multicellular macroconidia with both transverse and longitudinal septa

The answer is A. *Fusarium* is a genus of fungi that is pathogenic to plants. Commonly considered a contaminant, it is known to cause keratomycosis and mycetoma. Its colonies are cottony on Sabouraud's dextrose agar, with a lavender pigment at 4 days. Microscopically, it is a septate hyaline fungus that produces crescent-shaped septate macroconidia. Option B describes the member of *Zygomycetes, Rhizopus.* Option C describes the dermatophyte *Microsporum audouinii.* Option D describes the dematiaceous fungus *Alternaria.* (Koneman et al., pp. 94, 818)

34. An 8-year-old child presents with tinea capitis, thought to be caused by *Microsporum canis.* Suspicions can be confirmed by

A. direct examination of infected hair for fluorescence under a Wood's lamp
B. demonstration of endothrix invasion of hair
C. salmon-colored reverse of colony
D. production of abundant microaleuriospores on Sabouraud's dextrose agar

The answer is A. *M. canis* is a common agent of ringworm in domestic animals and of tinea capitis in children in the United States. Most human infections are acquired from cats and dogs. Hairs infected with a species of microsporum fluoresce a bright yellow-green under ultraviolet examination. Most other dermatophytes do not fluoresce. Many dermatophytes have a predilection for ectothrix—infection of hair evidenced by conidia forming a sheath around the surface of the hair shaft. Microsporum grows on Sabouraud's dextrose agar as a white, fluffy colony type with a chrome-yellow reverse. Microscopic examination of the colony reveals thick-walled, echinate, spindle-shaped macroaleuriospores, usually with an asymmetric terminal knob. *M. canis* can be differentiated from *Microsporum audouinii* by the ability of *M. canis* to grow and sporulate on polished rice grains. (Koneman et al., pp. 825–826, 799)

35. Which of the following pairings of yeast species with identifying characteristics is (are) correct?

A. *Cryptococcus neoformans:* urease-negative, encapsulated
B. *Candida albicans:* germ tube–negative, chlamydospore producer
C. *Torulopsis glabrata:* urease-positive, arthroconidia producer
D. *Geotrichum species:* hyphae-positive, arthroconidia producer

The answer is D. There are several approaches to laboratory identification of yeasts. Some key characteristics and preliminary tests are as follows:

Germ tube test: positive for *Candida albicans* in 2 h and negative for most of the yeast species in this time limit
Urease test: positive for *Cryptococcus* and *Rhodotorula* and negative for *Torulopsis, Geotrichum,* and *Candida* species, except for an occasional strain of *Candida krusei*
India ink test: positive for encapsulated yeast such as *Cryptococcus neoformans* and negative for nonencapsulated yeast species

Corn meal agar: detects formation of chlamydospores, arthroconidias, and blastoconidia; *Candida albicans* forms chlamydospores, *Geotrichum* forms hyphae and arthroconidia, and *Torulopsis* forms blastoconidia only

(Koneman et al., p. 838)

36. Which of the following is characteristic of *Dientamoeba fragilis?*

A. Easily recognized by its rapid, jerky motility
B. No known cyst stage, trophozoite shaped like an amoeba
C. Two-to-four nuclei have a small pindot karyosome
D. The size is typically smaller than *E. nana* cysts

The answer is B. As its name suggests, *D. fragilis* usually has two nuclei in the trophozoite form. In addition, it has no known cyst stage. *D. fragilis* moves like an amoeba with a slow, progressive, gliding motion. The nuclei contain a karyosome, which is often splintered into four parts. The size is typically larger than *E. nana* cysts. (Garcia et al., pp. 40–41)

37. A thick film has been prepared from a patient suspected of having malaria. It is stained with Wright's stain. Inclusions seen in the patient's erythrocytes are described as blue disks with red nuclei. The infected erythrocytes are generally enlarged and some of them have granules of brownish pigment. Many of the erythrocytes appear to have more than 15 nuclear masses in a single cell. Identify the parasite described.

A. *Plasmodium falciparum*
B. *Plasmodium malariae*
C. *Plasmodium ovale*
D. *Plasmodium vivax*

The answer is D. *P. vivax* is a *Plasmodium* species that prefers young erythrocytes (reticulocytes), which may be slightly larger than the average red cell on a peripheral smear. The typical appearance of the *Plasmodium* trophozoite on a Wrights-stained smear is the "signet ring," a blue ring with a red nuclear mass. Reddish or brown granules known as Schüffner's dots may be seen in red cells infected in either *P. vivax* or *P. ovale. P. vivax* commonly divides to produce a total of 12 to 24 nuclear masses within a single erythrocyte. *P. ovale* usually produces four to 12 merozoites during schizogony. (Garcia et al., p. 122)

38. The diagnostic stage of *Strongyloides stercoralis* infection is the

A. egg
B. cyst
C. larva
D. trophozoite

The answer is C. *Strongyloides* does not develop cyst or trophozoite stages. The female lays her eggs in the patient's intestinal mucosa. Ordinarily the eggs hatch in the mucosa and mature into the rhabditiform larvae, which appear in the feces. *Strongyloides* eggs do not appear in the stool except in very severe diarrhea. These eggs resemble the hookworm egg in general size and shape. The two are distinguished by the fact that *Strongyloides* ova are not embryonated when passed. (Garcia et al., p. 204–207)

Microbiology

39. Trematodes that mature in the lung and produce eggs that appear in the sputum or stool are probably

   A. *Fasciolopsis buski*
   B. *Schistosoma japonicum*
   C. *Paragonimus westermani*
   D. *Clonorchis sinensis*

The answer is C. Although all the parasites listed are flukes capable of infecting humans, only *Paragonimus* consistently invades the lung. *F. buski, S. japonicum,* and *C. sinensis* parasitize the intestine, blood vessels, and liver, respectively. (Garcia et al., p. 318)

40. A 15-year-old girl was admitted with severe headache and confusion. An examination of her spinal fluid revealed many small, motile amebae. The girl was visiting friends in Georgia and had been swimming and diving in a freshwater pond. The most likely genus and species of the organism is

   A. *Entamoeba histolytica*
   B. *Endolimax nana*
   C. *Iodamoeba bütschlii*
   D. *Naegleria fowleri*

The answer is D. Certain free-living water amebae can cause primary meningo-encephalitis. Fatalities have been reported in the United States, Belgium, Australia, England, and Czechoslovakia. Illness begins with headaches and mild fever, and sometimes, sore throat and rhinitis. While headache and fever increase over the next 3 days, vomiting and neck rigidity develop. Soon the patient becomes disoriented and may lapse into a coma and die. Most case studies to date have occurred following swimming and diving in warm ponds or pools containing water amebae. It is postulated that the amebae gain entrance through the nasal passages, invade along the olfactory nerves, and spread via the subarachnoid space. The ameba most frequently associated with primary amebic meningoencephalitis is *Naegleria fowleri. Hartmannella* and *Acanthamoeba* have also been reported, rarely, as causative agents. (Garcia et al., pp. 75–79)

41. The causative agent of Q fever is

   A. *Coxiella burnetii*
   B. *Rickettsia typhi (mooseri)*
   C. *Rickettsia rickettsii*
   D. *Rickettsia tsutsugamushi*

The answer is A. Three of the more important rickettsial diseases in the United States are Rocky Mountain spotted fever, Q fever, and murine typhus. *C. burnetii* causes Q fever. *R. mooseri* is the agent of murine typhus. *R. rickettsii* causes Rocky Mountain spotted fever, and *R. tsutsugamushi* causes scrub typhus. (Koneman et al., p. 1,047)

42. Cerebrospinal fluid from a 24-year-old man reveals a high number of mononuclear cells and a negative routine culture for bacteria. Spinal fluid, glucose, and protein values are normal. In addition, the patient has vesicular genital lesions. The most likely etiologic agent is

A. *Neisseria meningitidis*
B. Rotavirus
C. *Chlamydia trachomatis*
D. Herpes simplex virus

The answer is D. *N. meningitidis* does not cause vesicular lesions, and if infection of the meninges were involved, glucose levels would be below normal. Rotavirus is a common cause of infant diarrhea and is not known to cause skin lesions. *C. trachomatis* genital lesions are characteristically nonvesicular, whereas those caused by herpes simplex virus are vesicular. Herpes simplex genital infection may rarely progress to meningitis, which would result in a mononuclear infiltrate to the CSF but no change in the CSF glucose levels. (Koneman et al., p. 993)

43. A 20-year-old man with urethritis who had been treated with penicillin returns to the outpatient clinic the following week. A possible cause of his symptoms is *Chlamydia trachomatis,* which may be confirmed by

A. inoculating the specimen onto selective media
B. demonstrating inclusion bodies in the cell culture
C. performing a direct Gram's stain for gram-negative rods
D. performing a blind passage of cells

The answer is B. The recommended technique for in-vitro isolation of *C. trachomatis* is tissue culture. Many laboratories use the McCoy cell line. After incubation for 48 to 72 h, the cell monolayer is stained with iodine or an immunofluorescent stain. *C. trachomatis*-infected cell cultures are detected by iodine or fluorescent stained inclusions. *C. trachomatis* usually cannot be visualized by direct Gram stain. Direct specimens (e.g. cells from conjunctiva, urethra, cervix) will often be used for more rapid confirmation of *Chlamydia trachomatis* by Direct Fluorescent Antibody (DFA), by enzyme linked immunosorbent assays (ELISA), or by DNA probe methods. (Baron, et al., pp. 554–556)

44. Bacteriophage typing is of greatest value in

A. differentiating between the genera staphylococcus and micrococcus
B. distinguishing the different species of staphylococcus
C. detecting the source of nosocomial infections due to *Staphylococcus aureus*
D. determining strains of staphylococcus that have unique susceptibility patterns

The answer is C. Various strains of staphylococci can be segregated into specific types by identifying a unique marker to trace similar strains. When an outbreak of staphylococcal food poisoning or suspected nosocomial infection occurs, it may be desirable to detect the source of the outbreak. Although a variety of techniques have been used for epidemiologic typing, the established method is bacteriophage typing. This procedure involves comparing patterns of lysis produced by test strains of *S. aureus* to a battery of phages. Distinctive lytic patterns are observed that serve as traces among the various strains of the species. (Ballows et al., pp. 233–234)

45. A method of value in the epidemiologic study of outbreaks of infection due to *Pseudomonas aeruginosa* is

    A. antimicrobic susceptibility testing
    B. biotyping
    C. morphologic typing
    D. pyocin typing

The answer is D. Pyocin typing may be used to trace a source of *P. aeruginosa* in a nosocomial outbreak, although it generally is a reference technique. Antibiograms are usually quite resistant and do not serve to differentiate strains. Similarly, biotyping and morphologic features do not distinguish clearly between strains. Pyocin typing, serotyping, and bacteriophage typing have been used singly and in combination to trace strains of *P. aeruginosa*. (Ballows et al., p. 174)

46. Falsely decreased zone diameters on a Kirby-Bauer agar disk-diffusion test would most likely result from

    A. an inoculum that is less turbid than a 0.5 MacFarland standard
    B. use of disks with a higher-than-recommended concentration of antimicrobial
    C. a 2-h delay in placing the antimicrobial disks on the seeded plate
    D. a 2-h delay in incubating the plates after the disks have been applied

The answer is C. A 2-h delay in placing antimicrobial-containing disks on the seeded plate would allow the organism to multiply before the antimicrobial is applied. This factor will result in falsely small zone sizes. Other factors that may cause falsely decreased zone size include the use of Mueller-Hinton agar at a depth of greater than 4 mm, use of deteriorated disks, and an increase in the concentration of calcium or magnesium ions in the agar when testing *Pseudomonas aeruginosa* with the aminoglycosides. The use of a mixed culture may also cause falsely small zones in cases in which one organism is sensitive to a drug, and the other organism is resistant. If the inoculum is too sparse, fewer organisms will result in falsely increased zone diameters. Using antimicrobial disks with higher-than-recommended concentrations of antimicrobials enhances diffusion and allows more organisms to be inhibited. Delaying more than 15 min after disks are applied before incubating plates allows excess prediffusion of antibiotics. These factors result in falsely increased zone diameters. Other factors that may produce falsely large zones include use of Mueller-Hinton agar thinner than 4 mm and too light an inoculum. (Ballows et al., pp. 1,120–1,122)

47. In interpreting a minimal inhibitory concentration (MIC) by the macrobroth-dilution method, you determine that the first test tube that shows visible turbidity has a final dilution factor of 1 : 32. Since twofold serial dilutions are made from the working stock of 0.256 mg/mL, the MIC for this isolate is

A. 4 µg/mL
B. 8 µg/mL
C. 16 µg/mL
D. 32 µg/mL

The answer is C. Since the MIC end point is the lowest concentration of the antimicrobial at which no visible growth can be detected, the end point in this problem is the 1 : 16 dilution. To calculate the concentration of antimicrobial at this dilution, divide the stock concentration of 256 µg/mL by the dilution factor of 16. Thus, the MIC is 16 µg/mL. (Ballows et al., pp. 1,105–1,107)

48. In a synergy study, when drug A, drug B, and drug A + B act singly and in combination on a single population of growing bacteria in vitro as illustrated, the type of killing action signified is

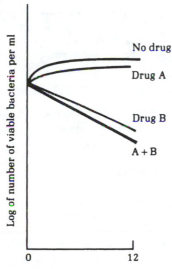

(Source: From J. A. Washington, *Laboratory Procedures in Clinical Microbiology.* New York: Springer, 1981, p. 725)

A. antagonism
B. indifference
C. synergism
D. not determinable from this representation

The answer is B. Synergy studies test the effect of combinations of antimicrobials on the rate of killing of microbes and may be indicated in the treatment of serious infections. The purpose is to determine if the two drugs in combination are *synergistic* (the effect of the two drugs together is greater than the sum of the effects of either drug alone), *indifferent* (the combined effect does not exceed the sum of the independent effects), or *antagonistic* (the combined drugs are less effective than one of the drugs alone). Examples of the three types of interactions are depicted in the following figure. (Koneman et al., pp. 651–654)

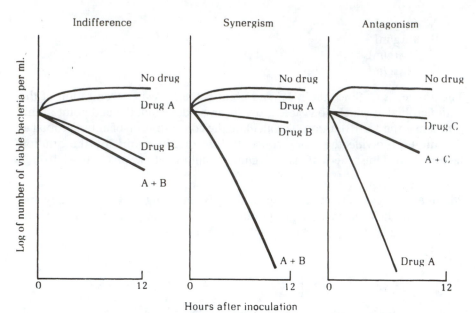

(Source: From J. A. Washington, *Laboratory Procedures in Clinical Microbiology.* New York: Springer, 1981, p. 725)

49. In the Kirby-Bauer agar-disk diffusion susceptibility test, a steady decrease in zone diameter of the penicillin disks obtained with the control organism *Staphylococcus aureus*, ATCC 25923, may be due to the fact that the

A. *S. aureus* control strain is too old
B. penicillin disks were not stored frozen
C. pH of the agar is less than 7.2
D. Mueller-Hinton agar is too thick

The answer is B. Since only the zones for penicillin are decreasing, a problem with the penicillin disks is probable. Antimicrobial disk cartridges that contain drugs belonging to the penicillin or cephalosporin family should be stored frozen to maintain their potency. A decrease in zone size with the control strain of *S. aureus* and the penicillin disks indicates that the disks are no longer fully potent. This may be due to improper storage conditions. Other factors that cause disk deterioration are humidity and contamination. (Koneman et al., pp. 658–659, 624)

50. "Clue cells" seen in a malodorous vaginal discharge are associated with a diagnosis of bacterial vaginosis; vaginal culture typically shows a predominance of:

A. *Gardnerella vaginalis*
B. *Haemophilus ducreyi*
C. *Lactobacillus* species
D. *Streptococcus agalactiae*

The answer is A. Bacterial vaginosis presents with a copious, foul-smelling vaginal discharge. Presumptive diagnosis can typically be made by demonstrating a discharge pH greater than 4.5, a "fishy" amine-like odor from addition of 10% potassium hydroxide to the discharge, and clue cells on direct wet mount or Gram's stain of the discharge. Clue cells are squamous epithelial cells coated with tiny gram-variable bacilli. *Gardnerella vaginalis* serves as one indicator organism of the syndrome, which also involves mixed anaerobic organisms. Gram stain (*not* culture) is viewed to be the most reliable diagnostic lab test for bacterial vaginosis. (Bailey and Scott, p. 570). *H. ducreyi* is the etiologic agent of chancroid, which displays with necrotic lesions. *Lactobacillus* species are normal female genital-tract microflora. *S. agalactiae* is carried in the vagina by many healthy females. (Koneman et al., pp. 499–500)

References

Ballows A, Hausler Jr W, Herrmann K, et al. *Manual of Clinical Microbiology* (5th ed). Washington DC: American Society for Microbiology, 1991.

Baron EJ, Peterson L, Finegold S. *Bailey and Scott's Diagnostic Microbiology* (9th ed). St. Louis: Mosby, 1994.

Garcia LS, Bruckner D. *Diagnostic Medical Parasitology* (2nd ed). Washington DC: American Society for Microbiology, 1993.

Koneman EW, Allen S, Janda W, et al. *Color Atlas and Textbook of Diagnostic Microbiology* (4th ed). Philadelphia: Lippincott, 1992.

Microbiology

5

Immunology

Section Editors   **Michelle S. Wright and Kathryn Doig**

CLT Review Questions

Contributors

Catherine Sheehan
Kathy Waller

1. In a radial immunodiffusion test for IgG, the results on the standards tested were as follows:

Standard	IgG concentration (mg/dL)	Ring diameter (mm)
1	2,300	10
2	1,000	6
3	250	2

If a patient sample were tested on the same plate and had a ring diameter of 12, the CLT should

A. dilute the patient serum with saline and run it again
B. extrapolate from the highest standard and report the result
C. report the IgG concentration of the patient as >2,300 mg/dL
D. divide the ring diameter of 12 by 2 (resulting in 6 mm), read the concentration from the standard curve and double the result, and report the patient result as 2,000 mg/dL

The answer is A. When the patient sample yields a precipitin ring with a diameter greater than that of the highest standard tested, the patient sample should be diluted 1 : 2 with normal saline and reassayed. The result in mg/dL must then be multiplied by the dilution factor (e.g., 2) and reported. (Sheehan, p. 127)

2. In immunoelectrophoresis, the antiserum is applied by

A. dissolving it in the agar-support medium while still liquid
B. placing it in a second well opposite the serum sample
C. placing it in a trough cut into the agar
D. placing it in a trenching dish in which the agar plate is soaked

The answer is C. The antiserum is placed in a trough cut into the agar between the control serum and the patient serum after separation by protein electrophoresis. The serum and antiserum are allowed to diffuse to form precipitin bands at the point of equivalent concentration. (Sheehan, p. 132)

3. A serum immunoelectrophoresis shows a dense, sharply peaked arc when reacted with IgG antiserum. This indicates

  A. an incorrect antigen/antibody ratio in the test system
  B. increased polyclonal IgG in the patient serum
  C. a monoclonal IgG in the patient serum
  D. the presence of kappa light chains

The answer is C. Normal polyclonal IgG produces a rounded arc. Monoclonal proteins, in this case IgG, produce sharply peaked arcs. The intensity of the band indicates the concentration of protein, not the clonality. (Miller et al., pp. 108–109)

4. An RPR card test performed on a spinal fluid sample was nonreactive. The physician was skeptical and asked for a repeat test of the spinal fluid. The RPR result was reactive 1 : 1 dilution. The result

  A. should be reported as nonreactive
  B. should be reported as reactive 1 : 1 dilution
  C. is inconclusive, and should be repeated on a new spinal fluid sample
  D. is unreportable; the RPR card test should not be performed on spinal fluid

The answer is D. The RPR card test is not recommended by the CDC to test spinal fluid. The VDRL is the method of choice. (Miller, pp. 204, 209)

5. The results of a quantitative VDRL test are as follows:

  1 : 1 1 : 2 1 : 4 1 : 8 1 : 16
  WR   R   R   WR   NR

This result is reported as

  A. reactive, titer 4
  B. reactive, titer 8
  C. weakly reactive
  D. weakly reactive, titer 16

The answer is A. The titer is reported when dilutions are performed in the VDRL test. The titer is defined as the greatest dilution to yield a reactive result. Weakly reactive sera are titered to eliminate errors due to prozone reactions as shown in this example; however, a weakly reactive result is not considered when determining the titer endpoint. (Miller, p. 204)

6. A common test kit for rheumatoid factor (RF) contains a saline diluent, positive and negative controls, and an IgG-coated latex particle reagent. In this procedure, which of the following statements is true?

  A. A positive reaction is indicated by agglutination of the latex particles
  B. RF inhibits the agglutination of the latex particles
  C. The RF in patient serum primarily represents IgG immunoglobulin
  D. The test is specific for rheumatoid arthritis

The answer is A. Most tests for RF are passive agglutination procedures in which antigen (IgG) is linked to latex particles or sheep RBCs. Serologically detectable RF, an IgM anti-IgG, will react with this IgG-particle complex. Specifically, the RF in the patient's serum combines through its Fab region to the Fc region of the IgG molecule of the IgG-coated latex particle reagent. Since the IgG is passively attached to latex, the latex particles will agglutinate. The test is not specific. False positives are seen in syphilis, lupus erythematosus, and other diseases. (Bryant, p. 271)

7. The results of an agglutination test for antibody detection using dilutions of patient serum are shown below. What do the results in tubes 1 through 5 represent?

Tube no.	1	2	3	4	5	6	7	8	9
Dilution	1:2	1:4	1:8	1:16	1:32	1:64	1:128	1:256	antigen control
Patient	0	0	0	0	0	+	+	+	0

+ = agglutination; 0 = no agglutination

   A. Agglutination was prevented by lack of complement activation
   B. Prozone due to antigen excess
   C. Prozone due to antibody excess
   D. Technical error; these results cannot occur when the procedure is correctly performed

The answer is C. These results represent the classic prozone phenomenon due to antibody excess. It is thought that excess of antibody relative to antigen prevents lattice formation. (Sheehan, pp. 124, 135)

8. Which of the following statements is true regarding C-reactive protein (CRP)?

   A. CRP is an immunoglobulin
   B. It can be elevated in postoperative patients
   C. It remains elevated in the serum after an inflammatory response has subsided
   D. It is diagnostic for active rheumatic fever

The answer is B. CRP is not an antibody but a protein produced by the liver. It is elevated when tissue injury occurs. The presence of CRP is not diagnostic for any specific disease but indicates necrosis and inflammation of numerous origins. Thus, CRP may be elevated postoperatively until inflammation has subsided. Although small amounts of CRP are seen in healthy persons, it is elevated only during the acute injury and disappears rapidly following recovery. (Miller, p. 143)

9. A 32-year-old white female presents with signs suggestive of systemic lupus erythematosus (SLE). The antinuclear antibody (ANA) screen by indirect immunofluorescence shows many evenly distributed spots of fluorescence over the entire nucleus. Which antibody is most likely present in the patient's serum?

   A. Anti-DNA
   B. Anti-DNP
   C. Anti-RNA
   D. Anti-Sm

Immunology

The answer is D. Anti-Sm is the only antibody listed that fluoresces in a speckled pattern. Anti-RNA fluoresces in a nucleolar pattern. Anti-DNA and anti-DNP yield either homogenous or peripheral fluorescence patterns. (Sheehan, p. 324)

10. A patient's serum sample is reactive at the 1 : 8 dilution when tested with the RPR card test. An FTA-ABS was subsequently performed according to the established laboratory protocol, which required heat inactivation of the serum and adsorption with the sorbent, yielding a 1 : 5 patient-serum dilution. The patient sample was nonreactive at the 1 : 5 sorbent dilution, and controls were satisfactory. The most likely explanation for this discrepancy is

    A. a biological false-positive reaction in the RPR
    B. a false-negative reaction in the FTA-ABS due to increased sensitivity
    C. the patient serum should also be run undiluted in the FTA-ABS
    D. the patient serum was not inactivated before performing the RPR

The answer is A. The FTA-ABS is a more specific confirmatory test most often run when a positive RPR screening test result is obtained. There are many causes of biologically false-positive RPRs. The 1 : 5 dilution of the sorbent is correct, and undiluted serum is not tested in the FTA-ABS. The protocol for the RPR card test does not include heat inactivation of the patient serum, since the addition of choline chloride replaces this step. (Miller, pp. 199, 205–212)

11. In an immunoassay, serum is added to a microtiter well coated with specific antibody. After incubation and washing, enzyme-labeled specific antibody is added. This procedure is

    A. a competitive-binding immunoassay
    B. an enzyme-multiplied immunoassay
    C. a homogeneous immunoassay
    D. a sandwich immunoassay

The answer is D. The specific antibody that coats the well is used to capture any corresponding antigen in the serum. Unreacted serum components are washed away. Then the enzyme-labeled specific antibody will bind to the captured antigen, sandwiching it between unlabeled and labeled antibody. The enzyme activity is then measured and is directly proportional to the amount of captured antigen. (Sheehan, pp. 166–167)

12. In an enzyme-multiplied immunoassay (EMIT), the patient sample showed high levels of enzyme activity. This indicates the presence in the patient serum of a

    A. high concentration of the antigen being measured
    B. high concentration of the antibody being measured
    C. low concentration of the antigen being measured
    D. low concentration of the antibody being measured

The answer is A. The concentration of the antigen being measured in the test is directly proportional to the level of enzyme activity measured in the test system. (Miller, pp. 71–72)

13. Which of the following is most likely to be associated with a false-negative urine pregnancy test performed by latex-particle agglutination immunoassay?

    A. Glycosuria (>500 mg/dL)
    B. pH (<7.5)
    C. Proteinuria (>1g/24h)
    D. Specific gravity (<1.010)

The answer is D. False-negative results in urine immunoassay procedures can result from dilute urine with very low specific gravity (<1.015) due to lack of measurable concentration of human chorionic gonadotropin. Other situations in which very low levels of hCG are found, such as very early pregnancy, may also result in a false-negative reaction. (Bryant, p. 331)

14. An antistreptolysin-O neutralization test was performed on the serum from a 5-year-old white female. The results were as follows:

Tube no.	1	2	3	4	5	6	7	8	9	10
Todd units	100	125	166	250	333	500	625	833	1,250	2,500
Patient	NH	NH	NH	NH	NH	PH	H	H	H	H

NH = no hemolysis; PH = partial hemolysis; H = hemolysis

Assuming that all controls were acceptable, the patient's titer is

    A. 625 Todd units
    B. 500 Todd units
    C. 333 Todd units
    D. >2,500 Todd units

The answer is C. The end point of the ASO neutralization test is the greatest dilution to exhibit no hemolysis. (Sheehan, p. 237)

15. In performing an ASO neutralization test, the streptolysin-O control is not hemolyzed. This indicates that the

    A. streptolysin-O reagent is working properly
    B. RBCs are of the incorrect ABO group
    C. streptolysin O has been oxidized
    D. test serum was heat inactivated

The answer is C. Streptolysin-O is oxygen labile. If the streptolysin-O control, which contains only the streptolysin-O reagent and group O RBCs, does not hemolyze, oxidation is a likely cause of reagent inactivation. (Miller, pp. 188–192)

16. A modified Davidsohn's differential rapid-slide test is set up as follows:

    Left side: patient serum + guinea-pig kidney reagent + horse cells
    Right side: patient serum + beef erythrocytes + horse cells

The reactions appear as follows:

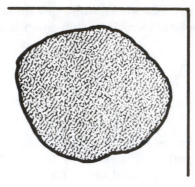 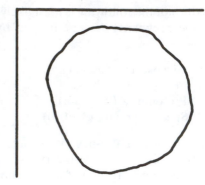

These findings indicate

A. infectious hepatitis
B. infectious mononucleosis
C. normal serum
D. serum sickness

The answer is B. On the left side of the slide, the antibody in the patient's serum is not absorbed by guinea-pig kidney. Therefore, the patient's heterophile antibodies are not neutralized and are available to react with horse cells to give agglutination. On the right side of the slide, the antibody in the patient's serum is absorbed by beef erythrocytes. Therefore, no antibody is left to react with horse cells, and no agglutination occurs. This is the expected reaction in infectious mononucleosis. (Sheehan, p. 230)

17. Which of the following is true of the antihyaluronidase test?

A. The antibody in the patient's serum neutralizes the hyaluronidase activity
B. The highest dilution which does *not* form a mucin clot is the end point.
C. Potassium hyaluronate combines with antihyaluronidase to form a mucin clot
D. The amount of antibody in the patient's serum is directly proportional to the intensity of the green color developed after overnight incubation

The answer is A. In this test, antihyaluronidase in the patient's serum will react with and neutralize hyaluronidase. This will prevent hyaluronidase from breaking down its substrate, potassium hyaluronate. When acetic acid is added, it will react with the intact potassium hyaluronate to form a mucin clot. The titer is the reciprocal of the last dilution in which a mucin clot is formed. (Sheehan, pp. 237–238)

18. A rubella antibody titer is to be performed. Doubling dilutions of the patient's serum are made in saline, with the first tube containing 0.2 mL of serum and 0.2 mL of saline, continuing through tube 10. Rubella antigen is added in a constant amount, negligible to the serum dilution. At this point, 0.3 mL of a 2%-suspension of RBCs is added to each tube. What is the final serum dilution, after addition of the red cells, in the third tube?

A. 1 : 5
B. 1 : 8

C. 1 : 13.3
D. 1 : 20

The answer is D. The initial dilution in the third tube is made by adding 0.2 mL of saline to 0.2 mL of the 1 : 4 dilution from the second tube, or 1 : 8. Since the dilutions continue, 0.2 mL of the 0.4 mL in the third tube are removed, leaving 0.2 mL of a 1 : 8 dilution. When 0.3 mL of RBCs are added, the new total volume in the tube is 0.5 mL. Since we are determining the dilution of the serum, the volume of the serum (0.2) is divided by the total volume (0.5) and multiplied by the initial dilution in the tube. 0.2/0.5 or 2 : 5 times 1 : 8 equals 2 : 40 or 1 : 20. (Miller, pp. 31–33)

19. A cold-agglutinin titer is performed. The results are as follows:

Dilution	1 : 2	1 : 4	1 : 8	1 : 16	1 : 32	1 : 64	1 : 128
Patient	4+	4+	3+	1+	1+	0	0

The patient's titer is

A. 8
B. 16
C. 32
D. 64

The answer is C. The end point of the cold-agglutinin titer is the greatest dilution to show agglutination. Cold-agglutinin titers must be confirmed by reversal of agglutination on warming. (Miller, p. 364)

CLS Review Questions

1. While reading a radial immunodiffusion (RID) plate, the CLS notices that one well has an irregularly shaped area of precipitation around one side. The most likely explanation for this result is

A. a high concentration of antigen in the sample
B. uneven distribution of monospecific antibody in the agarose
C. the well was not filled with sample
D. the well was nicked when filled with sample

The answer is D. If the well is nicked when filled, an irregularly shaped precipitin ring will form after incubation where the nick occurred. (Sheehan, p. 129)

2. In a serum immunoelectrophoresis, the precipitin arc formed for IgM is close to the trough. This indicates

A. high concentration of IgM in the test serum
B. low concentration of IgM in the test serum
C. the presence of monoclonal IgM
D. the test should be repeated; the electric current was inadequate

The answer is A. The closer the arc is to the trough, the higher the concentration of the immunoglobulin being measured in the test serum. Since the anti-

Immunology

IgM in the trough and the IgM in the electrophoresed sample are diffusing in all directions, including toward one another, the precipitin arc will form at the zone of equivalent concentrations. The reactant of higher concentration, in this case the serum IgM, will diffuse farther before becoming dilute enough to equilibrate with the anti-IgM and form a precipitin arc. Thus, the arc will form closer to the trough containing the reactant of lesser concentration, the anti-IgM. (Miller, p. 47)

3. Which of the following is characteristic of the Laurell or rocket technique of one-dimensional electroimmunoassay?

   A. Antigen is moved by electrophoresis rather than by diffusion
   B. Lines of identity and nonidentity can be distinguished easily
   C. It is performed in test tubes and similar to the Oudin test
   D. It is a qualitative rather than quantitative test

The answer is A. In rocket electroimmunoassay, the antigen is placed in a well, and antibody is incorporated into the agar. Current is then applied, moving the antigen by electrophoresis through the agar. Precipitation occurs along the edges of the antigen trail, resembling a rocket. The length of the rocket is directly proportional to the antigen concentration in the sample tested. (Sheehan, p. 134)

4. A Western-blot assay to detect HIV antibodies is performed according to established laboratory procedure. All controls are acceptable. The patient sample exhibits a p24 band only. The result that should be reported is

   A. positive for HIV
   B. negative for HIV
   C. indeterminate result; repeat assay
   D. false-positive for HIV; investigate for anti-HLA antibodies

The answer is C. The CDC recommends that sera exhibiting gp41 alone or gp41, gp120, or gp160 plus a second band should be reported as positive. A negative report should only be made when no bands appear. If a single band other than gp41 appears, the result is indeterminate, and the patient should be retested in 6 mo to allow for the possibility that the patient was in an early stage of infection. (Sheehan, p. 252)

5. A 25-year-old female suffering from systemic lupus erythematosus (SLE) and an ear infection is tested for syphilis using the RPR card test. The result is reactive; however, the patient denies any sexual activity. A repeat test 8 mo later is still reactive although the ear infection has resolved. The most likely explanation for these results is

   A. chronic biological false-positive due to SLE
   B. the patient has pinta or yaws
   C. the syphilis is in the incubation period
   D. transient biological false-positive due to the infection

The answer is A. Systemic lupus erythematosus, an autoimmune connective-tissue disease, is known to commonly cause chronic biological false-positive results in reagin tests lasting 6 mo or longer. It is possible that the ear infection could cause a transient false-positive; however, false-positives due to infections rarely last more than 6 months. (Henry, pp. 1,095–1,096; Miller, p. 199)

6. The results of a quantitative VDRL are reported to the physician as reactive, undiluted only. The results were recorded in the laboratory as follows:

1:1 1:2 1:4 1:8
WR NR NR NR

The supervisor checking the day's results should

A. change the report to weakly reactive
B. change the report to nonreactive
C. confirm the report as stated
D. perform a qualitative RPR test

The answer is A. The results have been incorrectly reported. Specimens that exhibit only weak flocculation are reported as weakly reactive unless a prozone reaction has been demonstrated. (Miller, p. 204)

7. The results below represent a viral hemagglutination-inhibition test for rubella. The titer of the first tube is 1 : 10; doubling dilutions are used thereafter. What interpretation of the results can be made?

Tube no.	1 2 3 4 5 6 7	8 virus control	9 serum control	10 RBC control
Results	0 0 0 0 0 + +	+	0	0

+ = agglutination; 0 = no agglutination

The results are

A. invalid due to the virus control pattern and should not be reported
B. invalid due to the serum control pattern and should not be reported
C. valid; a titer of 160 should be reported
D. valid; a titer of 320 should be reported

The answer is C. For this hemagglutination-inhibition test, the serum is diluted as 1 : 10, 1 : 20, 1 : 40, etc. A constant amount of virus preparation is added, followed by indicator red cells. The cells settle, and the pattern of sedimented cells is read. The end point is the highest dilution of serum that will inhibit hemagglutination by the virus. All controls are valid; the virus control (containing no serum) shows hemagglutination; the serum control (containing no virus) shows that the serum used had no antibodies to RBCs; the RBC control contains only RBCs and shows no spontaneous agglutination. The end point of the test is tube 5, representing a titer of 160. (Sheehan, p. 220)

8. A latex-agglutination test is set up to titer rheumatoid factor. The positive control is acceptable and the antigen control shows no agglutination. The patient serum has been diluted 1 : 20 in the first tube and in doubling dilutions thereafter. The patient's results are shown below:

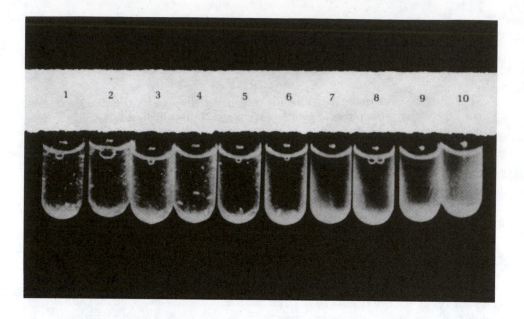

The results should be interpreted as

A. invalid and should not be reported
B. a titer of 320
C. a titer of 640
D. a titer of 1,280

The answer is C. The controls are all acceptable and the end point is seen in tube 6 of the photograph. Since the dilution in tube 6 is 1 : 640, the titer is the reciprocal of that dilution, or 640. (Miller, pp. 31–33, 50)

9. An antinuclear antibody screen exhibits diffuse, peripheral, and coarse-speckled fluorescence. All of the controls are acceptable. No other samples tested in the same run exhibit multiple patterns of fluorescence. The CLS should

A. concentrate the sample exhibiting multiple patterns and reassay
B. dilute the sample in question and reassay
C. report the types of fluorescence seen; this is not unusual
D. run an LE prep to confirm

The answer is C. Multiple ANAs are not unusual in many patients with rheumatic conditions. An LE prep is a less sensitive test than the ANA and is not used as a confirmatory procedure. (Miller, pp. 340–341)

10. An indirect fluorescent assay for *Toxoplasma gondii* is performed using commercially prepared *T. gondii* slides as the substrate. The test serum shows strong green peripheral staining under the fluorescent microscope. This should be interpreted as

A. negative
B. 1+
C. 4+
D. inconclusive

The answer is C. Strong apple-green fluorescence along the edge of the substrate organism is considered to be a 4+ result. No fluorescence is negative, and 1+ fluorescence would be a weak apple-green color around the edge of the organism. (Miller, p. 312)

11. A beta-subunit RIA test for human chorionic gonadotropin (hCG) yields a result of 615 mIU/mL. The patient's last menstrual period was 10 weeks ago. This is indicative of

    A. choriocarcinoma
    B. ectopic pregnancy
    C. hydatidiform mole
    D. normal intrauterine pregnancy

The answer is B. Low levels of hCG during the first trimester are indicative of ectopic pregnancy. Levels of hCG in normal pregnancy peak at 70 days after the last menstrual period. Choriocarcinoma and hydatidiform mole are trophoblastic tumors that secrete large amounts of hCG, usually >5,000 mIU/mL. (Sheehan, pp. 176–177)

12. A qualitative, enzyme-linked immunosorbent assay (ELISA) was performed as follows:

    1. Add patient serum to an antigen-coated microtiter well
    2. Incubate
    3. Wash
    4. Add horseradish peroxidase-labelled antihuman globulin
    5. Incubate
    6. Add peroxide and chromagen
    7. Stop the reaction

The resulting color development was extremely intense because

    A. incorrect substrate was added
    B. the patient's serum contained a large amount of antibody
    C. the patient's serum contained a small amount of antibody
    D. a step in the procedure was not performed

The answer is D. In ELISA procedures, a washing step must follow each reagent addition to remove unbound reagent. Failure to wash after step 5 results in no separation of bound from free reagent; therefore, falsely elevated values are obtained. Since the color development is directly proportional to the amount of bound reagent, intense color would be seen in this case. (Sheehan, pp. 171–172, 175)

13. An anti-DNase-B neutralization test was performed on the serum of an acutely ill 24-year-old female. The titer was 120. Two weeks later, a convalescent serum was obtained and tested by the same method in parallel with the acute specimen. The convalescent titer was 240; the titer on the acute specimen was again 120. These results indicate that the patient

    A. has not had a recent infection with group-A streptococcus
    B. has had a recent group-A streptococcal infection

C. is at risk for severe poststreptococcal glomerulonephritis

D. suffers from streptococcal pyoderma

The answer is A. The patient has exhibited less than a fourfold rise in titer between the acute and convalescent specimens; a fourfold rise in titer is indicative of a recent infection with group-A streptococcus. A fourfold increase is needed to detect a significant change in the antibody level. A twofold increase is a one tube difference and can be expected to be within the error of the method. (Sheehan, p. 239)

14. In an ASO test, the streptolysin-O control tube demonstrates no lysis. What might be the effect on the results of the test?

A. False elevated values

B. Falsely decreased values

C. No effect, since the end point is read as the highest dilution demonstrating hemolysis

D. No effect, since all tubes would be equally affected

The answer is A. The principle of the ASO test is as follows: streptolysin-O causes the lysis of erythrocytes. In the presence of a neutralizing antibody (ASO), however, hemolysis of cells is inhibited. The end point of the test is read as the greatest serum dilution showing no hemolysis. The absence of hemolysis in the streptolysin control tube indicates inactivation of the reagent. Thus, a falsely elevated value will be obtained, since the reagent streptolysin-O is not effective in hemolyzing erythrocytes. (Sheehan, p. 237)

15. A heterophile differential-absorption test was performed on serum from a patient suspected of having infectious mononucleosis. The patient serum reacted with horse RBCs initially and after absorption with beef erythrocytes, but not after absorption with guinea-pig kidney cells. This result is consistent with the presence of

A. Forssman antibodies

B. infectious mononucleosis antibodies

C. Mycoplasma-associated cold agglutinins

D. serum-sickness antibodies

The answer is A. The heterophile antibody known as the Forssman antibody reacts with beef erythrocytes and horse erythrocytes. Therefore, when the serum is absorbed with beef erythrocytes, the Forssman antibody attaches to these cells and is not available in the serum to react with the horse erythrocytes. (Sheehan, p. 229)

16. One mL of patient serum is added to 2 mL of saline in a test tube labeled tube 1. A total of 5 tubes are set up, with 1.5 mL of saline added to tubes 2 through 5. Next, 0.5 mL of the serum dilution from tube 1 is transferred to tube 2, mixed, and 0.5 mL is serially transferred to the remaining tubes. What is the dilution in tube 3?

A. 1 : 3

B. 1 : 12

C. 1 : 24

D. 1 : 48

The answer is D. The volume of the serum in tube 1 is divided by the total volume in tube 1, so the initial dilution is 1 divided by 3, or 1 : 3. Since 0.5 mL is then added to tube 2, the new dilution in tube 2 is 0.5 divided by the total volume in tube 2, which is now 2 mL (0.5 mL + 1.5 mL). The new dilution in tube 2 is 1 : 4. The new dilution must then be multiplied by the initial dilution, because we now have a 1 : 4 dilution of the 1 : 3 dilution in tube 1; so, $1/3 \times 1/4 = 1/12$, or 1 : 12. We again make a new 1 : 4 dilution in tube 3 (0.5 mL from tube 2 + the 1.5 mL saline). Since we have made a 1 : 4 dilution of the 1 : 12 dilution in tube 2, our dilution in tube 3 is $1/4 \times 1/12 = 1/48$, or 1 : 48. (Miller, pp. 31–33)

17. The following results are seen in an antistreptolysin-O (ASO) test on serum from a 35-year-old male. The red cell control shows no lysis, and the streptolysin control shows total hemolysis. The positive serum control is expected to be 333 Todd units.

Tube no.	1	2	3	4	5	6	7	8	9
Positive control	NH	NH	NH	NH	SH	TH	TH	TH	TH
Patient	NH	NH	NH	NH	SH	TH	TH	TH	TH
Todd units	100	125	166	250	333	500	625	833	1,250

NH = no hemolysis; SH = slight hemolysis; TH = total hemolysis

What conclusion can be drawn from this result?

A. The patient's ASO titer is within the normal range for an adult
B. The patient's ASO titer is elevated, suggesting a recent group-A strep-tococcal infection
C. The results are invalid due to partial hemolysis in some tubes
D. The results are invalid due to the control results

The answer is B. Low ASO titers are seen in the majority of the population, but the normal level varies widely with age and geographic locale. Levels for preschool youngsters and mature adults are generally less than 100 Todd units, whereas school-age children, teenagers, college students, and members of the armed services have slightly higher levels (e.g., 166 Todd units). It is important to remember that a low titer may be normal and that regional and hospital norms exist. Acute and convalescent ASO titers are desirable for good diagnostic workups. Significant elevations of titer (250 Todd units or greater) are indicative of recent group-A streptococcal infection. The control results are acceptable, and slight hemolysis can occur in some tubes (i.e., tubes that are between those showing no hemolysis and those showing total hemolysis). (Miller, pp. 190–192)

18. A fluorescent label commonly used in flow cytometric analysis is

A. auramine
B. Giemsa
C. phycoerythrin
D. Romanowsky

The answer is C. The three most commonly used fluorescent labels in flow cytometry are fluorescein isothiocyanate, phycoerythrin, and rhodamine. (Sheehan, p. 192)

Immunology

References

Bryant NJ. *Laboratory Immunology and Serology* (2nd ed). Philadelphia: Saunders, 1986.

Henry JB (ed). *Clinical Diagnosis and Management by Laboratory Methods* (18th ed). Philadelphia: Saunders, 1991.

Miller LE, et al. *Manual of Laboratory Immunology* (2nd ed). Philadelphia: Lea and Febiger, 1991.

Sheehan C. *Clinical Immunology: Principles and Laboratory Diagnosis.* Philadelphia: Lippincott, 1990.

6

Laboratory Practice

Section Editor   **Linda L. Seefried**

CLT Review Questions

Contributors

Suzanne W. Conner
Mary Ann McLane
Jean D. Holter
William B. Hunt
Barbara Snyderman
Rosemary Kuhn
Linda M. Ubelacker
Judy C. Jones

1. How should sodium hydroxide burns of the skin be treated?

   A. Flush with copious amounts of water
   B. Flush with 10% hydrochloric acid and copious amounts of water
   C. Flush with 5% ammonium hydroxide and copious amounts of water
   D. Rush the victim to the nearest emergency facility

The answer is A. For chemical burns of the skin, wash away the chemical with large amounts of water, using a shower or hose as quickly as possible and for at least 5 min. Remove the victim's clothing from the areas involved. (Sullivan, p. 770)

2. Which of the following procedures is most basic and effective in preventing the spread of infectious diseases in the hospital environment?

   A. Wearing face masks and gloves in the presence of patients
   B. Wearing laboratory coats in patient rooms
   C. Wearing laboratory coats in the laboratory
   D. Washing hands between each patient contact

The answer is D. It has been said that soap, water, and common sense are the best disinfectants. Although laboratory coats, masks, and gloves have their place and are important in certain situations, the single most effective means of reducing nosocomial infections is frequent and thorough hand washing between patient contacts. (Anderson et al., p. 25)

3. A clinical laboratory technician determines that a minimum of 85 mL of working reagent is needed for a procedure. To prepare a 1 : 5 dilution of reagent from a stock solution, one should measure

   A. 15 mL of stock solution and dilute to 85 mL
   B. 20 mL of stock solution and dilute to 100 mL
   C. 25 mL of stock solution and dilute with 125 mL
   D. 30 mL of stock solution and dilute with 125 mL

The answer is B. Dilution usually refers to the volume of concentrate in the total volume of final solution. If 20 mL of the stock are diluted to a total volume of 100 mL, 20 mL/100 mL = $1/5$. (Anderson et al., p. 18)

4. Polystyrene containers are unsuitable for specimen transport offsite because they

A. cannot be completely sealed
B. are not inert and may interact with the specimen
C. allow too much light exposure to the sample
D. may crack when exposed to freezing temperatures

The answer is D. Polypropylene and polyethylene are usually suitable for specimen transport. (Burtis et al., p. 78)

5. How many grams of sodium hydroxide are required to prepare a 200-mL solution of a 10% (weight per volume) solution? (Atomic weights: Na = 23; O = 16; H = 1)

A. 4 g
B. 10 g
C. 20 g
D. 40 g

The answer is C.

$10\% = 10$ g/100 mL

X g/200 mL = 10 g/100 mL

$100X = 2,000$

$X = 20$ g

(Anderson et al., p. 14)

6. A whole blood sample arrives at a laboratory with the following handwritten information. Which information is incorrectly included on the sample?

A. Sally Doe—604A, 253-01-0001
B. Isolation
C. 07/16/94—Dr. McLane
D. Call results ASAP   09:30 LLS

The answer is B. No specific labeling should be attached to patients with infectious diseases to suggest that these samples should be handled with special care. All samples should be handled with appropriate blood and body-fluid precautions. (Garza et al., p. 155)

7. 11.0 mg/dL of serum calcium is equivalent to which of the following? (Atomic weight of Ca = 40.)

A. 2.6 mmol/L
B. 2.75 mmol/L
C. 2.9 mEq/L
D. 3.15 mEq/L

The answer is B. Convert the weight per volume to weight per liter of solution. The weight per liter is divided by the atomic weight of the ion being calculated.

11 mg/dL = 110 mg/L

.040 g/L = 1 mmol Ca

$$\frac{110}{.040} = 2.75 \text{ mmol/L}$$

(Anderson et al., p. 17)

8. The normality of an unknown HCl solution is 7.2. Calculate the specific gravity of this HCl solution given the assay percentage of HCl (21.6%) and the atomic weight of HCl (36.5).

   A. 1.424
   B. 1.217
   C. 1.19
   D. 1.08

The answer is B. Normality is the number of gram equivalents of solute per liter of solution, and molarity is the number of grams of solute per liter of solution.

Density × 10 × percentage = g/L

7.2 eq/L × 36.5 g/eq = 262.8 g/L

Density × 10 = 21.6 × 262.8

Density = 1.217

(Anderson et al., p. 20)

9. What is the correct formula to convert degrees Fahrenheit to degrees centigrade?

   A. $5/9$ (°F + 32)
   B. $5/9$ (°F − 32)
   C. $9/5$ (°F + 32)
   D. $9/5$ (°F − 32)

The answer is B. The centigrade scale is divided into 100 degrees and is the unit in which most scientific study is expressed. (Anderson et al., p. 13)

10. Testing for occult blood in feces should be done on aliquots of excreted stools rather than on material obtained on the glove of a physician doing a rectal exam because

   A. the exam procedure may cause enough bleeding to produce a positive result
   B. glove powder has been shown to cause false-positive results
   C. glove powder has been shown to cause false-negative results
   D. there is a greater chance of urine contamination of the rectal exam specimen

The answer is A. Glove powder has no effect on occult blood testing. There is also a chance that the volume of stool on a glove may not be truly representative of the whole feces, possibly resulting in a false negative. (Burtis et al., p. 73)

11. To properly use a volumetric pipet calibrated "to deliver" (TD), one should

A. wipe the outside following delivery of the contents
B. drain the contents but do not blow out
C. rinse out the contents several times
D. drain the contents to the lowest etched mark on the volumetric pipet

The answer is B. The volumetric pipet is designed to deliver a fixed volume of liquid with the greatest accuracy and precision. The tip of the pipet is tapered to slow the flow of liquid to reduce drainage error. When the liquid has ceased to flow, the tip of the pipet is touched to the inner surface of the container and the residual fluid is allowed to flow out by capillary action. Any remaining liquid should not be blown out. (Anderson et al., p. 4)

12. Various blanks may be run during spectrophotometric analysis to correct for absorbance contributed by entities of the test system other than the actual color reaction. Which of the following blanks is used to compensate for absorption of the color of the test sample before reagents are added?

A. Reagent blank
B. Water blank
C. Alcohol blank
D. Serum blank

The answer is D. A water blank is used when no interfering absorbance is contributed by any part of the test system. A reagent blank is used if there is appreciable absorbance contributed by one or more reagents in the system. Alcohol can be a type of reagent blank. In this instance, a serum blank should be run if the color of the sample itself causes absorption at the wavelength being used. (Anderson et al., p. 157)

13. What is the total magnification produced when using a 10X ocular lens and a 40X objective lens on a light microscope?

A. 4,000X
B. 800X
C. 400X
D. Cannot be determined without additional information

The answer is C. Magnification power of a microscope is the product of the enlarging ability of the objective lens and that of the ocular lens. The resolving power of the microscope is provided by the objective lens, and the ocular lens magnifies the image coming from the objectives lens. (Walters et al., p. 30)

14. If a technician performing routine microscopic analysis on unstained urine sediment is to have sufficient contrast and resolution to identify important elements, the microscope must be adjusted by

A. lowering the condenser and reducing the light
B. lowering the condenser and increasing the light
C. raising the condenser and reducing the light
D. raising the condenser and increasing the light

The answer is A. To have the appropriate black-white contrast and sufficient resolution to identify important urine-sediment structures in unstained preparations, especially casts, the amount of light must be reduced. For most microscopes this can be done effectively by both lowering the condenser and decreasing the setting on the rheostat. (Walters et al., p. 31)

15. Which part of the microscope should be adjusted to increase brightness of a microscopic field?

    A. Condenser
    B. Iris diaphragm
    C. Light-source rheostat
    D. Prism

The answer is C. Misalignment of the light source and optical axis is probably the most common type of misuse of the microscope. Visible light from the bulb is internally reflected by a mirror into the optical axis of the microscope. This light must be collected and focused on the object of the stage. The condenser is a combination of lenses beneath the stage that focuses the light on the object at an optimal level. The iris diaphragm regulates the diameter of the light field relative to the numerical aperture of the objective lens. Neither the iris diaphragm nor the condenser should be used to control brightness since that would result in a loss of resolution, which is particularly critical at high magnifications. The purpose of the rheostat, normally included in the microscope base, is to control the brightness of illumination. (Walters et al., p. 30)

16. Applications for employment must conform to

    A. Better Business Bureau guidelines
    B. Clinical Laboratory Improvement Act of 1967 regulations
    C. Title VII of the Civil Rights Act
    D. National Labor Relations Act regulations

The answer is C. An employment application is considered a screening tool to eliminate unqualified people from consideration for employment and must not be discriminatory or have a disparate impact on minorities. Title VII of the Civil Rights Act (1964) guarantees equality to all persons. The act has been amended by the Equal Opportunity Act of 1972, the Pregnancy Discrimination Act of 1978, the Rehabilitation Act of 1973, and the Age Discrimination Employment Act of 1967. (Snyder et al., p. 181)

17. Which of the following statistics is determined by the formula shown below?

$$\sqrt{\frac{\Sigma (X - \overline{X})^2}{n - 1}}$$

    A. Mean
    B. Standard deviation
    C. Variance
    D. Confidence limits

The answer is B. The standard deviation is an attempt to represent a true or reproducible measure of dispersion in quantitative determinations. The first step is to note the amount by which the individual measurements differ from the mean and to calculate the average of these deviations. The deviations are squared to eliminate negative signs. The result to this point is called the *variance,* or the square of deviations. We then take the square root of the variance to convert the statistic to a workable form. The positive square root of the variance is known as the standard deviation. (Anderson et al., p. 45)

18. If a ground circuit in an instrument wire is *not* complete

A. the instrument will not work
B. current leakage may cause a shock to the operator
C. the fuse or circuit breaker will blow
D. a fire will result

The answer is B. To avoid shocks, all instruments must be grounded. The third wire is provided to drain leakage currents harmlessly to ground. A ground prong should never be cut off because the old receptacle only has two slots. If it is necessary to connect a three-prong plug to a two-slot receptacle, an adapter should be used and the ground wire of the adapter must be securely attached to the retaining screw of the receptacle coverplate to avoid shock. (Snyder et al., p. 324)

19. Which of the following has the highest incidence of infectious risk in the clinical laboratory?

A. Hepatitis
B. Infectious mononucleosis
C. Acquired immunodeficiency syndrome (AIDS)
D. Rubella

The answer is A. Viral hepatitis is the leading cause of laboratory-acquired infections. Human blood can transmit a number of infectious diseases such as hepatitis and AIDS and should be treated as a potentially infectious material. The risk of infection is directly related to the degree of contact with contaminated blood. Infection with the AIDS virus, HIV, has grave consequences, but the occurrence of hepatitis B is more common and hence the leading infectious risk in the clinical laboratory. (Koneman et al., p. 1,002)

20. Which of the following represents a diagram of a spectrophotometer?

A. Hollow cathode—Cuvette—Monochromator—Detector—Readout
B. Cuvette—Light source—Monochromator—Detector—Readout
C. Monochromator—Light source—Cuvette—Detector—Readout
D. Light source—Monochromator—Cuvette—Detector—Readout

The answer is D. The light source is usually a tungsten lamp; monochromators are either a diffraction grating, prism, or filter; cuvettes are made from glass, quartz, or plastic; detectors are barrier-layer cells or photomultiplier tubes; readout devices may be meters, digital devices, or microprocessors. (Anderson et al., p. 78)

21. Which of the following instruments is used to measure the speed of a centrifuge?

A. Volt-ohm-meter (VOM)
B. Refractometer
C. Tachometer
D. Potentiometer

The answer is C. An external tachometer of known accuracy should be used to calibrate the speed of a centrifuge; the tachometer should be used to check the speed of the centrifuge at least every 3 months for all speeds at which the centrifuge is routinely used. (Burtis et al., p. 26)

22. The wavelengths in the ultraviolet region are

    A. 620 to 700 nm
    B. over 700 nm
    C. 400 to 450 nm
    D. below 400 nm

The answer is D. Wavelengths visible to the unaided eye occur at approximately 400 to 700 nm. Ultraviolet light is not visible and occurs at wavelengths below 400 nm. Infrared wavelengths occur above 700 nm. (Anderson et al., p. 74)

23. Which gauge needle would be most appropriate for blood collection if the vein tends to be thready or collapse easily?

    A. 16
    B. 18
    C. 19
    D. 21

The answer is D. In such instances, choosing the smallest bore needle possible is advisable. The larger the gauge, the smaller the bore size. (Garza et al., p. 62)

24. Which of the following wavelengths of light are visible to the unaided eye?

    A. 300 to 700 nm
    B. 200 to 800 nm
    C. 400 to 700 nm
    D. 400 to 900 nm

The answer is C. Only electromagnetic radiation with a wavelength between approximately 400 and 700 nm is visible to the unaided eye. The color of light is determined by its wavelength, with red having the longest wavelength and blue the shortest. (Anderson et al., p. 74)

25. Flammable chemicals such as waste ether and chloroform

    A. may be flushed down the drain with copious amounts of water
    B. may be safely sent to a landfill with the regular trash
    C. should be incinerated
    D. should not be used in the clinical laboratory because of the danger

The answer is C. Flammable chemicals can fill the sewer vents with vapors that are a fire hazard. Such flammables should be incinerated or otherwise specially handled by an approved chemical waste hauler. (Snyder et al., p. 335)

26. One nanometer is equal to

    A. 10^{-2} meter
    B. 10^{-6} meter

Laboratory Practice

C. 10^{-9} meter

D. 10^{-12} meter

The answer is 2. Wavelength of light is the distance between peaks as the light travels in a wavelike manner. This distance is expressed in nanometers (nm). 1 nm = 10^{-9} m. (Anderson et al., p. 73)

27. Which of the following phlebotomy equipment is *not* used in an arterial puncture?

A. Tourniquet

B. Glass syringe

C. 18–20 gauge needle

D. Heparin solution

The answer is A. No tourniquet is required since the artery has a strong blood pressure of its own. (Garza et al., p. 115)

28. Storage of computer data may be done

A. with magnetic disc or tape

B. on a cathode ray tube (CRT)

C. in the central processing unit (CPU)

D. on a video display terminal (VDT)

The answer is A. Both a CRT and a VDT allow the operator to visualize the data as they are entered. A CPU is the computer chip through which all data flow before they are stored. The principal means of storing data is on magnetic disc or tape. Data retrieval is faster from disc than it is from tape. (Anderson et al., p. 127)

29. The following are examples of monochromators used in photometers *except* the

A. barrier-layer cell

B. prism

C. diffraction grating

D. interference filter

The answer is A. A barrier-layer cell is a type of detector found in simple photometers, whereas prisms, diffraction gratings (transmittance and reflectance), and interference filters are all examples of monochromators. (Henry, p. 31)

30. Chemicals such as sodium hydroxide and sulfuric acid should be labeled

A. poison

B. corrosive

C. biohazard

D. irritant

The answer is B. Corrosives used in the laboratory are defined as acids or bases that can etch flesh with first-, second-, or third-degree burns 24 h after contact. Some corrosives destroy live tissue immediately; others cause damage after they have penetrated into deeper tissues. Inhalation of corrosive vapors or ingestion of corrosives causes severe edema and extensive burning of the respiratory tract or mouth and throat. All containers of corrosive acids and bases should be labeled with a CORROSIVE label. Eye, respiratory, and skin protection should be worn when working with corrosives. (Anderson et al., p. 27)

31. Which of the following liquids has the lowest flashpoint and is therefore the most flammable?

    A. Class IA
    B. Class IC
    C. Class II
    D. Class III

The answer is A. The temperature at which a flammable or combustible liquid gives off enough vapor to form an ignitable mixture with air is called the flashpoint of a liquid. Class IA has a flashpoint below 23°C and is therefore the most volatile. (Burtis et al., p. 51)

32. Blood to be collected from an arm with an intravenous line on the dorsal side of the hand may be taken from which site on that arm without interference?

    A. Middle finger
    B. Lateral wrist
    C. Mid-forearm
    D. Anticubital fossa

The answer is A. A sampling site must be distal to that of the blood flow carrying the infusion. (Garza et al., p. 107)

33. Which of the following should be performed to determine the optimal wavelength at which to measure the absorbance of a colored solution?

    A. Calibration curve
    B. Wavelength calibration
    C. Spectral transmittance curve
    D. Molar absorptivity calculation

The answer is C. When various wavelengths are plotted vs. %T, a spectral transmittance curve will result which will peak at the wavelength where greatest absorbance or least transmittance occurs. This process can be used to determine the optimal wavelength of light to use for the analysis. This results in improved specificity, sensitivity, and linearity of spectrophotometric measurement. (Anderson et al., p. 76)

34. Which of the following does the most to minimize aerosol production during centrifugation?

    A. Using a refrigerated centrifuge
    B. Using centrifuge tubes with tapered bottoms
    C. Selecting centrifuge tube sizes that will fit securely into the centrifuge rack
    D. Using stoppered centrifuge tubes or a cover over the rotar chamber

The answer is D. Specimen-collection tubes should be left stoppered for centrifugation; if need arises to centrifuge an unstoppered tube, it should be covered with Parafilm or fitted snugly with a stopper. Alternately, a centrifuge with a rotar-chamber cover will contain any aerosols. (Burtis et al., p. 24)

35. From the following data, calculate the concentration of the analyte in a serum sample read at 560 nm.

Absorbance of the unknown sample = 0.325
Absorbance of a 200-mg/dL standard = 0.460

    A. 283 mg/dL
    B. 141 mg/dL
    C. 130 mg/dL
    D. 14.1 mg/dL

The answer is B. Beer's law states that concentration (conc) is directly proportional to absorbance (abs) if the analysis is linear. The calculation is as follows:

$$\frac{\text{abs unknown}}{\text{conc unknown}} = \frac{\text{abs standard}}{\text{conc standard}}$$

$$\frac{0.325}{x} = \frac{0.460}{200} = 141 \text{ mg/dL}$$

(Anderson et al., p. 77)

36. Application of a tourniquet for longer than 3 min during venipuncture will result in

    A. decreased hemoconcentration around the puncture site
    B. no changes in blood composition if fist pumping is avoided.
    C. significant decrease in total protein
    D. increased filtration pressure across capillary walls

The answer is D. Three-min stasis can lead to hemoconcentration, regardless of whether fist pumping is used, and up to 15% increase in the concentration of protein and protein-bound constituents. (Burtis et al., pp. 60–61)

37. If a timed urine specimen is required for analysis, the patient should be instructed to complete which of the following for the first voided specimen?

    A. Collect and save the sample
    B. Discard the first and the last sample
    C. Discard the first specimen and begin the timing of the urine collection
    D. It doesn't matter if the first specimen is collected as long as the timing is accurate

The answer is C. The first voided sample should be discarded and the timing of the urine collection begun. At the completion of the required time, the patient should void and add the last specimen to the collection container. (Burtis et al., p. 70)

38. A 4.0-mg/dL creatinine standard is needed. To prepare 100 mL of the working standard, how much stock standard of 1 mg/mL creatinine is needed?

    A. 0.1 mL
    B. 0.4 mL
    C. 4 mL
    D. 40 mL

The answer is C. To solve this problem, use the following formula:

$$\text{Volume}_1 \times \text{concentration}_1 = \text{Volume}_2 \times \text{concentration}_2$$

where volume$_1$ and concentration$_1$ represent the stock standard and volume$_2$ and concentration$_2$ represent the working standard. Units of concentration must be the same between the stock and working standards, so 1 mg/mL should be expressed as 100 mg/dL to be consistent with the working standard.

$$V_1 \times 100\ \text{mg/dL} = 100\ \text{mL} \times 4\ \text{mg/dL}$$

$$V_1 = \frac{100\ \text{mL} \times 4\ \text{mg/dL}}{100\ \text{mg/dL}}$$

(Campbell, pp. 121–124)

39. A pipet should be wiped off

    A. before lowering the meniscus to the calibration mark
    B. after lowering the meniscus to the calibration mark
    C. never if it is a volumetric pipet
    D. only if it is a TC (to contain) pipet

The answer is A. The pipet should be loaded, wiped, held vertically, then emptied until the meniscus touches the calibration mark. This applies to serologic, volumetric, and TC pipets. (Henry, pp. 17–18)

40. A laboratory fire ignited by faulty wiring in a chemistry analyzer and partially fueled by surrounding paper products is classified as

    A. Class B
    B. Class C
    C. Class A and B
    D. Class A and C

The answer is D. Paper and other ordinary combustibles constitute a class-A fire when ignited, and the burning-energized electric equipment characterizes a class-C fire. The situation described above is a combination class-A and -C fire. (Anderson et al., p. 26)

41. Which of the following precautions must be observed when working with corrosive materials in the laboratory?

    A. Work in a Class II biosafety cabinet
    B. Wear gloves and goggles
    C. Wear face protection and shoe covers
    D. Put corrosive material in container and add water

Laboratory Practice

The answer is B. When handling corrosive solutions, laboratory personnel should wear goggles or a face mask, do any stirring or mixing in a fume hood, avoid wearing contact lenses, and wear protective gloves. (Anderson et al., p. 30)

42. Which of the following has been prohibited from use on anything other than a temporary basis in the clinical laboratory?

A. Power strips
B. Portable floor fans
C. Extension cords
D. Multi-outlet boxes

The answer is C. In 1980, the National Committee for Clinical Laboratory Standards (NCCLS) standard on power requirements for clinical laboratories prohibited the use of extension cords except under certain temporary conditions. In such cases, cords must be less than 12 feet long, single-outlet, at least 16 AWG wire, and UL-approved. (Anderson et al., p. 32)

43. Following collection of a fingerstick blood sample and tube centrifugation, hemolysis of the serum is noted. The most likely cause is

A. the presence of alcohol at the site of puncture
B. failure to clean the finger before collection
C. the use of nonsterile collection materials
D. "milking" the finger prior to collection

The answer is A. Massage of the finger to stimulate blood flow may cause the sample to be contaminated with excess tissue fluid. (Burtis et al., pp. 63–64)

44. On linear coordinate graph paper, using the ordinate for absorbance and the abscissa for concentration, a straight line through the origin and three plotted standards indicates all of the following *except* the

A. concentration of the standard vs. the absorbance of the standards is linear
B. concentration of the standard vs. the %T is linear
C. test complies with Beer's law
D. concentration of the standard vs. the log %T is an inverse relationship

The answer is B. The standard curve described demonstrates Beer's law; i.e., the concentration is directly proportional to absorbance. Concentration is also inversely proportional to the logarithm of %T. The concentration of the standard does not have a linear relationship with %T. (Anderson et al., p. 75)

45. The function of a condenser on a microscope is to

A. regulate the amount of light passing through the objective
B. magnify the image
C. reverse the image
D. project and center the light through the specimen and objective lens

The answer is D. The condenser is a combination of lenses beneath the stage that focuses the light on the specimen and also provides a cone of light sufficient for the numerical aperture (NA) of the objective lens. The condenser should not be used to control brightness as it will result in loss of resolution. Brightness should be controlled by the rheostat on the light source. (Walters et al., p. 25)

46. When collecting a blood sample by means of a syringe, hemolysis can be avoided by

    A. using multiple syringes to permit small-volume collection
    B. keeping the needle on the syringe during transfer to other tubes
    C. using a small-bore needle for collection of the sample
    D. precooling the needle and syringe before collection

The answer is C. There is less turbulence of the blood when a small-bore needle rather than a larger bore needle is used. (Burtis et al., p. 61)

47. Beer's law states that the concentration of a substance is

    A. directly proportional to the amount of light absorbed
    B. inversely proportional to the concentration
    C. proportional to the logarithm of the transmitted light
    D. proportional to the square root of the concentration

The answer is A. The light absorption is proportional to the number of molecules of absorbing substance through which the light passes. If the absorbing substance is dissolved in a transparent medium, the absorption of the solution is proportional to its molecular concentration. (Anderson et al., p. 76)

48. The term *computer software* consists of

    A. the program and operating system
    B. memory, program, and printout
    C. CPU and program
    D. all the data stored in volatile memory

The answer is A. Software is the part of the computer system you cannot touch. Software gives the computer instructions as to how to carry out different tasks. It consists of programs and the operating system. (Anderson et al., p. 128)

49. When a blue filter is placed in the path of a white light source, the filter will

    A. transmit wavelengths other than blue
    B. transmit the red wavelengths
    C. absorb only the blue wavelengths
    D. absorb wavelengths other than blue

The answer is D. A solution will appear blue because it transmits wavelengths in the blue portion of the spectrum and absorbs light of other wavelengths. (Burtis et al., p. 122)

50. A control has a mean of 5.5 with a standard deviation of 0.5. If the laboratory is using a 95% confidence interval, the control values must fall between

A. 4.5 to 6.5
B. 5.0 to 6.0
C. 4.0 to 7.0
D. 5.0 to 6.5

The answer is A. A confidence limit or confidence interval of 95% is equal to the mean plus or minus 2 SDs. In this case it is equal to 5.5 ± 1 or 4.5 to 6.5. (Anderson et al., p. 45)

CLS Review Questions

1. Chemicals exist in varying degrees of purity. For quantitative measurements and preparation of accurate standard solutions, it is important to use pure chemicals labeled as

   A. technical grade
   B. reagent grade
   C. purified
   D. *United States Pharmacopeia (USP)*

The answer is B. For quantitative measurements and preparation of accurate standard solutions, it is important to use pure chemicals and to identify exact amounts of compounds or elements desired, as well as amount of contaminants. The use of *reagent-grade* chemicals, although more expensive than using less pure grades of chemicals, is essential to accuracy. Because several grades of chemicals are available, an awareness of the terms used widely is necessary. For the most highly purified chemicals, either *reagent grade, analytical grade,* or *ACS* (for having met standards of purity established by the American Chemical Society) should appear on the label or in the catalogue. Less pure chemicals are referred to as *purified* and *technical.* (Burtis et al., p. 5)

2. Which of the following statements does *not* apply to dry chemical fire extinguishers?

   A. They can be used on flammable liquid fires involving live electric equipment
   B. They can be used on class A, B, and C fires
   C. They can be used on fires in which a reignition source is present
   D. They contain ingredients that are nontoxic

The answer is C. Dry chemical fire extinguishers can be used on flammable liquid fires and fires involving live electricity (classes B and C) because the chemical does not conduct electricity. Because it rapidly extinguishes fire, dry chemical is also often used on fires involving combustible materials (class A). However, because the use of a dry chemical does not produce a permanently inert atmosphere above the fire surface, if there is any possibility of reignition, such as from hot surfaces or smoldering embers, additional appropriate extinguishing agents such as foam must be used. (Burtis et al., p. 53)

3. Monitoring the work area in which radioactive substances such as iodine 125 and carbon 14 are handled is an important aspect of maintaining safe

working conditions. Such monitoring may be performed in a number of ways, the most sensitive of which is

A. visual examination of the work area
B. survey of the work area with a thin-window Geiger-Müller counter
C. wipe-sample analysis of the work area
D. survey of the work area with a general, all-purpose, Geiger-Müller counter

The answer is C. The wipe-sample analysis is much more sensitive than the survey meter for most radionuclides. A Geiger-Müller counter, even with a thin window, is not sensitive enough to register low-level beta emissions such as those from carbon 14 and tritium. A laboratory using both gamma and beta emitters should be monitored by wipe-testing the work area, with the sample filters counted in a liquid scintillation counter. (Miller, p. 4)

4. The most environmentally acceptable method for disposal of most chemical waste products is

A. burial
B. disposal to a sewer system
C. incineration
D. listed in the appropriate Material Safety Data Sheet (MSDS)

The answer is D. For each chemical product, the appropriate disposal method should be referenced from the MSDS. (NCCLS, p. 32)

5. A 200-mg/dL solution was diluted 1 : 10. This diluted solution was then additionally diluted 1 : 5. What is the concentration of the final solution?

A. 2 mg/dL
B. 4 mg/dL
C. 20 mg/dL
D. 40 mg/dL

The answer is B. To calculate final dilutions, multiply the original concentration by the dilution, expressed as a fraction.

$$200 \text{ mg} \times \frac{1}{10} \times \frac{1}{5} = 4 \text{ mg/dL}$$

(Anderson et al., p. 19)

6. What is the molarity of an unknown HCl solution that has a specific gravity of 1.10 and an assay percentage of 18.5%? (Atomic weight: HCl = 36.5)

A. 5.6 mol/L
B. 6.0 mol/L
C. 6.3 mol/L
D. 6.6 mol/L

The answer is A. To solve this problem, it is necessary to convert the density and percentage strength of the strong acid to grams per liter (g/L) and then to molarity:

Density × 10 × percentage = g/L

Molarity = No. of grams of solute per liter of solution

therefore,

1.10 × 10 × 18.5 = 203.5 g/L × 1 mole/36.5 g = 5.6 mol/L

(Anderson et al., p. 20)

7. A method requires the use of an 8% (weight per volume) solution of NaOH. The available solutions are labeled 1N, 2N, 2.5N, and 10N. Which solution is equivalent to 8% NaOH? (Atomic weights: Na = 23; O = 16; H = 1)

A. 1N
B. 2N
C. 2.5N
D. 10N

The answer is B. The normality of a solution is equal to the number of gram equivalents of solute per liter of solution or the number of milligram equivalents (mEq) of solute per milliliter of solution.

mEq/L = (mg/100 mL) × 10 × valence/atomic mass

8% (w/v) = 8 g/100 mL or 8,000 mg/100 mL

mEq/L = (8,000 mg) × 10 × valence/40 = 80,000/40 = 2,000

N = 2,000 mEq/L/1,000 mL = 2N

(Anderson et al., pp. 14–17)

8. Quartz or plastic cuvettes of optical quality should be used when performing spectrophotometric assays in the ultraviolet (UV) region (i.e., less than 340 nm of the spectrum) because the usual borosilicate glass

A. refracts light at 340 nm
B. contributes to light scatter at 340 nm
C. absorbs light at 340 nm
D. emits light of a different wavelength

The answer is C. Regular glass cuvettes made of borosilicate glass should not be used for UV determinations because this material absorbs some of the incident light at these wavelengths, resulting in optical densities that are falsely elevated. (Henry, p. 32)

9. Which of the following best describes the relation of nephelometry to turbidimetry?

A. Nephelometry measures the amount of light absorbed by particles in solution, and turbidimetry measures the amount of light transmitted through a solution
B. Nephelometry directly measures the amount of light scattered by particles in solution, and turbidimetry measures the decrease in incident-light intensity

  C. Nephelometry measures the amount of light emitted by particles in
   solution, and turbidimetry measures the amount of light reflected by
   particles in solution
  D. Nephelometry measures the amount of light transmitted, and turbidimetry measures the amount of light absorbed

The answer is B. Turbidimetry is the measurement of the cloudiness of a
solution due to the number of particles suspended in solution. It is the decrease
in the amount of incident light that is transmitted through the sample that is
actually measured. Nephelometry measures directly the amount of light that
is scattered or reflected, rather than absorbed, by the particles in suspension.
(Burtis et al., p. 154)

10. Which of the following statements best describes the principle of dark-
  field microscopy?

  A. Transparent objects are rendered visible by changing the amplitudes
   of light waves as they pass through the objects under study
  B. Selective absorption produces a visible image because specimen detail
   appears as differences in color to which the eye is sensitive
  C. Light passes through the specimen at an angle, is diffracted, and enters
   the objective lens, producing a bright image
  D. A visible image is produced by the use of magnetic fields, making
   possible greater magnification and resolution

The answer is C. In dark-field microscopy an opaque disk built into the
condenser allows only peripheral rays of light to enter the condenser. These
rays pass through the specimen at an angle such that the field appears unillumi-
nated. Any particles in the field will diffract the light and appear bright against
a darkened background. Dark-field microscopy is useful in visualizing bacterial flagella and spirochetes, which are poorly defined by bright-field and
phase-contrast microscopy. (Brunzel, p. 20)

11. To obtain better separation of liquid and solid components by centrifugation,

  A. increase the speed of the head
  B. decrease the radius of the circle inscribed by the revolving head
  C. increase the length of the tube containing the specimen
  D. reduce the number of specimens in the centrifuge

The answer is A. The relative centrifugal force (rcf) is calculated using the
following formula:

$rcf = 0.00001118 \times r \times N^2$

 r = radius of centrifuge head in centimeters

 N = speed in rpm

Thus, rcf can be increased by increasing the speed or the radius of the head.
(Henry, p. 13)

Laboratory Practice

12. The term "contaminated sharps" means

   A. any contaminated object that can penetrate the skin
   B. needles only
   C. needles and lancets only
   D. dirty broken glass only

The answer is A. The OSHA bloodborne-pathogen standard defines a contaminated sharp as any contaminated object that can penetrate the skin, including, but not limited to, needles, scalpels, broken glass, broken capillary tubes, and exposed ends of dental wires. (Federal Register, pp. 64,004–64,182)

13. Ensuring reliability of all steps of a laboratory procedure requires

   A. use of a serum standard
   B. incorporation of preanalyzed control material
   C. duplicate patient testing
   D. use of a primary standard

The answer is B. The reliability of laboratory procedures is best ensured by incorporating a preanalyzed control in the run of patient specimens. In this way, all steps of the procedure and all variations therein are monitored through acceptance or rejection of the value of the preanalyzed control for the test. Standards may not be subject to all of the same test conditions as the unknowns, whereas the control material would be treated as an unknown. If the test result for the control falls within the preestablished acceptable limits of variation around the mean, the accuracy and precision, and consequently the reliability, of the entire test procedure is ensured. (Burtis et al., p. 561)

14. A hematology laboratory in a hospital has determined that the abnormal low RBC control has a mean value of 3.12 million red cells per mm^3. The 95% confidence limits include red cell count values from $3.06 \times 10^3/mm^3$ to $3.18 \times 10^6/mm^3$. One standard deviation for this control is equal to

   A. $0.01 \times 10^6/mm^3$
   B. $0.02 \times 10^6/mm^3$
   C. $0.03 \times 10^6/mm^3$
   D. $0.04 \times 10^6/mm^3$

The answer is C. Random errors occur in all laboratory measurements, creating the need for establishing acceptable ranges. When sufficient determinations are made, the distribution of values should follow the gaussian curve of normal distribution. Approximately 68% of the results should fall within 1 SD and 95% within 2 SDs. In the above situation, the laboratory personnel are confident that they can expect their low abnormal RBC control to fall between $3.06 \times 10^6/mm^3$ and $3.18 \times 10^6/mm^3$, 95% of the time. One SD is determined by subtracting the mean, 3.12, from the upper confidence limit, 3.18, and dividing by 2 to equal 0.03. (Burtis et al., p. 562)

15. In a normal distribution of results, the mean value ± 2 SDs will exclude

   A. 55% of the population
   B. 32% of the population

C. 5% of the population

D. 1% of the population

The answer is C. In a normal frequency curve, ±2 SDs *includes* 95% of the population; therefore, 5% are excluded. (Burtis et al., p. 391)

16. If a test has a specificity of 98%, it results in approximately

A. 98% false positives

B. 98% false negatives

C. 2% false positives

D. 2% false negatives

The answer is C. The index of specificity can be calculated using the following formula:

$$\text{Index of specificity} = \frac{\text{true negatives}}{\text{false positives} + \text{true negatives}} \times 100$$

Therefore, the index of specificity reflects the degree of true-negative results that would be expected from a normal population. A highly specific test produces a low incidence of false-positive and a high incidence of true-positive results. A test with low specificity produces a high incidence of false-positive and a low incidence of true-positive results. (Burtis et al., p. 496)

17. The coefficient of variation is the

A. square root of the variance from the mean

B. standard deviation expressed as a percentage of the mean

C. sum of the squared differences from the mean

D. confidence interval of the mean

The answer is B. The coefficient of variation (CV), or relative standard deviation, is a statistical tool used to compare variability in nonidentical data sets. To do this, the variability in each data set must be expressed as a relative rather than absolute measure. This is accomplished for each data set by expressing the standard deviation as a percentage of the mean:

$$CV = \frac{SD}{\overline{X}}(100)$$

The CV of each data set allows comparison of two or more test methods, laboratories, or specimen sets. (Burtis et al., p. 390)

18. A new method of glucose testing is compared to an accepted reference method by running split samples from 40 patients by each method. The least squares regression analysis is calculated. The type of error indicated by an upward shift of the line that does not intersect the origin is a

A. constant error

B. proportional error

C. random error

D. systematic error

The answer is A. In the comparison of methods experiment, a plot of data in which there are no analytic errors shows that all the points fall on a straight line that has a 45-degree angle and intersects the origin. Adding 2 mg/dL to the original values, simulating a constant type of systematic analytic error, results in a line that shifts upward by an amount that is constant throughout the range of the graph. The angle of the line is still 45 degrees, but the line does not intersect the origin. (Anderson et al., p. 66)

19. OSHA requires employers to have policies and procedures regarding precautions to take when working with blood and body fluids. This is called a(n)

A. universal precautions plan
B. chemical hygiene plan
C. exposure control plan
D. infectious disease plan

The answer is C. The 1991 rule issued by OSHA requires that an employer have an exposure control plan available to all employees at risk of infection from blood and body fluids. The rule requires that an employer supply personal protective equipment to the employee free of charge. It also requires the safe disposal of sharps and other biohazardous waste and requires that HBV vaccine and postexposure treatment be made available free of charge to all employees at risk of exposure. Annual training is also required that provides information on the risks of exposure, transmission, and necessary precautions to avoid exposure. The rule also addresses handwashing, specimen transport, use of pipet devices, spill cleanup, waste disposal, and decontamination of equipment. (Federal Register, pp. 64,004–64,182)

20. Collection of a 24-h urine includes which of the following procedural steps?

A. Inclusion of urine specimens at the beginning and end of the timed period
B. Discarding any urine specimen that is collected at the same time as a bowel movement
C. Collecting each void in a separate container without preservative and then emptying it into the larger container
D. Removal of aliquots for analysis before collection is complete as long as the volume removed is noted and corrected in the final total volume

The answer is C. The first urine during the collection period is discarded, and the final urine is collected. Precautions should be taken to prevent fecal contamination by a bowel movement, but such urines still need to be included. Aliquots are not permitted, because excretion of most compounds varies throughout the day. (Burtis, p. 70)

21. Carbon dioxide for extinguishers are suitable for use with the following hazards:

A. cloth and electrical
B. wood and flammable gas
C. flammable liquids and electrical
D. paper and natural gas

The answer is C. The only extinguisher to handle all three classes of fire is a dry-chemical type. (Burtis et al., p. 53)

22. Under a general NRC license, liquid ^{125}I waste from an RIA procedure is best disposed of by

A. letting it decay for 5 years
B. flushing it into the sanitary sewer
C. sending it to the sanitary landfill
D. sending it back to the manufacturer

The answer is B. A general license from the NRC is required for the use of RIA kits in the clinical laboratory, even when exempt material such as ^{125}I is used. Under these regulations, effluents from RIA in-vitro tests may be flushed into the sanitary sewer and diluted with large amounts of water. It is good practice to designate one sink for this purpose so the amount of radioactive material can be monitored and periodic wipe tests for contamination can be done. (Federal Register, pp. 64,004–64,182)

23. The term that means reproducibility among replicate determinations of a sample is

A. accuracy
B. precision
C. reliability
D. standard deviation

The answer is B. Precision refers to the magnitude of the random errors and the reproducibility of the measurements. The precision of a clinical method is measured by its variance or standard deviation. The smaller the variance, the greater the precision; if two methods are being compared, the method with the smaller variance is more precise. (Burtis et al., p. 511)

24. A physician requests the following tests on an EDTA-vacutainer sample: hemoglobin, hematocrit, BUN, sodium chloride, glucose, calcium, creatine kinase, and iron. Of the requested tests, which of the following combinations *cannot* be accurately analyzed on the EDTA specimens?

A. Hemoglobin, hematocrit
B. BUN, glucose
C. Hematocrit, sodium chloride
D. Creatine kinase, calcium

The answer is D. EDTA (Ethylenediaminetetraacetic acid) containing vacutainers are generally drawn for hematology testing because EDTA preserves the cellular components of blood. EDTA chelates calcium to prevent coagulation. As an anticoagulant, it has little effect on most chemistries except calcium, iron, alkaline phosphatase, creatine kinase, and leucine aminopeptidase. (Burtis, pp. 66–67)

25. What is the proper sequencing of steps for cleansing the venipuncture site when collecting a blood culture?

1. Rinse with sterile water
2. Allow to dry for 1–2 min
3. Wash with alcohol

4. Apply 1–2% tincture of iodine
5. Wash with green soap

A. 1, 2, 3, 4, 5
B. 5, 4, 3, 2, 1
C. 3, 5, 2, 4, 1
D. 5, 1, 4, 2, 3

The answer is D. Less than 3% of blood cultures should contain contaminating microorganisms from the skin. Therefore, the venipuncture site should be prepared as follows: 1) wash with green soap; 2) rinse with sterile water; 3) apply 1–2% tincture of iodine or povidone-iodine; 4) allow to dry 2–3 min; and 5) wash with 70% alcohol to remove the iodine. The iodine and alcohol must be used to disinfect the venipuncture site unless povidone-iodine is used; then, the 70% alcohol wash is omitted. (Koneman et al., pp. 30–33)

26. A laboratory has acquired a new piece of equipment, but there is no free outlet near the desired location. Which of the following would be temporarily allowed by the 1980 NCCLS standard on power requirements for clinical laboratories?

A. Receptacle extender at a nearby outlet that allows two cords to receive power
B. UL-approved 10-foot extension cord
C. Three-prong adapter attached to the new equipment's power cord
D. A power strip installed two feet below bench level

The answer is B. The cord should be less than 12 feet in length, have at least 16-AWG wire, and have only one outlet at the end. The power strip would be permitted as a permanent solution if it were mounted at least 3-in above the bench top and had its own circuit breaker or fuse. (Burtis, p. 52)

27. A substance-of-abuse specimen has been sent to the laboratory for cocaine analysis. If there is a possibility that this result will be used in a medical legal investigation, which of the following procedures should be used?

A. The phlebotomist draws the blood and takes the specimen to the nurses' station for delivery to the laboratory
B. A chain-of-custody form is completed and the specimen is sent to the laboratory with the other specimens from the floor
C. A chain-of-custody form is signed for each stage of specimen transfer, analysis, and reporting of the result
D. No special procedure is needed as long as the specimen is analyzed by the laboratory personnel collecting the specimen

The answer is C. Specimens that are analyzed for drugs of abuse and alcohol may have medical legal implications. Therefore, handling of these specimens must follow a chain of custody—procedures to account for the integrity of the specimen by tracking its handling from the time of collection to reporting of results. A chain-of-custody form is used to identify each individual in the chain of custody of the specimen. This form must be completed by each individual to document the date and purpose of handling the specimen. If the specimen is aliquoted, a chain-of-custody form must accompany the aliquot. (Henry, pp. 74–75)

28. Which of the following analytes requires anaerobic conditions during centrifugation to allow accurate measurement later?

A. Glucose
B. Creatine kinase
C. Ionized calcium
D. Free testosterone

The answer is C. Calcium is found as protein-bound or free (ionized). The balance between these two forms is pH dependent. Exposure of a blood sample to air can allow the escape of CO_2, which results in raising the blood pH. (Burtis, p. 76)

29. A patient with a presumptive diagnosis of primary liver disease has an LD-isoenzyme pattern performed on a fresh serum sample then again on the same sample the following day. Results are as follows:

| | **Percent of total LD** | | | | |
	LD-1	**LD-2**	**LD-3**	**LD-4**	**LD-5**
Normal control	26	36	20	10	8
Day 1	16	26	18	12	28
Day 2	24	34	20	9	13

The most plausible explanation of these results is that overnight the serum sample was

A. refrigerated or frozen
B. left at room temperature
C. left uncapped
D. diluted with distilled water

The answer is A. Lactate dehydrogenase isoenzymes 4 and 5 are more stable at room temperature than at 4°C. Both are rich in the M form, which bind NAD^+ more weakly, allowing dissociation and subsequent oxidation of the subunit's sulfhydryl groups when stored in the cold. (Burtis, pp. 76, 816)

30. If a patient is suspected of having whooping cough from *Bordetella pertussis,* which of the following is considered the best type of specimen to isolate the organism?

A. Throat swab
B. Nasopharyngeal swab
C. Cough plate
D. Any of the above will isolate *Bordetella pertussis* if present

The answer is B. Whooping cough is caused by *Bordetella pertussis.* The best method for isolating this organism is the use of a nasopharyngeal swab or throat washing. Throat swabs are not adequate to recover *Bordetella pertussis.* The cough plate is considered inferior to the nasopharyngeal swab. (Koneman, pp. 11–14)

31. A sample is drawn off-site for transport to a central lab, with glucose, urea nitrogen, and electrolytes. The anticoagulant of choice is

A. sodium fluoride
B. potassium citrate
C. lithium heparin
D. sodium iodoacetate

The answer is D. While fluoride salts have been used for preserving glucose in transported specimens, its presence inhibits urease (used in urea-nitrogen methods). Neither citrate nor heparin are antiglycolytic. Iodoacetate (2g/L) has no effect on urease, although it does inhibit creatine kinase. (Burtis, pp. 66–67)

32. Which federal law removed the exemption of nonprofit hospitals from engaging in collective bargaining with employees?

A. Occupational Safety and Health Act of 1970
B. Clinical Laboratory Improvement Act of 1967
C. Amendment to National Labor Relations Act, 1974
D. Amendment to Federal Labor Standards Act, 1963

The answer is C. Amendments in 1974 to the National Labor Relations Act (NLRA) removed the previous exemption of nonprofit hospitals that prevented employees from engaging in collective-bargaining activities. Employees in independent and physicians' office laboratories also have the right to engage in collective-bargaining activities if the laboratory brings in a certain amount of revenue. The Fair Labor Standards Act (FLSA) establishes minimum wages, maximum hours, and certain working conditions. The 1963 amendment to the FLSA eliminates sex-biased wage differentials. (Karni et al., p. 530)

33. The regulations from the Clinical Laboratory Improvement Act of 1967 apply to

A. all clinical laboratories in the United States
B. hospital laboratories only
C. laboratories engaged in interstate commerce only
D. independent laboratories only

The answer is C. The Clinical Laboratory Improvement Act of 1967 applies to any laboratory engaged in interstate commerce (i.e., receiving specimens from other states). The regulations require specific personnel, quality-control standards, participation in approved proficiency testing programs, and site inspections. A laboratory found to be in compliance with the regulations receives a license. (Karni et al., p. 510)

34. Calculate the creatinine-clearance rate using the following information:

Urine creatinine = 126 mg/dL
Plasma creatinine = 0.8 mg/dL
Collection time = 24 h
Volume collected = 1.6 L
Patients surface are = 1.6 sq. meters

A. 280 mL/min
B. 189 mL/min
C. 175 mL/min
D. 17.5 mL/min

The answer is B.

$$\text{Clearance} = \frac{UV}{P} \times \frac{1.73}{A}$$

$$\text{Clearance} = \frac{126 \text{ mg/dL} \times 1,600 \text{ mL/1,440 min}}{0.8 \text{ mg/dL}} \times \frac{1.73}{1.60} = 189 \text{ mL/min}$$

(Burtis et al., p. 1,536)

35. Which of the following must be done before a job description can be written?

A. Check with other departments in the institution to see if they have similar jobs
B. Establish a salary range
C. Perform a job analysis
D. Establish performance standards

The answer is C. Each job in an institution must be analyzed for tasks and responsibilities before a job description is written. Standards needed for successful performance of the tasks (performance standards) are established through job analysis. Job analysis is accomplished by observation, interviewing and completion of questionnaires by employees. (Karni et al., p. 172)

36. A device that allows computers to communicate via phone lines is a

A. modem
B. CPU
C. RAM
D. ROM

The answer is A. A modem (short for modulating-demodulating) is a device that is wired into the telephone line instead of using an acoustic coupler with a handset. The speed at which a computer communicates over the phone lines is measured in bauds (bits audio). (Snyder et al., p. 300)

37. The computer term used for capturing data from instruments and processing them without delay is

A. time-sharing
B. batch-processing
C. real time
D. distributed processing

The answer is C. Real time means that the computer receives the information as it comes from the instrument analyzing the substance and processes it for immediate retrival. (Snyder et al., pp. 301–303)

38. Which of the following is essential in stating the conditions of centrifugation in a procedure?

A. Revolutions per minute (rpm)
B. Voltage output of centrifuge
C. Relative centrifugal force (rcf)
D. Angle of centrifuge head

The answer is C. Conditions for centrifugation should specify both the time and the rcf. The rcf is a function of the radius between the axis of rotation and the center of the centrifuge tube and the number of revolutions per minute.

$$rcf = 0.00001118 \times radius \times rpm^2$$

(Burtis et al., p. 24)

39. A "dumb" computer terminal can be used to

   A. run programs to perform specific tasks at the work station
   B. accept data entry only if the main computer is operating
   C. download programs from the main terminal
   D. store data if the main computer is not operational

The answer is B. A dumb terminal requires that the main computer be operational at the time of use and is used for data entry only. In contrast, an "intelligent" terminal is capable of running programs independent of the main computer, downloading programs from a local network to perform tasks, and storing data until the main computer is operational. (Burtis et al., p. 531)

40. When developing a clinical teaching module, the instructor must

   A. provide the student with the opportunity to practice the procedure
   B. prepare a slide series to reinforce the technique
   C. plan to use at least three types of audiovisual techniques
   D. plan to limit the activity to less than one hour

The answer is A. As soon as possible after the clinical teaching activity, the student should be given the opportunity to practice the procedure. Ample time should be given to allow the student to become proficient and confident in the procedure. A more complex task will require more time to master. Each teaching event should be evaluated to include or exclude audiovisual materials. In the clinical teaching arena, the procedure manual, instrument, pipet, reagent, and sample all become the audiovisual material to reinforce the learning event. (Beck et al., p. 122)

41. How many milliliters of 0.75N HCl would be required to neutralize 280 mL of 1.25N NaOH?

   A. 168
   B. 262.5
   C. 467
   D. 560

The answer is C. The formula used to solve this problem is $N \times V = N \times V$.

$$(0.75N)(X) = (1.25N)(280) = 467 \, mL$$

(Burtis et al., pp. 33–35)

42. Calibration of micropipets

   A. must be verified each day of use
   B. should be performed gravimetrically with mercury

C. is unnecessary if the pipet is certified by the manufacturer
D. can be verified spectrophotometrically on a predetermined schedule

The answer is D. Accurate calibration of micropipets must be verified on a regular schedule. Verification should not be performed with mercury because of environmental and safety hazards. Although calibration verification can be done gravimetrically using water with a density correction, another alternative is to use a colored compound and spectrophotometric verification. (Burtis et al., p. 18)

43. Statements of observable learning outcomes are called

A. goal statements
B. performance standards
C. objectives
D. test questions

The answer is C. Educational objectives are statements of learning outcomes stated in terms of observable learner behaviors. Statements of general purposes are termed goals. Achievement of objectives can be measured by construction of test questions that relate back to them. Objectives can be classified into three domains: cognitive, psychomotor, and affective. (Beck et al., p. 34)

44. A test that is used to evaluate an individual's abilities against a predetermined standard is

A. norm-referenced
B. criterion-referenced
C. not valid
D. not reliable

The answer is B. A criterion-referenced test has a predetermined minimal-competence level set for passing. A norm-referenced test sets a passing score based on the performance of all the examinees taking the test at that time. A frequently calculated passing score for a norm-referenced examination is 1 SD below the mean. (Beck et al., p. 90)

45. Which of the following statements concerning type-I reagent grade water is true?

A. It is not covered by NCCLS specifications for reagent grade water
B. It is recommended for use in procedures requiring minimal interference and maximal precision and accuracy
C. It may be used for washing glassware if followed by a rinse of higher reagent grade
D. It may be stored for extended periods of time after production without affecting its reagent grade

The answer is B. The term *reagent grade water* is accompanied by a type I, II, or III designation. Type I has rigid specifications of purity established by the NCCLS and is recommended for those procedures requiring minimal interference and maximal precision and accuracy. These procedures include preparation of standards, as well as enzyme and electrolyte analyses. (Burtis et al., pp. 3–5)

46. In "dry" chemistry-technology systems, cells, proteins, or other interfering substances are removed by

A. dialysis
B. centrifugation
C. film membranes
D. column chromatography

The answer is C. Dialysis is used to remove interfering substances in "wet" chemistry systems such as the continuous-flow technology (SMAC). Centrifugation is used as a preanalytic preparation to remove some interferences. Column chromatography, gel filters, or ion exchange resins are used in wet chemistry systems such as the ACA (closed wet-pack technology). Film membranes are used in dry chemistry systems such as the Reflotron to exclude RBCs from the analytic procedure. (Burtis et al., p. 325)

47. An automated system that is used for many different analyte applications most frequently has a sample delivery system equipped with a

A. fixed pipet
B. variable pipet
C. selectable pipet
D. air-displacement pipet

The answer is B. A fixed pipet delivers only one set sample size and is used for limited applications. A variable pipet can usually deliver samples in volumes from 1 μL to 100 μL and may be adjusted based on the application required. A selectable pipet has a predetermined selection of sample sizes it can deliver; therefore, it widens the menu of applications. It is still not as versatile as a variable pipet. An air-displacement pipet is not generally used to pipet sample aliquots in an automated system, since the measure is affected by viscosity of the sample. Positive-displacement pipettes provide high reproducibility and increased accuracy compared to air-displacement pipettes. (Burtis et al., p. 329)

48. Given the following objective, determine the best audiovisual aid to augment learning:

"Following instruction, the student will be able to correctly interpret a Gram-stain slide on a sputum specimen."

A. Chalkboard
B. Overhead projector
C. Videotape
D. 35-mm slides

The answer is D. The chalkboard and overhead will not provide the color and discrimination the student will need to appropriately interpret a Gram's stain. A videotape may provide the color; however, the 35-mm slide is the best answer, since the slide is still and allows the student to determine the amount of time needed on each example. (Beck et al., pp. 65–70)

49. When there are five or six consecutive values that continue to increase or decrease on a Levey-Jennings chart, it is called a

A. shift
B. normal occurrence
C. trend
D. reliable measurement

The answer is C. A trend is a steadily increasing or decreasing control value. It occurs when the analytic method suffers a progressively developing problem. (Henry, p. 90)

50. The aperture diaphragm of a microscope

A. reduces stray light
B. gathers and focuses the illumination light onto the specimen
C. provides the secondary-image magnification of the specimen
D. regulates the angle of light presented to the specimen

The answer is D. The aperture diaphragm is located at the base of the condenser and regulates the angle of light presented to the specimen. The condenser gathers and focuses the illumination light onto the specimen for viewing. The ocular provides the secondary-image magnification of the specimen, and the field diaphragm reduces stray light. (Brunzel, pp. 2–3)

References

Anderson SC, Cockayne S. *Clinical Chemistry Concepts and Applications.* Philadelphia: Saunders, 1993.

Beck SJ, LeGrys VA. *Clinical Laboratory Education* (2nd ed.) American Society for Clinical Laboratory Science. Bethesda, MD. 1996.

Brunzel NA. *Fundamentals of Urine and Body Fluid Analysis.* Philadelphia: Saunders, 1994.

Burtis CA, Ashwood ER. (eds). *Teitz's Textbook of Clinical Chemistry* (2nd ed). Philadelphia: Saunders, 1994.

Campbell JB. *Laboratory Mathematics* (4th ed). St. Louis: Mosby, 1990.

Federal Register. *Occupational Exposure to Bloodborne Pathogens.* US GPO, vol. 56 (December 6, 1991).

Garza D, Becan-McBride K. *Phlebotomy Handbook* (2nd ed). Norwalk, CT: Appleton & Lange, 1989.

Henry JB (ed). *Clinical Diagnosis and Management by Laboratory Methods* (18th ed). Philadelphia: Lippincott, 1992.

Koneman EW, et al. *Color Atlas and Textbook of Diagnostic Microbiology* (4th ed). Philadelphia: Lippincott, 1992.

Karni K, Viskochil KF, Amos P. *Clinical Laboratory Management.* Boston: Little, Brown, 1982.

Miller B. *Laboratory Safety: Principles and Practices.* Washington DC: American Society for Microbiology, 1986.

Laboratory Practice

National Committee for Clinical Laboratory Standards (NCCLS). *Document G P 17-T*. Villanova, PA: NCCLS, 1989.

Snyder JR, Senhauser DA. *Administration and Supervision in Laboratory Medicine* (2nd ed). Philadelphia: Lippincott, 1989.

Sullivan JB. *Hazardous Materials Toxicology*. Baltimore: Williams & Wilkins, 1992.

Walters, Estridge, Reynolds. *Basic Medical Laboratory Techniques*. Albany: Delmar, 1986.

Review Tests

CLT Review Test

1. A patient who consistently has an abnormally high blood-glucose concentration *most likely* has defective or insufficient amounts of which hormone?

   A. Cortisol
   B. Epinephrine
   C. Glucagon
   D. Insulin

2. If a lipemic serum is centrifuged and the top creamy layer discarded before analysis, which of these errors will occur?

   A. The total cholesterol result will be falsely high
   B. The triglyceride result will be falsely low
   C. Both the total cholesterol and triglyceride results will be falsely high
   D. Both the total cholesterol and HDL cholesterol results will be falsely low

3. Serum total-protein results can be falsely increased if

   A. arterial blood is used
   B. hemolysis occurs
   C. a fasting specimen is used
   D. lipids are removed prior to analysis

4. An enzyme assay that shows substrate depletion should be repeated using

   A. less sample
   B. less substrate
   C. longer light path
   D. longer reaction time

5. In the Jaffe reaction, creatinine forms a colored complex that has an absorbance maximum at 485 nm. However, the reaction is usually read spectrophotometrically at ≈520 nm because

   A. acetoacetic acid interferes at 485 nm
   B. picric ion, present in excess, absorbs below 500 nm

183

C. spectrophotometers are more accurate at 520 nm than at 485 nm
D. noncreatinine chromogens that are not removed absorb below 500 nm

6. As a patient becomes acidotic, the plasma concentration of

A. total calcium increases
B. free ionized calcium increases
C. albumin-bound calcium increases
D. calcium complexed with ligands (e.g., phosphate) increases

7. An arterial-blood specimen is collected from a normal, healthy donor for blood-gas analysis. The specimen was improperly collected, and a large bubble of room air is present in the syringe. Which of the following changes can occur?

pH	PCO_2	PO_2
A. increase	decrease	increase
B. increase	increase	decrease
C. decrease	decrease	increase
D. decrease	increase	decrease

8. A purple color forms on the ketone reagent strip pad when urinary ketones react with

A. tetramethylbenzidine
B. diazotized sulfanilic acid
C. p-dimethylaminobenzaldehyde
D. sodium nitroprusside

9. Decreased serum levels of total thyroxine (T_4), thyroid-stimulating hormone (TSH), and tri-iodothyronine resin uptake (T_3RU) indicate

A. primary hypothyroidism
B. secondary hypothyroidism
C. euthyroidism with excess TBG
D. euthyroidism with decreased thyroxine-binding globulin

10. Select the pattern of test results *most* consistent with obstructive liver disease.

	Total Bilirubin	Conjugated Bilirubin	Total Alkaline Phosphatase
A.	increased	increased	increased
B.	increased	normal	increased
C.	normal	increased	decreased
D.	increased	normal	decreased

11. The glucose concentration in normal cerebrospinal fluid is

A. usually less than 40 mg/dL
B. 60 to 80% of the plasma-glucose concentration

C. equal to the plasma-glucose concentration
D. usually greater than 100 mg/dL

12. Which of the following is *not* required when calibrating a pCO_2 electrode on a blood-gas instrument?

A. The barometric pressure
B. A calomel reference electrode
C. Instrument temperature maintained at 37°C
D. Calibration gases at two different concentrations

13. The movement of buffer and some large, weakly charged proteins toward the cathode during electrophoresis is due to

A. electroendosmosis
B. a voltage that is set too high
C. bubbles trapped in the support media
D. evaporation during electrophoresis

14. Calculate the calibration set point for the pCO_2 electrode using the following:

Calibration gas concentration   10% CO_2
Temperature   37°C
Barometric pressure   750 mm Hg
Water vapor pressure (PH_2O)   47 mm Hg

A. 70 mm Hg
B. 75 mm Hg
C. 80 mm Hg
D. 100 mm Hg

15. Osmometers can determine osmolality using which one of these properties?

A. Boiling-point depression
B. Freezing-point depression
C. Osmotic-pressure depression
D. Vapor-pressure elevation

16. The following laboratory results are obtained on a patient:

Creatine kinase (CK): 213 U/L
CK-MB > 6%
LD-1 > LD-2

These laboratory findings are consistent with which of the following diagnoses?

A. Myocardial infarction
B. Duchenne's muscular dystrophy

C. Cirrhosis of the liver

D. Hepatic obstructive disorders

17. The plasma-urea concentration is increased by

A. urinary stasis

B. a vegetarian diet

C. an increase in diuresis

D. an increase in renal blood flow

18. A plasma sample was analyzed on an ISE, and electrolyte results were

$$Na^+ = 140 \text{ mmol/L}$$
$$K^+ = 14.0 \text{ mmol/L}$$
$$Cl^- = 112 \text{ mmol/L}$$
$$HCO_3^- = 18 \text{ mmol/L}$$

The most likely cause for these results is the

A. sample was hemolyzed

B. electrodes are protein-coated

C. sample was drawn in a tube with an improper anticoagulant

D. patient is on a high-potassium diet

19. A red-top tube was discovered on a phlebotomist's tray 3-1/2 h after it had been drawn. Which of the following sets of tests could still be run?

A. BUN, creatinine

B. Glucose, electrolytes

C. Total and direct bilirubin

D. Alkaline phosphatase, AST, ALT, LD

20. The following results were obtained for a patient:

total calcium = 2.1 mg/dL

phosphorus = 4.0 mg/dL

PTH = 85 pmol/L (<105)

These findings are consistent with

A. primary hypoparathyroidism

B. severe renal disease

C. hypermagnesemia

D. sample collection in an EDTA tube

21. A primary standard is defined as a solution

A. whose concentration is determined by repeated assays

B. whose solvent is Type-III water

C. of lyphilized serum with assayed values listed by the manufacturer

D. with an exact known concentration of an analyte

22. When preparing a sample for a sodium determination using a flame photometer, the serum sample is diluted with a solution containing a low concentration of a detergent and an internal standard such as

   A. lanthanum
   B. potassium dichromate
   C. lithium
   D. magnesium chloride

23. The linearity calibration of a spectrophotometer is best determined by using

   A. a didymium filter
   B. standard solutions of different concentrations
   C. a homium-oxide filter
   D. a calculation of the bandpass width

24. Which of the following dilutions should be performed to prepare a 1 : 8 dilution from a serum sample that has already been diluted 1 : 2?

   A. 1 mL of sample with 7 mL of diluent
   B. 1 mL of sample with 4 mL of diluent
   C. 0.5 mL of sample with 7 mL of diluent
   D. 0.5 mL of sample with 8 mL of diluent

25. Which of the following types of glassware should be used for the preparation of 25 mL of a 1-N solution of sodium hydroxide?

   A. A 25-mL graduated cylinder
   B. A 25-mL Erlenmeyer flask
   C. A 25-mL beaker
   D. A 25-mL volumetric flask

26. The measurement of which analyte provides the best indicator of renal function?

   A. Bilirubin
   B. Creatinine
   C. Creatinine kinase
   D. Total protein

27. When performing RID by the Mancini method for analysis of IgG levels, which of the following constitutes an error in the procedural performance?

   A. Adding antigen to wells
   B. Adding antibody to wells
   C. Incubating for 24 h at 25°C
   D. Plotting squared diameter of ring expansion versus standard concentration

28. Preanalytical variables that influence cholesterol results include all of the following *except*

A. age
B. gender
C. stress
D. fasting

29. A blood sample for blood-gas analysis was left exposed to air prior to analysis. Which of the following changes are likely to occur?

A. Increased pO_2
B. Decreased pO_2
C. Increased pCO_2
D. Decreased pH

30. Which of the following test methods is the *most* specific for measuring plasma glucose?

A. o-Toluidine
B. Hexokinase
C. Copper reduction
D. Dye-binding

31. Which of the following constitutes an error in the performance of an insulin assay by RIA using ^{14}C?

A. Counting the number of gamma emissions per min
B. Determining the time required to count a predetermined number of gamma emissions
C. Determining the gamma emissions using a solid scintillation counter
D. Determining the gamma emissions using a liquid scintillation counter

32. Two spectrophotometers are being considered for purchase. Instrument A has a bandpass of 20 nm and Instrument B has a bandpass of 10 nm. Which of the following interpretations can be made?

A. Instrument A has greater sensitivity and specificity
B. Instrument B has greater sensitivity and specificity
C. Instrument A has more sensitivity but less specificity than instrument B
D. Instrument B has more sensitivity but less specificity than instrument A

33. Which of the following statements is true regarding BUN and creatinine assays?

A. Creatinine is less affected by protein metabolism and is a more sensitive index of mild impairment of GFR
B. BUN is less affected by protein metabolism and is a more sensitive index of mild impairment of GFR
C. Creatinine is less affected by protein metabolism but is a less sensitive index of mild impairment of GFR

D. BUN is less affected by protein metabolism but is a less sensitive index of mild impairment of GFR

34. Which of the following tests provides the best index of a patient's average blood-glucose level over a 2-mo period?

A. Glucose tolerance test
B. Glycated serum proteins
C. Glycated hemoglobin
D. C-peptide

35. A patient is admitted to the emergency room complaining of severe chest pain. Physical examination reveals elevated blood pressure and heart rate. An electrocardiogram reveals tachycardia and arrhythmia. The attending physician will likely order (STAT)

A. CK, CK-MB, LD, and LD isoenzymes
B. AST, ALT, bilirubin, and ALP
C. serum amylase and lipase
D. acid phosphatase and CK-BB

36. A patient who is taking diuretics for congestive heart failure has blood drawn for a potassium level. The sample is centrifuged and analyzed as part of a large run. The value is 7.6 mmol/L. The original sample is pulled and is grossly hemolyzed. The CLT should

A. notify the physician immediately that the potassium is elevated
B. enter the data and handle as routine results
C. rerun the sample and report the results if they were similar to the first result
D. notify the physician that the sample hemolyzed and a new specimen needs to be collected

37. You obtain the following data on a cholesterol assay:

Sample	Absorbance (530 nm)	Concentration (mg/dL)
Standard	0.2	150
Normal control	0.2	100–200 (expected)
Abnormal control	0.6	250–300 (expected)
Patient	0.5	NA

After calculating the cholesterol concentrations of this test run for the normal and abnormal controls, you decide that

A. both are out of the expected range; the test results cannot be reported
B. the normal control is in range and the abnormal control is not; the test results can be reported
C. the normal control is in range and the abnormal control is not; the test results cannot be reported
D. the normal control is out of range and the abnormal control is in range; the test results cannot be reported

38. The following laboratory results were noted on a frail, elderly woman scheduled to begin renal dialysis:

Serum total calcium: low normal
Serum inorganic phosphorus: increased
Serum parathyrin (PTH): increased
Serum alkaline phosphatase: increased
BUN and creatinine: increased

These findings are consistent with a diagnosis of

A. primary hypoparathyroidism
B. secondary hyperparathyroidism
C. primary hyperparathyroidism
D. pseudohypoparathyroidism

39. Renal disease can be differentiated from lower urinary-tract disease when the microscopic examination of urine sediment reveals significant numbers of

A. yeast
B. granular casts
C. RBCs
D. WBCs

40. False-negative reagent-strip protein results can occur

A. if the urine pH is ≥ 9.0
B. if sufficient myoglobin is present
C. when a urine specimen is improperly stored
D. when free-sulfhydryl drugs are excreted in urine

41. A change in the glomerular filtration rate is *best* assessed using the

A. urea-clearance test
B. creatinine-clearance test
C. ammonium-chloride test
D. p-aminohippurate (PAH) clearance test

42. The following results are obtained on a urine specimen:

Reagent-strip protein test: negative
Sulfosalicylic-acid precipitation test: positive

These results can be caused by the increased urinary excretion of

A. albumin
B. microalbumin
C. Tamm-Horsfall protein
D. immunoglobulin light chains

43. A urine specimen collected from a diabetic inpatient with possible hepatitis was not refrigerated. It remained at room temperature for 4 h before being delivered to the laboratory for testing. It was not accepted by the laboratory, and the nursing station was called. The technician explained that the specimen should be recollected due to the likely occurrence of which of the following changes?

A. Odor increases; glucose increases
B. Clarity decreases; bilirubin decreases
C. Color decreases; urobilinogen increases
D. Specific-gravity decreases; ketones decrease

44. Both the reagent strip and the refractometry methods for specific gravity

A. detect large nonionic solutes
B. require corrections for protein and glucose
C. are used to assess renal concentrating ability
D. reflect the pK_a change of a polyelectrolyte

45. Select the urinalysis results that are contradictory:

A. Reagent strip blood—negative; microscopic exam—0–2 RBCs/HPF
B. SSA protein test—negative; microscopic exam—2–5 hyaline casts/LPF
C. Reagent-strip leukocyte esterase—negative; microscopic exam—5–10 WBCs/HPF
D. Refractometry specific gravity—1.015; microscopic exam—5–10 radiographic dye crystals/LPF

46. False-negative reagent-strip ketone results can occur

A. if sufficient ascorbic acid is present
B. when a urine specimen is improperly stored
C. if the β-hydroxybutyrate concentration is too low
D. when free-sulfhydryl drugs are excreted in urine

47. Which of the following entities is always indicative of disease when found in urine sediment, regardless of the number present?

A. fat globules
B. hyaline casts
C. granular casts
D. RBCs

48. Which of the following urine-specimen results needs to be investigated or confirmed before reporting?

A. Reagent strip bilirubin—negative; ictotest—positive
B. Reagent-strip protein—negative; reagent-strip pH—8.0
C. Refractometer specific gravity—1.045; microscopic exam—cholesterol crystals
D. Reagent-strip leukocyte esterase—negative; microscopic exam—5–10 WBCs/HPF

49. Which of the following situations will cause falsely elevated cyanmethemoglobin levels?

A. Hemoglobin-F levels of 6%
B. RBC count of 3.21×10^{12}/L
C. sulfhemoglobin
D. WBC count of 80×10^9/L

50. Using a calibrated Miller disc and counting eight successive fields, 163 reticulocytes were counted in square A and 500 RBCs were counted in square B. The reticulocyte count in percent is

A. 3.2%
B. 3.6%
C. 6.4%
D. 16.3%

51. Which of the following is the reason EDTA is the preferred anticoagulant for platelet counts?

A. It inhibits blood-clotting factors
B. It does not alter the pH of the test procedure
C. The ratio of blood-to-anticoagulant is not as critical as with other anticoagulants
D. It prevents platelet aggregation

52. A manual platelet count was performed using a 1 : 100 dilution, and a total of 200 platelets were counted in a 1-mm² area. This count best matches which of the following platelet slide estimates?

A. markedly decreased
B. slightly decreased
C. normal
D. markedly increased

53. A false-negative result for hemoglobin S in the whole-blood screening solubility test can be caused by

A. recent transfusion
B. increased chylomicrons
C. extreme leukocytosis
D. hyperglobulinemia

54. A cerebrospinal-fluid specimen collected from a 9-month-old female had a cell count of 25 cells/µL with 70% monocytes and 30% lymphocytes. These results suggest

A. viral meningitis
B. bacterial meningitis
C. a cerebral infarction
D. a normal cell count and differential

55. The crystals in a synovial-fluid sample appear strongly birefringent when viewed under polarized light. When aligned parallel with the slow vibration of light, the crystal is yellow. This crystal is

A. apatite
B. cholesterol
C. monosodium urate
D. calcium pyrophosphate

56. Your last 20 Wright-stained smears were all too pink in color. What is the best way to remedy this situation?

A. Make all blood smears thinner
B. Increase the methanol content of the stain
C. Shorten the staining (buffer) time
D. Increase the pH of the buffer

57. Secondary granules first appear in which stage of neutrophilic development?

A. Myeloblast
B. Promyelocyte
C. Myelocyte
D. Metamyelocyte

58. A supravital stain must be used to demonstrate the presence of

A. Howell-Jolly bodies
B. siderocytes
C. malarial parasites
D. reticulum

59. An erroneously high spun hematocrit can be caused by

A. reticulocytosis
B. hemolysis of the blood sample
C. reading the buffy coat as part of the packed-cell portion
D. macrocytosis

60. A patient has chronic liver disease due to alcoholism. The MCV is normal, but on the peripheral blood smear many macrocytes are seen. What is the most likely explanation for this discrepancy?

A. Many reticulocytes are present
B. The macrocytes are really codocytes
C. The cells are well filled with hemoglobin
D. The macrocytes are "thin," with an increase in diameter but normal cell volume

61. All dilution fluids for WBC counts must serve at least two purposes. One is to suspend and disperse the WBC; the other is to

A. lyse RBCs
B. serve as a conductor for aperture counts
C. lyse platelets
D. stain the nuclei

62. The ESR is affected by all of the following *except*

A. fibrinogen level
B. hematocrit
C. type of hemoglobin
D. anticoagulant-to-blood ratio

63. In a normal WBC differential from a 24-year-old male, there are usually more

A. lymphocytes than any other cells
B. monocytes than eosinophils
C. basophils than eosinophils
D. band neutrophils than lymphocytes

64. A specimen is collected in powdered EDTA and transported to the laboratory within 30 min. When the smear is stained and viewed, the platelets appear to be clumped around the periphery of granulocytes. The appropriate course of action would be to

A. redraw the specimen, taking care to get a free-flowing amount of blood
B. allow the original sample to mix for at least 10 min prior to making another smear
C. warm the sample to 37°C prior to testing
D. redraw the specimen using a microtechnique

65. A sample is stored for quality-control precision testing. After nearly 24 h at 4°C, the sample is

A. appropriate to use immediately
B. appropriate to use after warming and mixing for at least 5 min
C. inappropriate to use due to swelling of RBCs
D. inappropriate to use due to autolysis of WBCs

66. A sample of blood for a CBC with no differential is drawn at 7:00 am and brought to the laboratory by 8:00 am. At 2:00 pm, the physician telephones to request that differential also be done. The correct course of action is to

A. allow the blood to mix well prior to making the smear
B. make the smear only if the blood has been stored at 4°C
C. make the smear if the physician has a written order brought to the laboratory
D. inform the physician that a new sample of blood must be drawn

67. A clinical laboratory technician has made ten peripheral blood smears. All ten show the presence of large amounts of rouleaux. One possible explanation for this is

A. all ten patients have hypoglobulinemia
B. the drop of blood that was used was too big

C. the angle of the spreader slide was too high for the amount of blood that was put onto the slide
D. there was a prolonged time between the moment at which the blood contacted the spreader slide and the beginning of the push

68. During the automatic stainer's run, it was noticed that the slides were being washed of the buffer with a more vigorous action than necessary. One possible consequence to this instrument problem is

A. the slides are washed clean of the sample
B. the cells stain a deeper blue
C. the cells stain a brighter red
D. the cells appear faded

69. Peripheral blood smears with uneven edges may be caused by

A. too large a drop of blood
B. too small a drop of blood
C. changes in the speed of the spreader slide across the base slide
D. changes in the angle of the spreader slide across the base slide

70. Which of the following situations would falsely decrease the quantitation of hemoglobin using the cyanmethemoglobin (ferricyanide) method?

A. Large amounts of sulfhemoglobin
B. Large amounts of carboxyhemoglobin
C. Presence of hemoglobin S
D. Absence of hemoglobin A_2

71. Falsely elevated microhematocrits may be reported in

A. patients with pulmonary edema
B. patients with poikilocytosis sufficient to increase the percent of trapped plasma
C. prolonged centrifugation time due to a wearing away of the centrifuge's brushes
D. samples that have been over anticoagulated

72. A protein buildup in the orifice of the aperture of an impedance counter will result in a falsely increased

A. RBC count
B. MCV
C. RDW
D. MCHC

73. Which of the following coagulation tests would *not* be included in a routine preoperative coagulation-screening battery?

A. Factor-VIII assay
B. Bleeding time

C. Activated-partial-thromboplastin time (APTT)
D. Prothrombin time

74. A physician orders a factor-IX assay. The screening test that has probably been performed and found to be abnormal is

A. bleeding time
B. PT
C. APTT
D. both PT and APTT

75. A normal APTT with a prolonged PT would indicate a possible deficiency in factor

A. II
B. X
C. VIII
D. VII

76. The specimen of choice for platelet aggregation is whole-blood anticoagulated with

A. EDTA
B. heparin
C. sodium citrate
D. ammonium oxalate

77. After removal of the plasma from a centrifuged specimen of whole blood anticoagulated with sodium citrate, the clinical laboratory technician notices the presence of fine, thread-like filaments left in the remaining sample. He should

A. continue with the coagulation study
B. recentrifuge the remaining cells and plasma to remove more supernate
C. ask for a new specimen
D. warm the remaining sample at 37°C prior to testing

78. Specimens for prothrombin-time testing can be stored

A. uncentrifuged at 0°C for no longer than 1 h
B. uncentrifuged at 4°C for no longer than 2 h
C. centrifuged and separated at 10°C for no longer than 1 h
D. centrifuged and separated at 20°C for no longer than 2 h

79. When preparing reagents for the performance of activated-partial-thromboplastin times, it is important to incubate the $CaCl_2$ at 37°C

A. for at least 30 min
B. for 15 to 30 min
C. no longer than 2 min
D. with no specific time limit

80. A review of the quality-control chart for the past week suggests

Prothrombin time - normal control

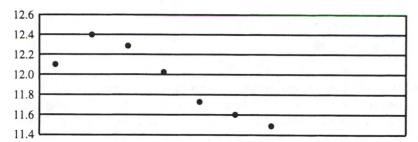

normal control mean: 12.0 sec
1 SD: 0.3 sec

A. a normal distribution of results
B. a trend starting on day 2
C. loss of control on day 6
D. deterioration of control noticeable throughout the week

81. In the performance of a bleeding time on a newborn, the blood pressure cuff should be set to

A. above 100 mm Hg
B. between 70 and 100 mm Hg
C. between 30 and 70 mm Hg
D. lower than 30 mm Hg

82. The normal APTT control has a mean of 28.5 sec with 1 SD of 1.0 sec. Today's result is 30 sec. The possible cause may be

A. thromboplastin deterioration
B. calcium chloride contamination
C. normal-control random error
D. instrument variability

83. Coagulation instruments using the electromechanical principle have difficulty in testing samples that

A. have a bilirubin of 4.0 mg/dL
B. have a plasma hemoglobin of greater than 2 mg/dL
C. produce a shorter than expected clotting time
D. produce fragmented fibrin

84. Potential sources of error in the operation of an electro-optical coagulation instrument do *not* include

A. crimped tubing
B. baseline readout delay due to optical rippling
C. insufficient reagent
D. erratic temperature levels

85. In the performance of a bleeding time, pressure exerted by the blood-pressure cuff should be maintained at

A. 20 mm Hg
B. 40 mm Hg
C. 80 mm Hg
D. 120 mm Hg

86. When performing controls for the morning run in coagulation, the normal control is within acceptable limits for both the prothrombin and activated-partial-thromboplastin times. The abnormal control is out of range for both procedures. Appropriate action would be to

A. continue with morning run and report out only those results that are in normal range
B. continue with morning run and report out only those results that are in abnormal range
C. continue with morning run and repeat controls at the end of the morning run
D. repeat abnormal controls on a new bottle of control material before proceeding with analysis of any samples

87. If platelet concentrates are to be prepared from whole blood collected at a mobile site, the whole blood should be stored at which of the following temperatures for no more than 8 h prior to separation of the platelet-rich plasma?

A. 1–6°C
B. 10–20°C
C. 20–24°C
D. 30–37°C

88. Platelet concentrates prepared from whole blood collected from donors who have ingested aspirin within 72 h of donation must be

A. discarded
B. held in quarantine for 24 h before release into routine inventory to allow the platelet function to recover
C. labeled to indicate the donor recently ingested aspirin
D. tested to determine that the platelet count is adequate

89. Which of the following persons would *not* qualify as a regular blood donor?

A. A healthy man taking isoniazid due to a recent positive skin test for tuberculosis
B. A man who had minor surgery 5 weeks ago
C. A woman with a history of convulsions during a childhood illness that included a high fever
D. A woman in the first trimester of pregnancy

90. Following FDA regulations, the clinical laboratory technician performed platelet counts on platelet concentrates from four separate donors collected and processed during the month. The counts were as follows:

Donor A: 5.3×10^{10}/bag
Donor B: 4.2×10^{10}/bag
Donor C: 5.7×10^{10}/bag
Donor D: 4.6×10^{10}/bag

Based on these results, the CLT should

A. investigate explanations for low concentrations in the platelet concentrates
B. investigate explanations for high concentrations in the platelet concentrates
C. investigate explanations for excess variability between concentrations in the four platelet concentrates
D. report acceptable quality-control results for platelet concentrates

91. The screening of a female blood donor yielded the following results:

weight   115 lbs
hemoglobin   13.0 g/dL
temperature   36.5°C
blood pressure 145/85 mm Hg

In addition, the woman had no recent surgeries; had a tattoo applied 6 months ago; had not traveled outside the U.S.; had no history of jaundice or hepatitis; and took no routine medications (although she had taken 2 aspirin for a headache 5 days ago).

This donor is

A. acceptable as a red cell donor only
B. acceptable as a whole blood donor
C. deferred for at least 6 months
D. deferred indefinitely

92. In addition to the full name and hospital number, a patient's sample for typing and compatibility testing must also be labeled with the

A. diagnosis
B. name of the attending physician
C. date of collection
D. initials of the phlebotomist

93. After centrifugation, an antibody screening tube is shaken to resuspend the cell button. The cells stream off the button with only occasional small agglutinates in a background of free RBCs. Once the cell button is completely dislodged, it should be graded as

A. 1+
B. 2+

C. 3+
D. 4+

94. Mrs. M. delivered a two-week premature infant. Her physician ordered postnatal testing due to the infant's jaundice. The results are given below:

Mrs. M's results		**Baby M's results**	
ABO group:	A	ABO group:	O
Rh type:	negative	Rh type:	negative
Autocontrol:	negative	DAT:	positive
Antibody screen:	positive		
Antibody ID:	anti-D		

What procedures should be performed next?

A. Acid elution of maternal cells and antibody identification on the eluate
B. Autoabsorption of anti-D from maternal serum using maternal cells
C. Autoabsorption using the infant cells and antibody identification on the absorbed serum
D. Heat elution of the baby's cells and repeat of Rh typing on the eluted cells

95. Which of the following techniques can be used to gain reliable antibody screen and crossmatch results for patients whose serum causes test-cell rouleaux?

A. Autoabsorption
B. Enzyme pretreatment of cells
C. Prewarm technique
D. Saline replacement

96. Saline reactive IgM anti-D reagent cannot be used for weak D (D^u) typing because

A. anti-D, like other Rh antibodies, is usually IgG
B. antiglobulin reagent reacts with the Fc fragment of IgG but not IgM
C. IgM reacts better at room temperature, and the weak D test is incubated at 37°C
D. IgM will elute from the red cells during the washing procedure preceding the AHG phase of testing

97. Serum from the majority of group A individuals contains

A. anti-A
B. anti-A,B
C. anti-B
D. anti-D

98. Given the reactions below, the patient's group and type are:

	Anti-A	Anti-B	Anti-A,B	Anti-D	Rh control
patient cells	4+	0	4+	3+	0

	A_1 cells	B cells
patient serum	0	4+

A. Group A, Rh-negative
B. Group A, Rh-positive
C. Group B, Rh-negative
D. Group B, Rh-positive

99. Based on the following red cell reactions, the only Rh genotype that is *not* a possibility is

Antiserum	Reaction
anti-C	+
anti-D	+
anti-E	+
anti-c	+
anti-e	+

A. R^1r''
B. R^2r'
C. R^1R^2
D. R^0r''

100. Which of the following cells would be an appropriate positive control cell for antigen-typing procedures using commercially prepared anti-Jk^a?

A. ce, Fy(a−b+), Jk(a+b+), Le(a−b−)
B. Cce, Fy(a+b−), Jk(a−b+), Le(a−b+)
C. CDEe, Fy(a+b+), Jk(a−b+), Le(a−b+)
D. Ce, Fy(a+b−), Jk(a+b−), Le(a+b−)

101. The following reactions are obtained on ABO testing of a patient's blood sample. What is the most likely ABO group?

Patient cells +	Anti-A	Anti-B	Anti-A_1 lectin
	3+	0	0

Patient serum +	A_1 cells	A_2 cells	B cells	O cells
	2+	0	4+	0

A. A_1
B. A_3
C. A_2 with anti-A_1
D. A_2B with anti-A_1

102. All of the following antibodies are considered to be clinically significant *except*

   A. anti-Le^b
   B. anti-K
   C. anti-Jk^a
   D. anti-A

103. During interpretation of antibody cell panels, it is important to remember that M, N, and P$_1$ antibodies are most often identified:

   A. at room temperature, 18°C or 4°C
   B. by acidifying the patient's serum
   C. after the antiglobulin test
   D. after enzymatic treatment of red cells

104. Which of the following antibodies is enhanced by acidification of the patient's serum?

   A. Anti-Fy^a
   B. Anti-K
   C. Anti-M
   D. Anti-E

105. Given the following abbreviated cell panel, determine the most probable antibody(ies) in the patient's serum.

	C	D	E	c	e	K	M	N	S	37°C LISS	AHG	Check cells
1.	+	0	0	+	+	0	+	+	+	0	0	2+
2.	+	+	0	0	+	0	+	0	+	0	0	2+
3.	+	+	0	0	+	0	+	+	+	0	0	2+
4.	0	+	+	+	0	+	+	0	+	0	1+	NA
5.	0	0	+	+	+	0	+	+	0	0	0	2+
6.	0	0	0	+	+	+	+	+	0	0	1+	NA

   A. Anti-E
   B. Anti-c
   C. Anti-K
   D. Anti-E and anti-c

106. What reagent would be most useful in separating anti-C from anti-Fy^a?

   A. Ficin
   B. 2-Aminoethylisothiouronium (2-AET)
   C. 2-Mercaptoethanol (2-ME)
   D. Low-ionic-strength saline (LISS)

107. Given the following panel, what is the most likely specificity of the antibody(ies) in the serum tested?

	D	C	E	c	e	K	Fy^a	Fy^b	Jk^a	Jk^b	37°C LISS	AHG	Check cells
1.	+	+	+	0	+	0	+	+	0	+	0	4+	NP
2.	+	+	0	0	+	0	+	+	0	+	0	4+	NP
3.	+	0	+	+	0	0	+	0	0	+	0	4+	NP
4.	+	0	0	+	+	0	+	0	+	+	0	4+	NP
5.	0	+	0	+	+	0	+	0	+	+	0	2+	NP
6.	0	0	+	+	+	0	+	0	+	0	0	2+	NP
7.	0	0	0	+	+	+	0	+	+	+	0	0	2+
8.	0	0	0	+	+	0	+	0	0	+	0	2+	NP

A. Anti-Fy^b and anti-c
B. Anti-K
C. Anti-Fy^a
D. Anti-Fy^a and anti-D

108. A serum has been tentatively determined to contain anti-c and anti-K. A selected cell panel is composed as shown below. The serum is reacted with the selected cell panel producing the results shown.

	Antigens on cells		Serum reactions	
	K	c	AHG	Check cells
1.	+	0	2+	NP
2.	0	0	0	2+
3.	0	+	2+	NP
4.	+	0	2+	NP
5.	+	0	2+	NP
6.	0	0	0	2+
7.	0	+	2+	NP
8.	0	+	2+	NP
9.	0	0	0	2+

These results indicate that

A. there is a third alloantibody present in the serum
B. the serum contains anti-K but not anti-c
C. the serum contains only anti-K and anti-c
D. the serum does not contain anti-c but contains anti-K and another unidentified alloantibody

109. How long after transfusion must a sample from the donor unit be retained in the transfusion service?

A. 24 h
B. 48 h
C. 3 days
D. 7 days

110. A common cause of a positive autocontrol is

    A. ABO discrepancy
    B. Rh discrepancy
    C. *in-vivo* coating of cells with antibody
    D. unexpected serum alloantibody

111. An incompatibility in the immediate spin phase of pretransfusion-compatibility testing suggests a/an

    A. ABO mismatch
    B. anti-Fy^a
    C. positive donor antibody screen
    D. Rh antibody

112. A group O, Rh-positive patient experienced a delayed transfusion reaction. The postreaction specimen demonstrated anti-c. Select the most appropriate donor genotype for further red cell transfusions.

    A. R^{1}R^1
    B. r′r′
    C. R^{0}r
    D. rr

113. A group A, Rh-negative patient has a transfusion record identifying anti-Jk^a two years ago. Current antibody screens are negative. The best red cell phenotype for transfusion to this patient is

    A. group A, Rh-negative, Jk(a+)
    B. group A, Rh-positive, Jk(a−)
    C. group O, Rh-positive, Jk(a−)
    D. group O, Rh-negative, Jk(a−)

114. A 46-year-old male is expected to need 3–5 units of blood for surgery. He is group O, Rh-positive and has a negative antibody screen. His transfusion history reveals a delayed transfusion reaction 5 years ago. The antibody identified at that time was anti-e. Which of the following is an appropriate protocol for pretransfusion testing on this patient?

    A. Immediate spin-only crossmatch on random donors
    B. Immediate spin-only crossmatch on e-negative donors
    C. Crossmatch random donors through the antiglobulin phase
    D. Crossmatch e-negative donors through the antiglobulin phase

115. Below are the results of an antibody screen and crossmatches on the serum of a patient scheduled for surgery.

	IS	37°C LISS	AHG	Check cells
screen cell I	0	0	0	2+
screen cell II	0	0	0	2+
donor A	0	0	0	2+
donor B	0	0	0	2+
donor C	0	0	0	2+

These results should be interpreted as

A. negative antibody screen and compatible crossmatches
B. negative antibody screen and incompatible crossmatches
C. positive antibody screen and compatible crossmatches
D. positive antibody screen and incompatible crossmatches

116. When performing a direct antiglobulin test using polyspecific AHG, no agglutination is detected using IgG-coated red cells (check cells). This test should be considered

A. negative and reported
B. invalid; repeat using a monospecific reagent
C. positive and reported
D. invalid; repeat using a polyspecific reagent

117. In a Kleihauer-Betke test, the fetal cells

A. appear as "ghosts"
B. stain blue
C. stain light red
D. lyse and are not visible

118. Below are the ABO groups, Rh types, and gestational ages for four pregnant women. Which of them is eligible for antenatal Rh-immune globulin?

A. Group O, Rh-positive, 32 wk
B. Group A, Rh-negative, 25 wk
C. Group B, Rh-negative, 28 wk
D. Group AB, Rh-positive, 24 wk

119. Below are the results of pre- and posttransfusion testing on four patients suspected of having transfusion reactions.

	DAT		Serum hemolysis	
	pre	post	pre	post
Patient 1	0	0	0	1+
Patient 2	0	2+	0	0
Patient 3	0	0	0	0
Patient 4	0	0	1+	1+

Which demonstrate(s) evidence of a possible hemolytic reaction?

A. Patients 1 and 2
B. Patients 3 and 4
C. Patients 1 and 4
D. Patient 2 only

120. A group O, R^2R^2 woman delivers an infant with a positive DAT. The infant's father is group O (rr). Which of the following antibodies is most likely causing the infant's positive DAT?

A. Anti-A,B
B. Anti-D
C. Anti-c
D. Anti-e

121. Cryoprecipitated antihemophilic factor (AHF) being thawed for transfusion must be thawed at temperatures between

A. 1–6°C
B. 10–20°C
C. 20–24°C
D. 30–37°C

122. The minimum testing required for blood-group confirmation of an AB-positive plasma is

A. typing with anti-A, anti-B, and anti-A,B
B. typing with anti-A, anti-B, anti-A,B, and anti-D
C. testing against A and B cells
D. no testing required

123. A unit of packed red cells was returned to the transfusion service unused. Examine the data below to determine whether the unit can be reissued.

unit was not entered   —
time out of the laboratory: 14:53
time returned to the laboratory: 15:38
appearance of plasma: clear
segments attached: 3

A. The unit can be reissued
B. The unit cannot be reissued based on the amount of time out of the laboratory
C. The unit cannot be reissued based on the appearance of the plasma
D. The unit cannot be reissued based on the number of segments attached

124. Which of the following blood components returned within 30 min of issue can be returned to the transfusion service inventory and reissued to another patient?

A. A unit of fresh-frozen plasma (FFP) thawed two days ago
B. A unit of cryoprecipitated antihemophilic factor (AHF) with a spike in one port

C. A unit of RBCs returned with a temperature of 6°C
D. A unit of platelet concentrate that has been refrigerated

125. Gram-positive cocci in pairs and clusters are isolated from a superficial skin lesion. The isolate is beta-hemolytic on sheep-blood agar. Further testing reveals that the isolate is catalase-positive and coagulase-positive. The definitive identification of this organism is

A. *Staphylococcus aureus*
B. *Staphylococcus epidermidis*
C. *Streptococcus agalactiae*
D. *Streptococcus pyogenes*

126. A transtracheal aspirate yields a pure culture of an alpha-hemolytic gram-positive coccus that is catalase-negative. A test to perform in the subsequent identification process is

A. CAMP reaction
B. coagulase
C. susceptibility to bacitracin
D. susceptibility to ethylhydrocupreine hydrochloride (optochin)

127. A child presents with a typical paroxysmal "whoop"-type cough and lymphocytosis. The most appropriate primary culture medium to isolate the suspected etiologic agent is

A. charcoal yeast-extract agar
B. chocolate agar
C. Bordet-Gengou agar
D. Tinsdale agar

128. A gram-negative diplococci that is a normal inhabitant of the human nasopharynx, but is known to cause serious systemic illness in children and young adults is

A. *Haemophilus influenzae*
B. *Listeria monocytogenes*
C. *Neisseria meningitidis*
D. *Streptococcus pneumoniae*

129. Most members of the genus Pseudomonas are gram-negative rods that are

A. glucose-fermenters & motile
B. oxidase-positive & motile
C. oxidase-negative & nitrate-positive
D. glucose-fermenters & nitrate-negative

130. A microorganism resembling *Escherichia coli* is isolated from an infected traumatic wound. After additional tests the organism is identified as *Aeromonas hydrophila*. The single best test to differentiate *A. hydrophila* from *E. coli* is

A. Gram's stain
B. glucose fermentation
C. lactose fermentation
D. oxidase production

131. A STAT Gram's stain is requested on the purulent sputum specimen of a 55-year-old patient. Microscopic examination of the stained smear shows numerous polymorphonuclear cells with a purple cast. Also noted are many gram-positive cocci in pairs. The next step for the clinical laboratory technician is to

A. phone the report to the physician, indicating findings of 4+ GPCs in pairs
B. set up a sputum culture with "P" disk to confirm the presence of suspected *Streptococcus pneumoniae*
C. examine the smear more carefully to rule out other potential pathogens
D. repeat the Gram's stain with a thinner smear, taking care to decolorize adequately

132. Which of the following specimens should not be routinely processed for anaerobic evaluation?

A. blood
B. clean, voided urine
C. synovial fluid
D. transtracheal aspirate

133. Chocolate agar is usually used as primary plating medium for

A. spinal fluid
B. throat
C. stool
D. urine

134. Several vacationers at a Gulf Coast seaside resort complain of severe abdominal pain and diarrhea after ingesting raw oysters. The media that is most appropriate for screening these patients' stools is

A. bismuth sulfite
B. cellibiose arginine lysine
C. cycloserine cefoxitin fructose
D. thiosulfate citrate bile salts sucrose

135. The reagent(s) used to detect a positive indole reaction for the *Enterobacteriaceae* is(are)

A. alpha-naphthylamine and sulfanilic acid
B. alpha-naphthol and potassium hydroxide
C. paradimethylaminobenzaldehyde
D. tetramethylparaphenylenediamine dihydrochloride

136. Which pair of organisms provides an appropriate quality-control check for the biochemical reactions on eosin-methylene blue agar (EMB) and on Hektoen enteric (HE) agar?

 A. *Escherichia coli, Klebsiella pneuomniae*
 B. *Salmonella enteritidis, E. coli*
 C. *Shigella sonnei, E. coli*
 D. *Providencia rettgeri, K. pneumoniae*

137. A saprobic fungus whose micromorphology can be easily confused with that of the mycelial phase of *Histoplasma capsulatum* is

 A. *Fusarium*
 B. *Pseudoallescheria*
 C. *Chrysosporium*
 D. *Sepedonium*

138. A direct microscopic examination of an exudate from the lung reveals large spherules with endospores. The thick-walled spherules should alert the technologist to the possibility of

 A. Cryptococcosis
 B. Coccidioidomycosis
 C. Candidiasis
 D. Blastomycosis

139. A quality-control regimen is to be selected for the following tests:

 Phenylalanine deaminase (PAD)
 Indole production
 Voges-Proskauer (V-P)

 Which pair of stock culture organisms would you select as suitable to verify the performance of these three tests?

 A. *Klebsiella pneumoniae, Proteus vulgaris*
 B. *P. vulgaris, Escherichia coli*
 C. *E. coli, Enterobacter aerogenes*
 D. *E. aerogenes, K. pneumoniae*

140. Which of the following parasites are most likely to be overlooked on a wet preparation and detected on a permanent-stained slide?

 A. Protozoa
 B. Larvae
 C. Helminth eggs
 D. Proglottids

141. Several cysts and trophozoites are seen on trichrome stain-permanent mount and on iodine preparation from stool concentrate. Which of the following are characteristic of *Entamoeba histolytica?*

 A. Cysts with five to eight nuclei and chromatoid bodies with splintered ends

B. Trophozoites with one nucleus with an eccentric karyosome
C. Cysts with two to four nuclei characterized by small, round karyosomes
D. Granular vacuoles containing bacteria and debris

142. Which of the following organisms would most likely be seen in a urethral discharge?

A. *Balantidium coli*
B. *Enteromonas hominis*
C. *Giardia lamblia*
D. *Trichomonas vaginalis*

143. Which of the following situations would most likely produce falsely decreased zones of inhibition on a Kirby-Bauer disk-diffusion susceptibility test?

A. Use of an antimicrobial disk with a higher-than-recommended concentration of an antimicrobial
B. Use of an inoculum that is too light
C. Use of Müeller-Hinton agar thinner than 4 mm
D. Use of Müeller-Hinton agar thicker than 4mm

144. In a broth dilution test, the lowest concentration of an antibiotic that produces an irreversible killing of the organism is called the minimal

A. antibiotic concentration
B. bactericidal concentration
C. inhibitory concentration
D. susceptible concentration

145. The test that would most likely be ordered for a patient who develops diarrhea after being hospitalized for an upper urinary-tract infection for five days is

A. stool culture for enteric pathogens
B. stool for parasite exam
C. fecal fat (qualitative)
D. stool for *Clostridium difficile*

146. To help distinguish fungal elements in a direct wet preparation of a suspected ringworm infection, the recommended preparation is

A. india ink
B. Gram's stain
C. 10% potassium hydroxide
D. acid-fast stain

147. Germ-tube production within 3 h of incubation of the organism in bovine serum at 37°C is indicative of

A. *Cryptococcus neoformans*
B. *Candida albicans*

C. *Torulopsis glabrata*
D. *Trichosporon beigelii*

148. Rheumatic fever and glomerulonephritis are diseases commonly associated with which organism?

A. *Staphylococcus aureus*
B. *Streptococcus agalactiae*
C. *Enterococcus faecalis*
D. *Streptococcus pyogenes*

149. A 19-year-old college student was seen for the continuation of a purulent urethral discharge despite treatment for suspected gonorrhea. Symptoms resolved after a course of tetracycline. Etiology of his urethritis was most likely

A. *Chlamydia trachomatis*
B. Herpes simplex
C. *Neisseria* species
D. papillomavirus

150. The bacterial enzyme tryptophanase breaks down the amino acid tryptophan to produce

A. phenylpyruvic acid
B. indole
C. acetylmethylcarbinol
D. urea

151. The duodenal-aspirate and Enterotest-capsule techniques may be used to recover

A. *Ascaris lumbricoides*
B. *Iodamoeba bütschlii*
C. *Giardia lamblia*
D. *Entamoeba histolytica*

152. A direct antigen detection test is a presumptive means for identifying which organism in cerebrospinal fluid?

A. *Cryptococcus neoformans*
B. *Rhodotorula* species
C. *Candida albicans*
D. *Naegleria* species

153. In suspected cases of tularemia caused by *Francisella tularensis*, the preferred plating medium is

A. Thayer-Martin
B. Sabourand
C. Bordet-Gengou
D. cystine blood agar

154. A small, microaerophilic, curved, gram-negative rod was isolated from a diarrhea stool specimen. Further characterization revealed the organism to be oxidase positive, resistant to cephalosporin, susceptible to nalidixic acid, and hippurate-hydrolysis positive, and it grew at 42°C. Identification of this organism is

A. *Yersinia enterocolitica*
B. *Campylobacter jejuni*
C. *Bacillus cereus*
D. *Salmonella typhi*

155. *Helicobacter pylori* is associated most commonly with

A. traveler's disease
B. Crohn's disease
C. arthritis
D. gastric ulcer

156. Stool cultures from children with a day-care outbreak of diarrhea revealed an oxidase-negative, nonlactose fermenting, nonmotile, gram-negative rod. These characteristics presumptively indicate

A. *Salmonella* species
B. *Shigella* species
C. *E. coli* 0157:H7
D. *Campylobacter* species

157. The first screening test of choice for human immunodeficiency virus (HIV) antibodies is the

A. ELISA
B. fluorescent antibody
C. cell culture technique
D. RPR

158. A beta-hemolytic, gram-positive rod was isolated from the cerebrospinal fluid of a baby with signs of meningitis. The isolate, which grew on sheep-blood agar, demonstrated tumbling motility. The presumptive identity of the isolate is

A. group-B streptococcus
B. *Haemophilus influenzae*
C. *Streptococcus pneumoniae*
D. *Listeria monocytogenes*

159. A modified acid-fast smear of the diarrheic stool of a dairy farmer revealed red spherical structures averaging 6 μm in diameter. These findings are consistent with

A. giardiasis
B. cryptosporidiosis
C. pneumocytosis
D. ascariasis

160. The Epstein-Barr virus is associated with which of the following?

    A. Hepatitis
    B. Infectious mononucleosis
    C. *Exanthem subitum* (roseola)
    D. Chicken pox

161. An organism growing on Martin-Lewis media is proven to be a gram-negative diplococci, oxidase positive, with a carbohydrate utilization pattern as follows:

    Glucose: positive
    Maltose: negative
    Sucrose: negative
    Lactose: negative

    This isolate produces beta-lactamase by cefinase method. The clinical laboratory technician must do the following to complete this report:

    A. comply with the policies governing reporting of communicable diseases
    B. perform a complete susceptibility test before reporting
    C. repeat the carbohydrate testing to verify the identification
    D. perform additional testing to differentiate pathogen from non-pathogen

162. The biological-safety cabinet is used during the processing of specimens for virus cultures primarily to

    A. prevent having to use latex gloves in handling specimens
    B. protect technicians from potential aerosols
    C. protect the viral specimens from other types of bacterial or fungal agents
    D. prevent excessive decontamination of work-area surface

163. An IgG RID plate was set up on Friday afternoon and read on Monday morning. What type of graph paper should be used to construct the standard curve?

    A. Log-log
    B. Semi-log
    C. Logit
    D. Linear

164. A serum immunoelectrophoresis from a 71-year-old female shows a very faint IgG arc close to the serum well. The normal control arc is denser and midway between the well and the trench. This result suggests

    A. incomplete electrophoresis
    B. the normal control was applied to the well twice
    C. the patient has a monoclonal IgG
    D. the patient has decreased IgG levels

165. In immunoelectrophoresis, a monoclonal protein will usually produce an arc that is

    A. thick and close to the trough
    B. less dense and more diffuse than the control
    C. close to the well
    D. broad and elliptical in shape

166. A serum VDRL test was performed on a patient with a rash on his body and a recent painless mouth lesion. The test was performed as follows:

    0.5 mL of fresh patient serum was mixed with 1/60 mL of VDRL antigen prepared in VDRL-buffered saline in the ceramic ring of a slide. The slide was rotated for 4 min at 180 rpm. Microscopically, the test showed no clumping. Controls were acceptable.

    The CLT should

    A. report the result as nonreactive
    B. repeat the assay with freshly prepared VDRL antigen
    C. repeat the assay with heat-inactivated serum
    D. report the result as reactive

167. The laboratorian opening a new lot of RPR-antigen suspension notices that all of the bottles contain suspension that is white. The most likely explanation for this observation is

    A. charcoal was omitted from the suspension
    B. choline chloride was omitted from the suspension
    C. flocculation has occurred spontaneously
    D. the cardiolipin has agglutinated

168. The source of I antigen in the cold agglutination assay is

    A. adult group O cells
    B. cord group O cells
    C. horse red cells
    D. sheep red cells

169. In a latex-agglutination test for bacterial antibodies, serum from a 35-year-old cattle breeder yields a *Brucella* titer of 640 and a *Francisella* titer of 160. These results suggest

    A. cross-reaction of *Brucella* antibodies with *Francisella tularensis* antigen
    B. cross-reaction of *Francisella* antibodies with *Brucella* antigen
    C. the patient is infected with both *Brucella abortus* and *Francisella tularensis*
    D. the patient is suffering from a severe case of tularemia

170. When performing a cold-agglutination assay, the CLT noticed that the temperature of the refrigerator was 20°C following incubation. How will this affect the results of the assay?

A. The temperature is acceptable; the results will be unaffected
B. The results will not be affected if the assay is reincubated at −20°C
C. False-negative results will occur
D. False-positive results will occur

171. In the FTA-ABS, the organisms appeared to be staining with a smooth linear pattern of green fluorescence. This suggests

A. a biologic false-positive result
B. circulating immune complexes
C. specific antibody to *Treponema pallidum* is present
D. the presence of antibody that reacts with cardiolipin

172. In the indirect immunofluorescence assay to detect antibody to nuclear antigens, the nuclei in resting cells appeared to stain evenly and the chromosomes in dividing cells also stained evenly. The antibody present reacts with

A. ss-DNA
B. deoxyribonucleoproteins (DNP)
C. ribonucleoproteins (RNP)
D. extractable nuclear antigens

173. In the test for anti-DNase B, the patient's serum is diluted in buffer and incubated with DNase B at 37°C. If the patient has anti-DNase B, the antibody will

A. agglutinate the DNase B antigen
B. hemolyze the DNase B coated RBCs
C. neutralize the DNase B enzyme
D. compete with DNase B for antigen binding sites

174. A heterogeneous immunoassay to detect rubella antibody will

A. detect both IgG- and IgM-class antibody
B. require a step to separate free from bound label
C. require calibration with a World Health Organization standard
D. be an automated assay

175. In a noncompetitive enzyme immunoassay to detect ferritin, the absorbance of the negative control was greater than the absorbance of the positive control. What should be done?

A. This is expected; report the absorbance values
B. This is expected; calculate the concentration of the unknowns
C. This is unexpected; repeat the assay with new controls
D. This is unexpected; repeat the assay with new patient samples

176. In a radioimmunoassay to detect the beta subunit of human chorionic gonadotropin (hCG), the patient counts per minute (CPM) were greater than the CPM of the highest standard. The next step is to

A. concentrate the patient sample and reassay
B. dilute the patient sample and reassay
C. dilute the standards and reassay
D. extend the standard curve and read the extrapolated patient result in mIU/mL

177. An ASO neutralization test shows no hemolysis in any of the patient dilutions. The serum control, cell control, and streptolysin-O control show no hemolysis. The positive control shows no hemolysis at any dilution. These results suggest

A. the patient serum contains no antistreptolysin-O
B. the patient serum contains a titer of antistreptolysin-O equal to the control titer
C. oxidation of the streptolysin-O reagent
D. deterioration of the serum control sample

178. An antihyaluronidase test is performed on serum from a 14-year-old female. The results are as follows:

dilution	1:64	1:128	1:256	1:512	1:1,024
patient	clot	clot	clot	threads	no clot

The patient's titer is

A. 64
B. 256
C. 512
D. 1,024

179. The following results were obtained when a differential absorption to detect the antibody for infectious mononucleosis was performed:

Left side of slide: Patient's serum + guinea pig reagent + horse cells: Agglutination

Right side of slide: Patient's serum + beef erythrocytes + horse cells: No Agglutination

The best interpretation of these test results is

A. an invalid test result
B. a normal serum reaction
C. a positive test for serum sickness
D. a positive test for infectious mononucleosis

180. In the cold-agglutinin assay to detect postinfection antibody, the end point is

A. the last dilution of patient serum in which no agglutination is present
B. the last dilution of patient serum in which agglutination is present
C. the first dilution of patient serum in which there is agglutination
D. the first dilution of patient serum in which there is no agglutination

181. A fluorescence assay requires that the initial screening serum dilution be 1 : 40. Which preparation will produce that dilution?

A. 1 μL serum plus 3.9 mL diluent
B. 1 μL serum plus 39 μL diluent
C. 1 μL serum plus 40 μL diluent
D. 1 μL serum plus 3.9 μL diluent

182. Which dilution is considered a doubling dilution?

A. 0.5 mL of serum plus 0.5 mL of diluent
B. 2 mL of serum plus 1 mL of diluent
C. 1 mL of serum plus 2 mL of diluent
D. The desired volume must be known before this can be calculated

183. Which of the following formulas may be used to convert absorbance (Abs) to percent transmittance (%T)?

A. Abs = 1 + log %T
B. Abs = 2 − log %T
C. %T = log T + logA
D. Abs = 1 − log %T

184. The purpose of the didymium filter used with the broad-bandwidth spectrophotometer is to

A. align the galvanometer beam
B. produce monochromatic light
C. adjust the concentration range of the solution
D. check the wavelength calibration

185. Needles must be discarded

A. in an autoclavable bag
B. with the needle recapped
C. in a puncture-resistant container
D. after they are cut with a needle-cutting device

186. A microscope has the following marks on the objective lens: 10 × .25NA and a 10 × ocular. What is the total magnification?

A. 100×
B. 1,000×
C. 25×
D. 250×

187. The agency that issues a license to users of radionuclides and sets down rules for handling and disposal of radionuclides is the

A. NRC
B. OSHA

C. EPA
D. CLIA-88

188. You are a phlebotomist and must draw a blood sample from a trauma patient in the emergency room. The patient has an IV in his left wrist and a cast on his right arm. Which of the following sites should be used to obtain blood for a glucose analysis?

A. Vein in the left hand
B. Left median cubital vein
C. Right median cubital vein
D. Earlobe

189. The source of a class-C fire is

A. electric
B. organic solvents
C. paper or trash
D. combustible metals

190. Which of the following terms identifies the chemical reagent with the highest purity?

A. Analytic grade
B. Chemically pure
C. Technical
D. Commercial

191. The following data are obtained from a spectrophotometric analysis that follows Beer's law up to 300 mg/dL:

Absorbance of standard = 0.250
Absorbance of unknown = 0.100
Concentration of standard = 100 mg/dL
Dilution of unknown = 1 : 10

What is the concentration of the unknown?

A. 250 mg/dL
B. 400 mg/dL
C. 2,500 mg/dL
D. Cannot calculate because it exceeds the limits of Beer's law

192. Products that may be discharged into a sanitary sewer system and flushed with copious amounts of water include

A. any liquid infectious-waste product
B. any liquid infectious waste except when designated "From Isolation"
C. suctioned fluids, urine, and small amounts of unclotted blood
D. no infectious waste product should be discharged into a sanitary sewer system

193. You have been informed by central receiving that the stock of EDTA vacutainer tubes is depleted. The company cannot ship these tubes until next week. Which of the following, if any, would be an alternative choice for CBCs in the hematology laboratory?

   A. Sodium fluoride
   B. Iodoacetate
   C. Heparin
   D. There is no suitable substitute for EDTA vacutainers

194. Which of the following parameters *cannot* be predicted in method-evaluation studies?

   A. Reference range
   B. Sensitivity and specificity
   C. Random error
   D. Systematic error

195. A "discrete analyzer" that allows random access

   A. enables parallel analysis to be performed
   B. provides for a group or batch of samples to be run together
   C. allows the operator to select both method and order of test performance
   D. allows the operator to select the method to be performed on each sample sequentially

196. Calculate the concentration in milliequivalents per liter for a solution of 80 mg/dL NaOH. (Atomic weights: Na = 23; O = 16; H = 1)

   A. 2 mEq/L
   B. 8 mEq/L
   C. 20 mEq/L
   D. 40 mEq/L

197. A procedure calls for an incubation of 30°C. Your water bath has a thermometer that only reads in degrees Fahrenheit. What should the thermometer read when the water bath is at the correct temperature for this procedure?

   A. 22°F
   B. 36°F
   C. 62°F
   D. 86°F

198. When a blood sample is drawn by a syringe, the order for filling vacutainer tubes should be

   A. red, blue, purple
   B. blue, purple, red
   C. purple, blue, red
   D. red, purple, blue

199. The disinfectant of choice during a biological-spill cleanup is

    A. bleach (undiluted)
    B. bleach (1 : 10 dilution)
    C. sodium hydroxide (1 : 10 dilution)
    D. benzidine (1 : 10 dilution)

200. When there are five or more consecutive values distributed on one side of the mean, it is known as a

    A. shift
    B. normal occurrence
    C. trend
    D. reliable measurement

Key to the CLT Review Test

#	Ans	#	Ans	#	Ans	#	Ans
1.	D	36.	D	71.	B	106.	A
2.	D	37.	C	72.	B	107.	D
3.	B	38.	B	73.	A	108.	C
4.	A	39.	B	74.	C	109.	D
5.	B	40.	B	75.	D	110.	C
6.	B	41.	B	76.	C	111.	A
7.	A	42.	D	77.	C	112.	A
8.	D	43.	B	78.	D	113.	D
9.	B	44.	C	79.	D	114.	D
10.	A	45.	D	80.	B	115.	A
11.	B	46.	B	81.	D	116.	D
12.	B	47.	A	82.	C	117.	C
13.	A	48.	C	83.	D	118.	C
14.	A	49.	D	84.	B	119.	A
15.	B	50.	B	85.	B	120.	D
16.	A	51.	D	86.	D	121.	D
17.	A	52.	C	87.	C	122.	D
18.	C	53.	A	88.	C	123.	B
19.	A	54.	D	89.	B	124.	C
20.	D	55.	C	90.	A	125.	A
21.	D	56.	D	91.	C	126.	D
22.	C	57.	C	92.	C	127.	C
23.	B	58.	D	93.	A	128.	A
24.	B	59.	C	94.	D	129.	B
25.	D	60.	D	95.	D	130.	D
26.	B	61.	A	96.	B	131.	D
27.	A	62.	C	97.	C	132.	B
28.	A	63.	B	98.	B	133.	A
29.	A	64.	D	99.	D	134.	D
30.	B	65.	B	100.	A	135.	C
31.	D	66.	D	101.	C	136.	B
32.	B	67.	D	102.	A	137.	D
33.	C	68.	D	103.	A	138.	B
34.	C	69.	D	104.	C	139.	A
35.	A	70.	A	105.	C	140.	A

141.	C	156.	B	171.	C	186.	A
142.	D	157.	A	172.	B	187.	A
143.	D	158.	D	173.	C	188.	A
144.	B	159.	B	174.	B	189.	A
145.	D	160.	B	175.	C	190.	A
146.	C	161.	A	176.	B	191.	B
147.	B	162.	B	177.	C	192.	C
148.	D	163.	D	178.	B	193.	C
149.	A	164.	D	179.	D	194.	A
150.	B	165.	A	180.	B	195.	C
151.	C	166.	C	181.	B	196.	C
152.	A	167.	A	182.	A	197.	D
153.	D	168.	A	183.	B	198.	B
154.	B	169.	A	184.	D	199.	B
155.	D	170.	C	185.	C	200.	A

CLS Review Test

1. The following are fasting results from a 45-year-old male:

Glucose: 180 mg/dL   Cortisol: elevated
BUN: 8 mg/dL   Aldosterone: normal
Na^+:   135 mmol/L   ACTH: elevated
K^+:   3.0 mmol/L
Cl^-:   100 mmol/L
HCO_3^-:   24 mmol/L

The most likely cause for these results is

A. Cushing's syndrome
B. glucagon producing tumor
C. pituitary hypofunction
D. Type-II diabetes mellitus

2. A lipemic serum separates into a thick creamy layer above clear serum after overnight refrigeration. Analysis gives these results (reference value in parentheses):

Triglyceride: 200 mg/dL (40–160)
Cholesterol: 250 mg/dL (140–220)
HDL cholesterol: 20 mg/dL (30–70)
Lipoprotein electrophoresis shows markedly elevated chylomicrons

Which of the following is an appropriate interpretation?

A. The cholesterol result should be much higher
B. The HDL cholesterol result should be much higher
C. The triglyceride result should be much higher
D. The lipoprotein electrophoresis should show more abnormalities

3. Serum chemistry results on a 53-year-old female are AST, 120 U/L (5–34); ALT, 185 U/L (<55); ALP, 785 U/L (<165); GGT, 225 U/L

(5–24), total bilirubin, 10.8 mg/dL; direct bilirubin, 8.6 mg/dL; urine bilirubin, positive; urine urobilinogen, decreased. These results are consistent with a diagnosis of

A. hemolytic anemia
B. hepatitis
C. Dubin-Johnson syndrome
D. biliary obstruction

4. The two most significant sources of error in accurate ammonia determinations are sample handling and

A. ammonia contamination in the laboratory
B. short shelf life of the test reagents
C. inability to automate the test procedure
D. need for age-dependent reference ranges

5. Methods for determining creatinine levels have been developed based on each of the following reactions *except*

A. enzymatic conversion to creatine coupled with a reaction catalyzed by creatine kinase to measure the creatine
B. conversion to urea by urease, then measurement of the urea
C. enzymatic production of ammonia from creatinine followed by quantitation of ammonia
D. reaction with alkaline picrate, then measurement of the orange chromogen formed

6. Prolonged vomiting, mineralocorticoid excess, diabetic ketoacidosis, or chronic gastric suction can each lead to a patient developing

A. hyperkalemia
B. hypochloremia
C. hypoxia
D. metabolic acidosis

7. Semen zinc levels can be used to evaluate prostate function. The method of choice for clinical analysis of semen zinc is

A. spectrophotometry
B. fluorescence polarization
C. gas chromatography
D. atomic absorption

8. A blood ethanol level of 100 mg/dL indicates

A. the detection threshold for assay by gas chromatography
B. a probable false value if serum ketones are present
C. probable impairment of cognitive or motor skills
D. a lethal concentration in most adults

9. Which of these patterns of results is consistent with primary hyperparathyroidism?

	Serum Ca	Serum P	Urine Ca	Urine P
A.	↑	↑	↑	↓
B.	↑	↓	↑	↑
C.	↓	↑	↓	↑
D.	↓	↓	↓	↓

10. A serum-protein electrophoresis is performed. The clinical laboratory scientist suspects that the sample used is *not* serum but plasma because of a characteristic peak in the

A. alpha$_1$ region
B. alpha$_2$ region
C. beta region
D. gamma region

11. Electrophoretic separation of proteins in concentrated spinal fluid is often requested for the diagnosis of

A. bacterial meningitis
B. multiple myeloma
C. multiple sclerosis
D. intracerebral hemorrhage

12. National published guidelines for laboratory assessment of increased risk of coronary artery disease indicate borderline HDL-Cholesterol levels fall between

A. 35–54 mg/dL
B. 130–159 mg/dL
C. 200–249 mg/dL
D. 250–500 mg/dL

13. If the amount of labeled ligand added to a competitive protein-binding assay is accidentally twice as much as the method calls for, the amount of

A. bound labeled ligand will decrease
B. bound labeled ligand will increase
C. free patient ligand will decrease
D. free and bound labeled ligand will not be altered

14. A moderately hemolyzed serum sample will result in falsely elevated results for each of the following analytes *except*

A. potassium
B. AST, LD, CK
C. bilirubin
D. phosphorus

15. Which of these isotopes can be measured in a gamma scintillation counter?

A. ^{14}C
B. ^{3}H

C. ^{125}I

D. ^{16}O

16. Each of the following methods is used for performing wavelength calibration on a spectrophotometer *except*

A. using pure solutions with characteristic absorption peaks
B. adding lanthanum to the measured solution
C. a holmium-oxide filter
D. a didymium filter

17. A solution whose concentration is said to have one equivalent weight of an element in one liter of solution will be a

A. 1-normal solution
B. 1-molar solution
C. 1-molal solution
D. 1% solution

18. Given the following fluorometric readings, calculate the value of the unknown:

	Reading
Standard	45
Standard blank	5
Unknown	50
Unknown blank	10

Concentration of the standard = 10.0 mg/dL

A. 9.0 mg/dL
B. 10.0 mg/dL
C. 11.1 mg/dL
D. 12.5 mg/dL

19. What weight of sodium chloride (MW = 58.5) is needed to prepare 500 mL of a 20% w/v solution?

A. 15 mg
B. 20 mg
C. 10 g
D. 20 g

20. One unit (U) of enzyme activity is defined at a specific temperature and pH as the amount of enzyme that catalyzes the reaction of

A. one mole of substrate per sec
B. one millimole of substrate per sec
C. one millimole of substrate per min
D. one micromole of substrate per min

21. Calculate using Beer's Law (A = abc) the concentration of analyte X in the patient sample described on next page:

Absorptivity coefficient of analyte X: $0.20 \text{ L} \times \text{mmol}^{-1} \times \text{cm}^{-1}$
Spectrophotometer path length: 1.0 cm
Absorbance reading of patient sample: 1.000

A. 0.005 mol/L
B. 0.50 mmol/L
C. 2.0 mol/L
D. 5.0 mol/L

22. Analytical methods are evaluated by determining and monitoring the amount of random and systematic error present. Which of the following is a characteristic of random error?

A. It is an indicator of a method's accuracy
B. It is an indicator of a method's precision
C. It occurs in one direction, i.e., either high or low but not both
D. It often occurs gradually and is noticed over time

23. The temperature control for a blood-gas instrument is malfunctioning and is currently at 39°C. Blood-gas determinations using this instrument would give falsely

A. decreased pH, increased pO_2, and increased pCO_2 results
B. decreased pH, decreased pO_2, and increased pCO_2 results
C. increased pH, increased pO_2, and decreased pCO_2 results
D. increased pH, decreased pO_2, and decreased pCO_2 results

24. A patient has consumed a mixture of barbiturates. Which of the following assay techniques is *best* able to identify the specific barbiturates ingested?

A. Gas chromatography (GC)
B. Radial immunodiffusion (RID)
C. Enzyme-multiplied immunoassay technique (EMIT)
D. Flourescence-polarization immunoassay (FPIA)

25. Chloride quantitation can be performed by the coulometric titration or by potentiometric methods. If a bromide-containing medication is being taken by a patient, the serum-chloride values obtained on this patient's specimen will be

A. accurate by either method
B. falsely increased by both methods
C. falsely increased by the coulometric-titration method
D. falsely increased by the potentiometric method

26. A slightly hemolyzed plasma sample was analyzed on an ISE, and electrolyte results were as follows:

$Na^+ = 140$ mmol/L
$K^+ = 14.0$ mmol/L
$Cl^- = 112$ mmol/L
$HCO_3^- = 18$ mmol/L

What should be done next?

A. Report the critically high potassium result to the physician immediately
B. Check the linearity range to determine if the sample must be diluted and rerun for the potassium result
C. The sample was too hemolyzed to use; request a new sample
D. Check the sample tube to see if improper anticoagulant was used for collection (improper tube drawn)

27. The following results were obtained from a heparinized blood-gas sample (the patient was breathing room air):

pH = 7.50
pCO_2 = 20 mm Hg
pO_2 = 138 mm Hg
HCO_3^- = 15 mmol/L
Na^+ = 138 mmol/L
K^+ = 3.9 mmol/L
Cl^- = 107 mmol/L
TCO_2 = 24 mmol/L

The most likely cause for these results is the

A. sample was not delivered on ice promptly to the lab
B. sample contained air bubbles
C. patient is in a state of partly compensated metabolic alkalosis
D. patient is in a state of partly compensated respiratory alkalosis

28. A bubble of room air is trapped in the pO_2 and pCO_2 measuring chambers of a blood-gas instrument. A sample assayed while these bubbles are present can produce falsely

A. decreased pO_2 and decreased pCO_2 results
B. decreased pO_2 and increased pCO_2 results
C. increased pO_2 and decreased pCO_2 results
D. increased pO_2 and increased pCO_2 results

29. A 19-year-old male is to have a 3-h glucose-tolerance test performed. He enters the outpatient clinic and tells the CLS he has eaten whatever he wanted the last few days—"mostly fast foods"—and has not eaten anything since dinner last night "except for a granola bar a half-hour ago." What should be done next?

A. Draw a fasting blood-glucose sample; if the result is less than 140 mg/dL, perform the OGTT
B. Wait 2 h and draw a blood sample for a 2-h postprandial baseline result; then begin the OGTT if the 2-h postprandial result is <200 mg/dL
C. Send the patient home and call his physician to explain the dietary noncompliance
D. Send the patient home after explaining the need to be nonfasting and reschedule the test for the next day

30. You are given the following data:

Total cholesterol: 200 mg/dL
High-density lipoprotein cholesterol (HDL-C): 20 mg/dL
Triglyceride: 150 mg/dL

Calculate the low-density lipoprotein cholesterol (LDL-C).

A. 150 mg/dL
B. 30 mg/dL
C. 45 mg/dL
D. 180 mg/dL

31. Which of the following enzyme determinations may be helpful in establishing the presence of seminal fluid?

A. Lactate dehydrogenase (LD)
B. Isocitrate dehydrogenase (ICD)
C. Acid phosphatase (ACP)
D. Alkaline phosphatase (ALP)

32. A dexamethasone-suppression test was performed on an individual later determined to have minimal endocrine function. In this patient, which of the following hormones would be decreased after injection of dexamethasone?

A. CRF
B. ACTH
C. Estrogen
D. TSH

33. A patient was admitted to the emergency room complaining of chest pain. The physician ordered a cardiac panel of tests to rule out a heart attack. The results of the tests indicated a healthy heart except for a very slight elevation in CK-MB. The patient was admitted and after two days of evaluation, his physician concluded that no heart attack had occurred. In this case, how would the initial CK-MB elevation be viewed as an indicator of myocardial infarction?

A. True positive
B. False positive
C. True negative
D. False negative

34. A 30-year-old female is being evaluated for amenorrhea. A pregnancy test is negative, and her serum prolactin is normal. Additional laboratory results include

Serum estradiol: low
Serum LH: elevated
Serum FSH: elevated

Which of the following conditions are consistent with this patient's laboratory results?

A. Dwarfism
B. Primary ovarian failure
C. Secondary ovarian failure
D. Addison's disease

35. A 46-year-old female complained of fatigue, cold intolerance, and dry skin. A weight gain of eight pounds without decreasing her activity or increasing her food intake was also mentioned. Thyroid function tests were ordered. The results of these tests were as follows:

Total T_4:   decreased
TSH: decreased
Free T_4 index: decreased
THBR: decreased

TSH was administered and a specimen was later drawn for determination of total T_4. The total T_4 level of the postinjection specimen was increased over the previous levels. Based on these results, which of the following glands would be ruled out as the cause of the hypothyroidism?

A. Thyroid gland
B. Pituitary gland
C. Hypothalamus
D. Ovary

36. A 65-year-old woman experienced sharp chest pain, pain radiating down the left arm, and nausea. Thinking the pain was due to indigestion, she did not seek immediate medical attention. Four days later, she decided to visit her doctor. A cardiac-enzyme profile was ordered. What would you expect her serum-enzyme profile to look like at this time?

A. Elevated CK-MB
B. Elevated total LD
C. Elevated total CK
D. Elevated LD-5

37. The protein concentration of a cerebrospinal fluid (CSF) specimen was found to exceed the linearity of level of the procedure. A dilution was made by adding 0.5 mL of CSF to 1.0 mL of saline. The dilution was analyzed and determined to be 24 mg/dL. What was the protein concentration of the CSF?

A. 48 mg/dL
B. 72 mg/dL
C. 96 mg/dL
D. 120 mg/dL

38. Four laboratories performed replicate analyses on the same lot number of control serum. Based on the results shown, which laboratory appears to have the best accuracy?

	Lab A	Lab B	Lab C	Lab D
SD	0.18	0.23	0.14	0.27
CV%	3.1	4.3	2.8	4.4
BIAS	+1.0	+0.2	+3.0	−1.1

A. Lab A
B. Lab B
C. Lab C
D. Lab D

39. The following urine values are obtained:

urine specific gravity = 1.004
urine osmolality = 180 mOsm/kg
24-h urine volume = 3 L

These data suggest the condition of

A. dysuria
B. isothenuria
C. oliguria
D. polyuria

40. Oval fat bodies, fatty casts, and free-floating fat droplets can be found
in the urine sediment during

A. nephrotic syndrome
B. acute tubular necrosis
C. acute interstitial nephritis
D. acute glomerulonephritis

41. The urine collection best suited for a reagent-strip nitrite test is a

A. random collection
B. 24-h timed collection
C. first morning collection
D. 2-h postprandial collection

42. Hyperfunctioning of the adrenal gland can lead to increased renal tubular
reabsorption of sodium and potassium excretion due to

A. decreased renin secretion
B. increased aldosterone secretion
C. decreased angiotensin secretion
D. increased antidiuretic hormone (ADH) secretion

43. A patient's urine specimen is known to be contaminated with radiographic contrast media. Which of the following specific-gravity methods
is able to assess this patient's renal concentrating ability using this
specimen?

A. urinometer
B. refractometer
C. reagent strip
D. densitometry

44. While using a negative control sample and multiconstituent reagent strips, all test pads produce negative results except for protein. A trace protein result is obtained. Selection the action that should be taken:

    A. Document and resolve the protein result before testing patient samples
    B. Resolve the protein result, then document only the acceptable result obtained before testing patient samples
    C. Document the results, but because the color-block change is difficult to read, a slightly positive protein result is acceptable for a negative control
    D. This is acceptable performance because the reaction is within ±1 color block of its expected value

45. The following routine urinalysis results are obtained:

    pH: 5.0   glucose: neg
    blood: small   ketone: neg
    protein: 300 mg/dL   nitrite: neg

    Significant microscopic findings include RBCs—2–5/HPF, dysmorphic; casts—hemoglobin, granular. These findings are most consistent with a diagnosis of

    A. acute cystitis
    B. nephrotic syndrome
    C. acute pyelonephritis
    D. acute glomerulonephritis

46. Select the microscopic technique that best differentiates hyaline casts from mucus threads.

    A. brightfield microscopy
    B. polarizing microscopy
    C. phase-contrast microscopy
    D. fluorescence microscopy

47. Select the statement that best explains the following results:

    Leukocyte esterase test: negative
    Microscopic exam: 5–10 WBCs/HPF

    A. The WBCs present are lymphocytes
    B. The amount of leukocyte esterase present is below the test's specificity
    C. The cells are squamous epithelial cells that were misidentified as WBCs
    D. Ascorbic acid is interfering, causing the leukocyte esterase to be falsely negative

48. A urine specimen is delivered to the lab for routine analysis. The collection time is not noted on the label. The following results were obtained:

Color: yellow-brown
Turbidity: slightly cloudy
Specific gravity: 1.029
pH: 6.5
glucose: negative
ketones: negative
protein: negative
hemoglobin: negative
bilirubin: negative
urobilinogen: negative
leukocyte esterase: negative
nitrite: negative
Ictotest: negative

The results are reported to the physician, who questions the results since the patient appears jaundiced and the urine is yellow-brown. A likely explanation is the

A. specimen was labeled with the wrong patient's name
B. specimen is not fresh and the bilirubin and urobilinogen have degraded, giving false-negative results
C. urinalysis was not carefully performed
D. Ictotest was outdated

49. A heparinized specimen is received in the hematology laboratory. Which procedure would be acceptable on this specimen?

A. Peripheral blood smear
B. WBC count
C. Osmotic fragility
D. Platelet count

50. An EDTA specimen received in the laboratory is noted to contain a very small clot. For what procedure(s) is this specimen acceptable?

A. Platelet count only
B. ESR only
C. No procedures will be accurate
D. Hemoglobin and hematocrit if they are performed by manual methods

51. A clinical laboratory scientist makes peripheral blood smears that are consistently too short and too thick. Which of the following actions should be taken to improve the quality of the smears?

A. Lower the angle of the spreader slide
B. Increase the angle of the spreader slide
C. Maintain the same angle on the spreader slide and increase the size of the drop
D. Maintain the same angle and increase the pressure on the spreader slide

52. All of the peripheral blood smears stained with a Romanowsky stain have bluish erythrocytes, and the nuclei of the leukocytes appear deep purple. What is the probable cause?

    A. Excess buffer for stain solution
    B. Smears are too thin
    C. Buffer is too alkaline
    D. Insufficient staining time

53. An average of 7 platelets per oil-immersion field are seen on a peripheral blood smear prepared by the wedge method. What is the approximate platelet count/mm³?

    A. 11,000–14,000
    B. 50,000–70,000
    C. 105,000–140,000
    D. 500,000–700,000

54. A hemoglobin value of 10.3 g/dL would correlate with a microhematocrit of

    A. 0.31 L/L
    B. 0.34 L/L
    C. 0.36 L/L
    D. 0.39 L/L

55. A hemoglobin and hematocrit are ordered on an EDTA specimen with lipemic plasma. In performing the manual cyanmethemoglobin procedure using spectrophotometry, the clinical laboratory scientist should

    A. centrifuge the hemoglobin dilution and read the supernatant
    B. dilute the sample 1 : 2 with distilled water; read and multiply results by 2
    C. add 0.01 mL of patient plasma to 5 mL of cyanmethemoglobin reagent and use this as the test blank
    D. add 0.02 mL of patient plasma to 10 mL of cyanmethemoglobin reagent; read and multiply result by 2

56. The following results are obtained on an EDTA blood specimen:

    RBC = 2.50×10^{12}/L
    Hb = 10.0 g/dL
    Hct = 0.30 L/L

    RBC indices calculated from these values best correlate with which of the following morphologies on the peripheral blood smear?

    A. Microcytic, hypochromic
    B. Microcytic, normochromic
    C. Normocytic, normochromic
    D. Macrocytic, normochromic

57. To obtain accurate results on a Westergren ESR, blood kept at room temperature should be set up within a maximum of how many hours?

A. 1
B. 2
C. 4
D. 8

58. A reticulocyte count is performed on an EDTA sample from a 45-year-old male with an RBC count of 3.80×10^{12}/L, Hb of 11.5 g/dL, and Hct of 0.35 L/L. The reticulocyte count is 0.9%. The corrected reticulocyte count (corrected for anemia) is

A. 0.4%
B. 0.6%
C. 0.7%
D. 0.8%

59. A patient is admitted to the emergency room with extensive burns. Expected erythrocyte morphologic features would include

A. microspherocytes
B. hypochromia
C. codocytes
D. drepanocytes

60. A patient has a WBC count of 60.0×10^9/L. On the 100-cell differential, 5% of the cells have dark blue cytoplasm with red granules that cover the nucleus. The nucleus has a fine chromatin pattern and is slightly off center. Several of these cells have nucleoli. These cells are most likely

A. myeloblasts
B. promyelocytes
C. myelocytes
D. atypical lymphocytes

61. Laboratory tests on a 4-year-old boy yielded the following results:

Hb:	11.0 g/dL	WBC:	7.6×10^9/L
Hct:	0.37 L/L	polys:	57%
RBC:	5.21×10^{12}/L	bands:	2%
RDW:	13.5%	lymphs:	38%
		monos:	3%

Codocytes and occasional basophilic stippling were seen on the peripheral blood smear. Based on these initial findings, which procedure would be indicated next?

A. Test for infectious mononucleosis
B. Serum lead and free-erythrocyte protoporphyrin
C. Hemoglobin electrophoresis and Hb A_2 quantitation
D. Serum B_{12} and folate levels

62. A patient has a WBC count of $20.0 \times 10^9/L$. There are 45 nucleated RBCs per 100 WBCs. The corrected WBC is

A. $7.3 \times 10^9/L$
B. $13.8 \times 10^9/L$
C. $19.9 \times 10^9/L$
D. $20.0 \times 10^9/L$

63. A screening solubility test for sickling hemoglobins is ordered on a patient with a hemoglobin of 5.0 g/dL. Which of the following will provide the most accurate results?

A. Add 0.02 mL of blood to 2.0 mL of dithionite reagent
B. Decrease sample volume to 0.01 mL
C. Add 0.02 mL of blood and increase reagent volume to 4.0 mL
D. Increase sample volume to 0.04 mL

64. The following results were obtained on an osmotic fragility test:

NaCl (% solution)	Patient (% hemolysis)	Control (% hemolysis)
0.00	100	100
0.10	100	100
0.20	100	100
0.30	100	97
0.35	100	89
0.40	100	60
0.45	100	10
0.50	97	0
0.55	96	0
0.60	92	0
0.65	75	0
0.70	35	0
0.85	0	0

These results indicate

A. increased fragility of the patient's erythrocytes
B. normal results for patient and control
C. decreased fragility of the patient's erythrocytes
D. invalid results due to inaccurate control results

65. RBCs seen on a peripheral blood smear stained with Wright's stain contain inclusion bodies that are thought to be iron. Which confirmatory stain should be done?

A. New methylene blue
B. Feulgen
C. Prussian blue
D. Crystal violet

66. The following results were obtained on a well-controlled leukocyte alkaline phosphatase stain:

Score	No. of cells
0	3
1	20
2	41
3	24
4	12

These results indicate

A. chronic myelogenous leukemia
B. acute lymphocytic leukemia
C. paroxysmal nocturnal hemoglobinuria
D. leukemoid reaction

67. A cerebrospinal fluid is diluted 1 : 10. A *total* of 160 WBCs is counted using the 4 corner squares on *both* sides of the hemocytometer. What is the WBC/mm^3?

A. 200
B. 400
C. 2,000
D. 4,000

68. On a cytospin preparation from a pleural fluid, 50% of the cells have the following characteristics:

uniform, regular arrangement
some cells resemble a "fried egg"
may be multiple nuclei
smooth nuclear outline and homogeneous chromatin
when present in clumps, there are clear spaces between the cells ("windows")

How would these cells be classified?

A. Atypical (reactive) lymphocytes
B. Mesothelial cells
C. Tumor cells
D. Ependymal cells

69. Which of the following is an acceptable preservative for bone-marrow biopsy specimens?

A. EDTA
B. Sodium citrate
C. Zenker's solution
D. Xylene

70. Examination of a Wright's-stained bone-marrow smear reveals many large cells (20–80 μm) with globular cytoplasmic inclusions. The cytoplasm has fine marks in it that resemble chicken scratches or crumpled tissue paper. Cytochemical analysis of the cell contents confirms the presence of glucocerebroside. The cells are suggestive of

A. multiple myeloma
B. Gaucher's disease
C. Niemann-Pick disease
D. Chediak-Higashi syndrome

71. A 70-year-old male with a diagnosis of pneumonia has the following results on an electronic cell counter which uses the principle of electronic impedance:

WBC: 15.0×10^9/L
RBC: 3.24×10^{12}/L
Hb: 14.8 g/dL
Hct: 0.39 L/L

What action should be taken by the clinical laboratory scientist?

A. Report results as obtained as quickly as possible
B. Perform a manual hemoglobin using a plasma blank
C. Perform a manual hemoglobin; spin down before reading % transmittance
D. Warm the specimen and rerun it

72. The following results are obtained on controls on an electronic cell counter:

Assay value (published)
Normal WBC $8.2 \pm 0.6 \times 10^9$/L
Abnormal WBC $15.5 \pm 0.9 \times 10^9$/L
Normal RBC $4.58 \pm 0.09 \times 10^{12}$/L
Abnormal RBC $1.54 \pm 0.12 \times 10^{12}$/L

When plotted on a Levy-Jennings quality control chart ($\pm$2SD), values for the last 8 shifts are represented below:

Laboratory Values

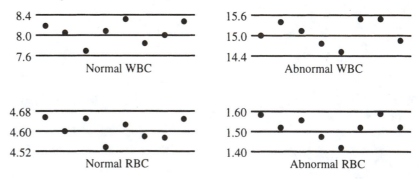

These data indicate that the

A. instrument is in control
B. diluent has become contaminated
C. controls have deteriorated
D. lysing agent has expired

73. A nontraumatic venipuncture using a vacuum system was performed on a patient who had been stabilized on coumadin. A blue-top tube (citrate) was collected first followed by a lavender top (EDTA) tube for a CBC. The citrate tube was centrifuged for 1,000 g. The prothrombin time performed 30 min after collection of the blood was significantly shorter than the previous month, lowering the patient's INR value below the therapeutic range. Both controls were within acceptable limits. The CBC was normal. From the above information, what could have caused the PT to be shortened erroneously?

A. The ratio of blood-to-anticoagulant was incorrect
B. Collection of the blue-top tube first introduced tissue thromboplastin
C. A lupus inhibitor may be present
D. Too much time elapsed between collection and testing

74. Blood collected for a test for serum fibrin(ogen)-degradation products (FDP) was collected in a red-top tube instead of the tubes provided with the FDP kit. What effect will this have on the outcome of the test?

A. No difference; serum FDP can also be measured from a red-top tube
B. Decreased value due to lack of fibrinogen in serum
C. Increased value due to additional fibrin lysis occurring after specimen collection
D. Decreased value due to residual fibrinogen present in patients with incomplete clotting

75. In addition to calcium ions, what major substance is necessary in the prothrombin time reagent?

A. Tissue thromboplastin
B. Reptilase venom
C. Platelet phospholipid substitute
D. Negatively charged particles

76. Which of the following tests may be used to confirm a positive screening test for a lupus anticoagulant (antiphospholipid antibody)?

A. activated partial thromboplastin time
B. platelet neutralization test
C. prothrombin time
D. protamine sulfate test

77. Which test system is used to evaluate the adequacy of fibrinogen in heparinized patients?

A. Stypven time
B. Reptilase time
C. Thrombin time
D. Functional fibrinogen

78. In establishing the normal range for prothrombin time, a laboratory analyzed samples from ten healthy donors (five women and five men).

One donor was analyzed each day. All specimens were handled in the same manner and analyzed with the same lot number of reagent. One donor fell three standard deviations from the mean and was eliminated. What in this laboratory's protocol might bias the results of the normal range?

A. Both healthy and ill donors should have been assayed to get a more accurate result
B. The donor that was an outlier should not have been eliminated from the data
C. The sample size was too small
D. All of the specimens should have been analyzed on the same day

79. The results of a patient's prothrombin time is 12 sec (mean normal, 11.9 sec). The activated partial thromboplastin time is 65 sec. The APTT showed no correction on a 1 : 1 mix with fresh normal plasma. What condition can cause these results?

A. Factor-VIII deficiency
B. Factor-IX deficiency
C. Lupus inhibitor
D. Heparin therapy

80. Coagulation and liver-enzyme testing were ordered on a jaundiced patient diagnosed with hepatitis B. Using appropriate precautions and a vacuum-collection system, the phlebotomist collected a red-top tube followed by a blue-top tube. The tests were performed on a photooptical instrument. The PT was 9.8 sec (normal range, 10.8–12.2 sec), and the APTT was 19.8 sec (normal range, 24–30 sec). Normal and abnormal controls were within acceptable limits. What caused the subnormal results for the patient PT and APTT?

A. Tissue juices transferred from the red-top tube speeded up the clot formation
B. Bilirubin in the plasma triggered the optical system too early
C. Turbulence in the vacuum collection created hemolysis that enhanced clotting
D. Hepatitis-B antigen acts as a negative surface for activation of factors VII and XII

81. A delta check on an 8-year-old male who was on no medications revealed that the prothrombin time had changed from 12 sec preoperatively to 16 sec one day following appendectomy. Which is the most appropriate action for the laboratory?

A. Notify the attending physician of the 25% increase immediately
B. Repeat the prothrombin time, and if it is the same, notify the physician
C. Repeat the controls only, and if they are in range, report the PT
D. Make new PT reagent and repeat all PTs for the day

82. A 6-year-old male presents with a history of bruising and frequent episodes of mild bleeding. The results of lab tests are

platelet count: $260 \times 10^9/L$ $(150\text{--}450 \times 10^9/L)$
template bleeding time: 18 min (2–9 min)
PT: 11.8 sec (11.0–12.0 sec)
APTT: 28 sec (24–30 sec)

What further testing is indicated?

A. Platelet-aggregation studies
B. Factor-IX assay
C. Factor-VIII assay
D. Thrombin time

83. A patient has a history of repeated spontaneous abortion. Coagulation studies reveal an elevated APTT, normal PT, normal platelet function, and normal clotting time. Shistocytes were seen on the peripheral blood smear. Which test should be performed to determine if the prolonged APTT is due to a lupus inhibitor?

A. Mixing studies with normal plasma
B. Mixing studies with factor-deficient plasma
C. Antinuclear-antibody test
D. Platelet-neutralization test

84. A patient presents with the following laboratory results:

PT: 12.5 sec (N = 12–14)
APTT: 80 sec (N = 25–35)
platelet count: $180 \times 10^9/L$ (N = $150\text{--}450 \times 10^9/L$)

The APTT is corrected by normal plasma, factor-IX deficient plasma, but not by factor-VIII deficient plasma. What factor assay should be performed?

A. None; a platelet disorder is indicated
B. Factor V
C. Factor VIII
D. Factor IX

85. What is used to set the 100% baseline reading on a platelet-aggregation instrument?

A. The patient's platelet-rich plasma
B. The aggregation reagent
C. Saline
D. The patient's platelet-poor plasma

86. To prevent shortened times when using an electrofibrometer, what should routinely be done between tests?

A. Clean the electrodes with 1% phosphoric acid and distilled water
B. Reset the cam that turns the moving electrode
C. Rinse the fibrocup with distilled water before using again
D. Realign the electrodes to be horizontal to each other

87. Which of the following does *not* affect platelet storage?

    A. Type of plastic bag
    B. Storage temperature
    C. Irradiation
    D. Agitation method

88. Exceptions to regular blood-donation requirements can be made for

    A. paid donors
    B. pregnant women
    C. healthy athletes
    D. autologous donations

89. A female donor weighing 98 lbs. (44.5 kg) comes into the donor center to make a directed donation for a family member. Determine the amount of blood that can be drawn from this donor.

    A. 400 mL
    B. 405 mL
    C. 450 mL
    D. 495 mL

90. One unit in a run has an HIV 1/2 screening test result just above the cutoff. The next step should be to

    A. repeat the test in duplicate
    B. order a Western blot test
    C. inform the donor of the positive test and ask additional history questions
    D. add the donor to the permanent deferral list

91. Which of the following donors would be investigated as a "look back" case?

    A. A donor newly diagnosed with HIV who previously tested negative
    B. A donor with a repeatedly positive test for HIV 1/2
    C. A donor with an indeterminate Western blot confirmatory test for HIV
    D. A donor with a screening test for HIV 1/2 with a value twice the cutoff value

92. Twenty mL of a 5% RBC suspension are needed for a test procedure. What is the total packed red cell volume required to prepare the volume of cells needed?

    A. 0.1 mL
    B. 1.0 mL
    C. 0.5 mL
    D. 1.5 mL

93. After performing an antibody-identification panel, the presence of anti-Sd^a and possibly another alloantibody were suspected. To perform further testing and identify the second antibody, the CLS decided to eliminate the possible interference of the anti-Sd^a by

A. destroying the Sd^a antigens on the panel cells with ficin
B. absorbing the anti-Sd^a with hydatid-cyst fluid
C. neutralizing the anti-Sd^a with Sd(a+) urine
D. performing an autoabsorption

94. As part of a new reagent evaluation, the CLS performed a titration. The results are recorded below. The titer is recorded as the reciprocal of the dilution. The strength represents the strength of the agglutination reaction observed. The score is the value assigned to the agglutination strength. What titer and total score should the CLS record for this reagent?

Titer	1	2	4	8	16	32	64	128	256	512
Strength	4+	4+	3+	3+	3+	2+	1+	0	0	0
Score	12	12	10	10	10	8	5	0	0	0

A. Titer 64; score 64
B. Titer 128; score 320
C. Titer 64; score 67
D. Titer 128; score 67

95. A lectin that, when appropriately diluted, has anti-A$_1$ characteristics is

A. *Bandeiraea simplicifolia*
B. *Ulex europeaus*
C. *Dolichos biflorus*
D. *Arachis hypogea*

96. In performing an antigen phenotype using anti-Fy^a, the best phenotype to use as a positive control is

A. Fy(a−b+)
B. Fy(a+b+)
C. Fy(a−b−)
D. Fy(a+b−)

97. Below are the results of ABO grouping and Rh typing on a patient for whom a type and hold order has been received:

Patient cells +	Anti-A	Anti-B	Anti-D	Patient serum +	A cells	B cells
	0	3+ mf	2+		3+	0

These results are most consistent with

A. the reactions of a subgroup of B
B. the typical mixed-field reaction of an A$_3$ subgroup
C. the weak reaction of an acquired B antigen
D. transfusion of group O cells to a group B patient

98. A 72-year-old woman with a history of ulcerative colitis entered the emergency room with severe abdominal pain and a hemoglobin level of 6 g/dL. The attending physician ordered four units of blood. The results of pretransfusion testing are recorded below:

Patient cells +	Anti-A	Anti-B	Anti-A,B	Anti-D	Rh control
	4+	1+	4+	3+	0

Patient serum +	A cells	B cells	O cells	Autocontrol
	0	4+	0	0

The next step taken to resolve this problem should be to

A. acidify the reagent-B antisera and regroup the patient's cells
B. identify the extra antibody with an antibody panel
C. immediately crossmatch the patient's serum with group-A donor cells
D. perform an autoabsorption using patient cells and serum

99. A 91-year-old male fell and broke a hip, which requires surgery to pin the fracture. Two units of blood were ordered. The patient's pretransfusion testing results are recorded below:

Patient cells +	Anti-A	Anti-B	Anti-A,B	Anti-D	Rh control
	0	0	0	0	0

Patient serum +	A cells	B cells	O cells	Autocontrol
	0	0	0	0

The next step taken to resolve this discrepancy should be to

A. crossmatch the patient's serum with O positive donor cells
B. open a new lot of reagent A and B cells; retest the patient's serum
C. place the reverse grouping tubes and the autocontrol in a 4°C refrigerator for 15 minutes, spin, and read
D. draw a new sample from the patient because two patient specimens must have been mixed up

100. A 44-year-old man needs 3 units of packed red cells for back surgery. The patient's cells fail to react with anti-A and anti-B; his serum reacts with A, B, and O cells. The next logical step to resolve this problem is

A. crossmatch the patient's serum with random donor cells at 37°C
B. identify the antibody(ies) using a panel of group O cells
C. perform an autoabsorption using the patient's own cells
D. titer the serum against the autologous control as well as random donor units. Compare the results and choose the least incompatible units

101. The antibody least likely to show dosage is

A. anti-D
B. anti-M

C. anti-Fy^a
D. anti-Jk^a

102. A request for 3 units of packed red cells is made for a male patient, aged 80 years, who will undergo surgery to repair a broken hip. He is group O, Rh-negative and has a positive antibody screen in the AHG phase of testing. A transfusion history indicates that he received 2 units of whole blood in 1979. The results of the antibody panel are given below:

Cell no.	C	D	E	c	e	K	k	Fy^a	Fy^b	Jk^a	Jk^b	M	N	S	AHG	Check cells
1	+	0	0	+	+	0	+	0	+	+	0	+	+	+	1+	NP
2	+	+	0	0	+	0	+	+	+	+	0	+	0	+	1+	NP
3	+	+	0	0	+	0	+	0	+	0	+	+	+	+	0	2+
4	0	+	+	+	0	+	+	0	+	+	+	+	0	+	1+	NP
5	0	0	+	+	+	0	+	+	+	+	+	+	+	0	1+	NP
6	0	0	0	+	+	+	0	+	0	0	+	0	+	0	0	2+

The antibody in the patient's serum is most likely

A. anti-C
B. anti-D
C. anti-Jk^a
D. anti-Jk^b

103. Which of the following sets of reactions would be most consistent with the presence of anti-I? Testing was carried out at 4°C.

	Patient serum + patient cells	Patient serum + normal adult cells	Patient serum + cord blood cells
A.	4+	4+	0
B.	4+	4+	4+
C.	1+	4+	4+
D.	1+	2+	1+

104. The antibody screen and both crossmatches on a patient serum were positive at the immediate-spin phase of testing. All other phases of testing performed (LISS 37°C and AHG) gave no reactions. A ten-cell panel was tested. Seven of the ten cells reacted with the serum at immediate spin and room temperature but not at AHG. The autocontrol was negative at all phases of testing. The most likely specificity of the antibody is

A: anti-K
B. anti-N
C. anti-I
D. anti-c

105. The antibodies in a patient's serum have been tentatively identified as anti-M and anti-K. To be 95% certain that these two antibodies are both present and that no other antibodies are present, a selected-cell panel should be tested. Which cells from the panel below should be selected for this purpose?

Cell no.	D	C	E	c	e	K	k	M	N	S	s
1	+	+	0	0	+	0	+	0	+	+	+
2	+	+	0	0	+	+	+	0	+	+	0
3	+	0	+	+	0	0	+	+	+	0	+
4	+	0	0	+	+	0	+	+	0	+	+
5	0	0	0	+	+	0	+	+	0	+	+
6	0	0	+	+	+	0	+	+	+	+	0
7	0	0	0	+	+	+	+	0	+	+	+
8	0	0	0	+	+	+	+	0	+	0	+
9	0	0	0	+	+	0	+	+	0	+	0
10	0	0	0	+	+	0	+	0	+	+	+
11	+	0	+	+	+	0	+	0	+	+	+

A. Cells 1, 2, 3, and 6
B. Cells 1, 2, 4, 5, 7, 8, 9, 10, and 11
C. Cells 2, 3, 4, 6, 7, 8, 9, 10, and 11
D. Cells 1, 10, and 11

106. Given the following pattern of reactivity, select the antibodies most likely present in the serum.

Cell no.	D	C	E	c	e	K	k	M	N	S	s	Fy^a	Fy^b	AHG	Check cells
1	+	+	+	+	+	+	0	+	0	+	+	0	+	4+	NP
2	+	+	0	0	+	0	+	+	+	0	+	+	+	0	2+
3	0	0	0	+	+	+	+	0	+	+	0	+	0	1+	NP
4	+	0	+	+	0	0	+	+	+	+	+	0	0	2+	NP
5	+	+	0	+	+	0	+	0	+	0	+	+	+	0	2+
6	0	0	0	+	+	0	+	0	+	+	+	0	+	0	2+

NP = not performed

A. Anti-C and anti-M
B. Anti-E and anti-K
C. Anti-Fy^a and anti-M
D. Anti-C and anti-E

107. The major crossmatch tests patient serum against

A. donor cells
B. patient cells
C. group A_1 and B cells
D. screening cells

108. Upon testing a patient for a presurgical workup, the CLS determines that the patient is group B, Rh-negative and has a negative antibody screen. During surgery the next day, 2 units of packed cells are ordered STAT. The crossmatch with one unit is incompatible at the AHG phase. The CLS crossmatches two more units; they are both compatible. The most likely cause of the incompatibility with one unit is

A. the patient has a positive DAT
B. the patient is Rh-positive and has been mistyped

C. the donor has a positive DAT
D. the donor has an unexpected antibody in the serum

109. Additional units of blood have been ordered on a patient transfused 3 days ago with two units of packed red cells. Pretransfusion testing now demonstrates incompatible crossmatches and a positive antibody screen at the immediate-spin and antiglobulin phases of testing. Polyspecific antiglobulin serum was used in the AHG phase. Anti-I was identified. Which of the following procedures would be most useful in finding compatible units?

A. Select I-negative units for the crossmatch
B. Cold autoabsorption
C. Enzyme pretreatment of donor cells
D. Prewarmed crossmatch

110. A patient is group O, Rh-positive. The patient's serum contains no unexpected antibodies. Which of the following donor units can be expected to be compatible in the crossmatch?

A. A-negative
B. B-negative
C. O-negative
D. AB-positive

111. A patient's sample gives the following reactions on pretransfusion testing:

Patient cells +	Anti-A	Anti-B	Anti-D	Rh-control
	4+	0	0	0

Patient serum +	A_1 cells	B cells	Screen cell I	Screen cell II
	1+	4+	0	0

Which of the following red cell units would be acceptable for transfusion if blood is needed urgently without time for further testing?

A. A-positive
B. A-negative
C. AB-negative
D. O-negative

112. Pretransfusion testing on a patient gives the following reactions:

Patient cells +	Anti-A	Anti-B	Anti-D	Rh-control
	0	0	3+	0

Patient serum +	A cells	B cells	Auto-control
	4+	4+	0

Antibody screen	IS	37°C LISS	AHG	Check cells
cell I	0	1+	2+	NP
cell II	0	0	0	2+

NP = not performed

These results are consistent with

A. acquired B antibody
B. autoantibody
C. rouleaux
D. unexpected alloantibody

113. After examining a patient, the physician ordered a DAT. The nurse used a red-top tube to obtain the specimen, permitted the blood to clot, and centrifuged and refrigerated the tube overnight before sending the specimen to the laboratory for testing the next day. The results of the DAT are given below:

	Polyspecific AHG	Monospecific IgG	Monospecific anti-C3
DAT	1+	0	1+
check cells	NP	2+	NP

NP = not performed

These results indicate

A. in-vivo sensitization with complement
B. in-vitro sensitization with complement
C. in-vivo sensitization with IgG
D. in-vitro sensitization with IgG

114. A DAT on the cells of a patient taking medications for hypertension is found to be 3+ positive. The patient's serum reacted with all panel cells at the AHG phase. The *best* procedure to use to prepare the serum for subsequent testing, assuming the patient has not been recently transfused, is

A. absorption with drug-treated cells
B. autoabsorption using AET-treated cells
C. absorption using selected cells
D. autoabsorption after ZZAP treatment of cells

115. A group O, Rh-negative mother delivers a group A, Rh-negative infant with a negative DAT. The mother's antibody screen and identification demonstrate a weakly reactive anti-D. The CLS should

A. issue Rh-immune globulin for the mother
B. indicate that the mother is not a candidate for Rh-immune globulin
C. investigate the origin of the anti-D
D. repeat the infant's DAT

116. Which of the women below is *not* a candidate for Rh-immune globulin (RhIg), assuming that all of the women have delivered Rh-positive infants?

    A. O, Rh-negative, weak D(D^u)-positive, negative antibody screen
    B. A, Rh-negative, weak D(D^u)-negative, negative antibody screen
    C. A, Rh-negative, weak D(D^u)-negative, positive antibody screen, anti-K identified, antenatal RhIg administered
    D. B, Rh-negative, weak D(D^u)-negative, positive antibody screen, anti-D identified, antenatal RhIg administered

117. Which of the following cases would most likely result in an immediate hemolytic transfusion reaction?

    A. Group O packed cells transfused to a group A patient
    B. Group B packed cells transfused to a group O patient
    C. Group A packed cells transfused to a group AB patient
    D. Group O packed cells transfused to a group B patient

118. Below are the results of preliminary tests done to investigate a possible transfusion reaction:

	DAT	Serum/plasma hemolysis
pretransfusion patient sample	0	absent
posttransfusion patient sample	1+	absent
pretransfusion donor segment	0	absent
posttransfusion blood bag	0	absent

These results are consistent with

    A. febrile transfusion reaction
    B. nonhemolytic transfusion reaction
    C. hemolytic transfusion reaction
    D. absence of a transfusion reaction

119. A physician has requested a unit of blood for exchange transfusion of a 1,000-g acidotic infant with hyperbilirubinemia born to a mother whose CMV antibody status is unknown. Which of the following blood components would be best used to prepare the resuspended whole blood for this transfusion?

    A. Directed donation, CMV-negative, collected 16 days earlier
    B. Irradiated, CMV-negative unit outdating in 28 days
    C. frozen, deglycerolized unit processed 18 h earlier
    D. freshly collected, irradiated, hemoglobin-S–negative unit

120. An intrauterine-exchange transfusion is ordered for the fetus of an A positive mother with a strongly reactive anti-Fy^a. Which of the following red-cell units would be appropriate for the transfusion?

A. A positive, Fy(a−)
B. A negative, Fy(a−)
C. O positive, Fy(a+)
D. O negative, Fy(a−)

121. Which of the following observations suggest bacterial contamination of a unit of RBCs?

A. A yellow color in the segments
B. A green hue to the supernatant fluid, although the cells appear normal
C. A dark purple unit compared to the segments
D. White debris at the supernatant/red-cell interface

122. Seven percent of the inventory of a transfusion service is usually O-negative. 500 units of red cells are used in an average month. If at least four units of O negative are necessary at all times for emergencies, what is the number of O negative units needed per day?

A. 4
B. 5
C. 6
D. 8

123. A unit of red blood cells is returned to the transfusion service unused. The unit has not been entered, was issued at 09:13 and returned at 09:30, has clear plasma, and no segments remain attached. Based on this information, determine whether the unit can be reissued.

A. The unit can be reissued
B. The unit cannot be reissued based on the time out of the laboratory
C. The unit cannot be reissued based on the appearance of the plasma
D. The unit cannot be reissued based on the number of segments attached

124. During issuance of a unit of packed red cells, the floor nurse picking up the blood reads the following information to the CLS who is checking the records for issue:

Thompson, Michael J.   133660
Donor type: B negative

The records being checked by the CLS reveal the following:

Thompson, Michael J.   133666
Patient type: B positive

Can this unit be released?

A. Yes
B. No; the Rh types do not match
C. No; the patient names do not match
D. No; the patient numbers do not match

125. An isolate from a urinary tract infection grows as a porcelain-white, butyrous colony that is nonhemolytic on sheep-blood agar. The isolate is a catalase-positive, gram-positive coccus. Biochemical testing reveals the following reactions:

Tube coagulase:	negative	Mannitol:	acid
Acid from anaerobic glucose:	acid	Trehalose:	acid
Novobiocin sensitivity:	resistant		

This isolate is best identified as

A. *Micrococcus* species
B. *Staphylococcus epidermidis*
C. *Staphylococcus saprophyticus*
D. *Stomatococcus* species

126. A sputum culture yields predominantly alpha-hemolytic, flat colonies on sheep-blood agar that on Gram's stain reveal gram-positive cocci in pairs. Which biochemical tests will aid in the identification of this isolate?

A. Bacitracin and sulfamethoxazole-trimethoprim susceptibility
B. Bile esculin hydrolysis and 6.5% NaCl tolerance
C. Catalase test and CAMP reaction
D. Optochin susceptibility or bile solubility

127. A catalase-negative nonhemolytic gram-positive coccus isolated from a urine specimen from a 42-year-old woman hydrolyzes bile esculin and grows in the presence of 6.5% NaCl. This isolate could be

A. *Streptococcus bovis*
B. *Enterococcus faecalis*
C. *Streptococcus pneumoniae*
D. alpha-hemolytic *Streptococcus viridans* group

128. To establish a definitive diagnosis of diphtheria, which of the following must be confirmed?

A. Biochemical test results
B. Methylene-blue micromorphology
C. Tellurite reduction
D. Toxin production

129. The following results are obtained from a nonlactose-fermenting, gram-negative rod isolated from a urinary tract infection:

Triple sugar iron:	alk/acid	Citrate:	negative
H_2S:	negative	Phenylalanine deaminase:	positive
Indole:	positive	Urease:	positive
Motility:	positive	Ornithine:	positive

The identity of this organism is

A. *Morganella morganii*
B. *Proteus mirabilis*

C. *Providencia alcalifaciens*
D. *Providencia stuartii*

130. A green colony type with black center on Hektoen agar is inoculated to a stool screen using triple sugar iron (TSI) agar, lysine iron agar (LIA), and Christensen's urease. The following reactions develop:

TSI: alkaline/acid and gas, H₂S-positive
LIA: lysine-positive, H₂S-positive
Urease: negative

These results are consistent with a species of

A. *Citrobacter*
B. *Escherichia*
C. *Proteus*
D. *Salmonella*

131. A patient diagnosed as having bacterial vaginosis complains of malodorous vaginal discharge. A direct smear of the vaginal exudate on Gram's stain reveals epithelial cells that are covered with masses of small gram-variable coccobacillary rods suggestive of "clue" cells. This finding is indicative of

A. *Chlamydia trachomatis*
B. *Gardnerella vaginalis*
C. *Neisseria gonorrhoeae*
D. *Lactobacillus* species

132. Laboratory diagnosis of primary atypical pneumonia is established by

A. serological tests
B. culturing the causative agent on sheep-blood agar
C. acid-fast staining of sputum smears
D. the use of tissue culture techniques

133. From a sputum specimen, an acid-fast bacillus grows on Löwenstein-Jensen medium for 18 days at 35°C capneic incubation. Initially, the colonies are buff, raised, and rough when grown in the dark. After exposure to light, no change in pigmentation is detectable. On examination under 10× magnification and on stain, serpentine cording is seen. Which of the following characteristics confirm the identify of the most likely etiologic agent?

A. Niacin-positive, nitrate-positive
B. Niacin-negative, nitrate-positive
C. Niacin-positive, nitrate-negative
D. Niacin-negative, nitrate-negative

134. A gram-negative rod is inoculated into nitrate broth and incubated for 24 h. After equal amounts of alpha-naphthylamine and sulfanilic acid are added, no color develops. Zinc dust is added and still no color develops. What action should you take?

A. Make up new reagents and check with quality-control stains
B. Repeat the nitrate test after 48 h of incubation
C. Interpret the results as negative
D. Interpret the results as positive

135. Sodium polyanetholsulfonate is added to blood culture media to

A. prevent clotting
B. activate complement activity
C. enhance phagocytosis
D. enhance the growth of fastidious pathogens

136. Which of the following bacterial species is unacceptable for performing quality-control testing of anaerobic jars or glove boxes?

A. *Prevotella melaninogenicus*
B. *Clostridium novyi*
C. *Clostridium tertium*
D. *Peptostreptococcus anaerobius*

137. *Blastomyces dermatitidis* can be differentiated from the saprobic species of *Chrysosporium* and *Pseudoallescheria* by

A. rapid growth of the colony
B. single conidia produced directly from hyphae or conidiophores
C. ability to convert to a yeast phase at 35°C–37°C
D. inability to grow on media containing cycloheximide and chloramphenicol

138. Persistent athlete's foot plagues a local baseball team in training season. A study is undertaken to identify the organism from each team member with typical signs of the fungal disease. The organism grows out in 12 days on Sabouraud's dextrose agar and Sabouraud's with chloramphenicol and cycloheximide as a snowy-white, velvety colony with a yellow reverse. Rare long, narrow, smooth-walled macroconidia are seen on microscopic preparation. Thin, clavate, teardrop-shaped microconidia are borne laterally. Based on these data, a likely etiologic agent is

A. *Microsporum audouinii*
B. *Microsporum canis*
C. *Trichophyton mentagrophytes*
D. *Trichophyton rubrum*

139. The purpose of the iodine solution used in the direct-preparation technique for screening stool specimens is to

A. enhance morphologic detail of organisms
B. check for motility of trophozoites
C. precipitate fecal material
D. stain debris and background material

140. An important cause of pneumonia in patients with acquired and congenital immunologic disorders is the organism that in a lung impression smear stained with a monoclonal antibody flourescent stain reveals clusters of cysts in a "honeycomb" appearance. The identity of this organism is

A. *Toxoplasma gondii*
B. *Pneumocystis carinii*
C. *Babesia*
D. *Sarcocystis*

141. *Babesia* may infect humans and multiply in red cells; however, it can be differentiated from malarial agents because *Babesia*

A. has crescent-shaped gametocytes
B. forms hemozoin pigment in red cells
C. also occurs in leukocytes
D. develops ring forms and maltese cross forms

142. A patient with a mild pneumonia that is suggestive of ornithosis would be infected with

A. *Chlamydia psittaci*
B. *Chlamydia trachomatis*
C. *Mycoplasma pneumoniae*
D. Rhinovirus

143. Cell-culture media have antimicrobials as ingredients to

A. enhance cell penetration
B. sterilize the medium
C. increase the cytopathic effect
D. reduce bacterial contamination

144. To develop a minimum inhibitory concentration (MIC) procedure by macro-broth-tube dilution you need to determine the required concentration of antimicrobial for preparation of working-stock solution. The highest concentration of antimicrobial to be tested will be 128 µg/mL. Two milliliters of stock are transferred directly to the first tube, and twofold serial dilutions are prepared in subsequent tubes. One milliliter of standardized inoculum is added to each tube. Based on these parameters, the concentration of antimicrobial in the working stock solution must be

A. 256 µg/mL
B. 512 µg/mL
C. 1,024 µg/mL
D. 2,048 µg/mL

145. The following results are obtained from a gram-positive coccus isolated from a patient with urinary tract infection:

catalase: negative   Resistant to vancomycin
PYR hydrolysis: negative   Leucine aminopeptidase: negative
Bile esculin: negative   Growth in 6.5% NaCl: negative

This isolate is best identified as

A. *Enterococcus faecium*
B. *Aerococcus*
C. *Pediococcus*
D. *Leuconostoc*

146. A direct wet smear of stool demonstrated bile-stained, mammillated, thick-shelled eggs in 1-cell stage. The presence of these eggs would indicate a(n) infection with

A. *Enterobius vermicularis*
B. *Ascaris lumbricoides*
C. *Necator americanus*
D. *Strongyloides stercoralis*

147. The following results are obtained from a slender, gram-negative rod isolated from an intra-abdominal abscess:

no growth in the presence of 1-mg kanamycin disk
growth in the presence of 5-mg vancomycin disk
no growth in the presence of 10-mg colistin disk
indole: positive
lipase: negative

The identity of this organism is

A. *Bacteroides fragilis*
B. *Bacteroides gracilis*
C. *Fusobacterium nucleatum*
D. *Fusobacterium necrophorum*

148. Organisms that grow best with greater carbon-dioxide concentrations than are found in ambient air are called

A. microaerobic
B. capnophilic
C. humidophilic
D. anaerobic

149. Specimens for viral isolation

A. should be incubated at 37°C for 2 h prior to inoculation
B. should be placed on ice and transported at once to the laboratory
C. should be frozen and transported at once to the laboratory
D. should be incubated at room temperature for 2 h prior to inoculation

150. Mycobacteria that are pigmented in the dark are termed

A. nonphotopigmented
B. nonphotochromogens
C. scotochromogens
D. photochromogens

151. The standard inoculum of bacteria to be used in antimicrobial-susceptibility testing (disk method) can be determined by the use of a

A. 0.5 McFarland standard
B. 1.0 McFarland standard
C. 1.5 McFarland standard
D. 2.0 McFarland standard

152. Which of the following primary-media combinations is appropriate for initial subculture of blood cultures?

A. Sheep-blood agar, MacConkey agar, Hektoen enteric agar
B. Sheep-blood agar, MacConkey agar, thioglycolate broth, chocolate agar
C. Sheep-blood agar, MacConkey agar, chocolate agar
D. Sheep-blood agar, MacConkey agar, chocolate agar, CDC-anaerobic blood agar

153. The ability of an organism to degrade the amino acid tryptophan as a result of the enzyme tryptophanase can be measured by

A. the citrate-utilization test
B. the phenylalanine-deaminase test
C. the Voges-Proskauer test
D. the indole test

154. *Bacteroides* species can be selected by using which of the following media?

A. CDC sheep-blood agar
B. Kanamycin-vancomycin laked-blood agar
C. Phenylethyl-alcohol, sheep-blood agar
D. Thioglycolate medium

155. A stool specimen from a five-year-old patient with bloody diarrhea is received by the laboratory. Which of the following media would be used to detect *Escherichia coli* 0157:H7?

A. MacConkey-sorbitol agar
B. Phenylethyl-alcohol agar
C. Xylose-lysine desoxycholate agar
D. Brilliant-green agar

156. Microscopic examination of a stool specimen for ova and parasites revealed spherical, thick-shelled eggs (31 × 43 μg) with prominent radial striations. The eggs possessed three pairs of hooklets within the embryonated oncosphere. The identity of this parasite is most likely

A. *Taenia saginata*
B. *Hymenolepis diminuta*
C. *Hymenolepis nana*
D. *Diphyllobothrium latum*

157. Lyme disease is caused by the bite of a tick infected with

A. *Borrelia vincentii*
B. *Borrelia recurrentis*
C. *Borrelia burgdorferi*
D. *Borrelia hermsii*

158. *Cryptosporidum* and *Isospora* species are difficult to detect without special staining. Which of the following stains may be used to demonstrate these organisms?

A. Trichrome stain
B. Chlorazol-black E stain
C. Iron-hematoxylin stain
D. Modified Kinyoun's acid-fast stain

159. The specimen of choice for darkfield examination to detect *Treponema pallidum* is

A. blood
B. urine
C. spinal fluid
D. fluid from a chancre

160. All members of the Enterobacteriaceae are

A. oxidase-negative
B. mannitol-positive
C. citrate-positive
D. sucrose-negative

161. An isolate from an animal bite gave the following results:

gram-negative coccobacillus   Catalase: positive
growth on blood agar   indole: positive
oxidase: positive   penicillin disk: susceptible

This isolate is best identified as

A. *Kingella kingae*
B. *Pasteurella multocida*
C. *Eikenella corrodens*
D. *Actinobacillus actinomycetemcomitans*

162. The following are reported on a given work day:

1. Observation of AFB organisms on a direct smear of a sputum
2. Identification of *Neisseria gonorrhoeae* from a genital specimen of a female outpatient

3. Positive findings of *Entamoeba histolytica* trophozoites and cyst forms
4. Oxacillin resistance noted in a *Staphylococcus aureus* isolate from an inpatient

What additional steps, if any, are required?

A. No. 1 requires follow-up of AFB cultures before reporting
B. No. 4 requires repeat testing to confirm this unusual susceptibility pattern
C. All reports require communication with epidemiology or infection-control personnel
D. No. 3 requires serologic testing for invasive strains to confirm diagnosis of amoebiasis

163. The following are concentrations and ring diameters for an IgA radial immuno-diffusion (RID) plate:

Standard 1   420 mg/dL   8.8 mm
Standard 2   220 mg/dL   7.9 mm
Standard 3   50 mg/dL   5.4 mm
Standard 4   22 mg/dL   3.8 mm
Unknown   —   2.2 mm

What is the appropriate action?

A. Dialyze the serum to concentrate it, then reassay
B. Extend the standard curve through the origin and read the results for 2.2 mm
C. Perform the assay on a low-level IgA plate
D. Repeat the assay, applying the unknown sample to the RID plate twice

164. Immunoelectrophoresis was performed using serum from a 62-year-old female. When her serum reacted with anti-total immunoglobulin antiserum, broad, elliptical arcs were seen corresponding to IgA and IgG controls, and a sharply peaked, very dense arc was seen corresponding to the IgM control. These results are consistent with

A. IgG and IgA gammopathy
B. free-light chains in the serum
C. an IgD reacting in concert with IgM
D. a monoclonal IgM in the patient's serum

165. An immunofixation electrophoresis yielded a dense, dark-staining band when patient serum reacted with IgM antiserum. A band with the same electrophoretic mobility and similar density was seen when patient serum reacted with kappa antiserum. These results indicate

A. an IgM-kappa monoclonal protein
B. contamination of the kappa antiserum
C. increased polyclonal IgM-kappa
D. normal levels of IgM-kappa

166. What is the correct order for performing a Western-blot assay for HIV?

   A. Electrophorese the HIV lysate on polyacrilamide gel; transfer to nitrocellulose strips; apply unknown serum; add enzyme conjugate; add substrate
   B. Electrophorese the unknown serum on polyacrilamide gel; transfer to nitrocellulose strips; apply HIV lysate; add enzyme conjugate; add substrate
   C. Electrophorese the HIV lysate on nitrocellulose gel; transfer to polyacrilamide gel; apply unknown serum; add substrate; add enzyme conjugate
   D. Electrophorese the unknown serum on nitrocellulose gel; transfer to polyacrilamide gel; apply HIV lysate; add substrate; add enzyme conjugate

167. A 45-year-old inmate in a correctional facility has a nonreactive RPR and a positive FTA-ABS. He has no signs or symptoms of syphilis. What is the most likely explanation for these results?

   A. The inmate currently has syphilis
   B. The inmate has had syphilis in the past but is not currently infected
   C. The FTA result is inaccurate; it should be negative if the RPR is non-reactive
   D. The RPR is inaccurate; it must be reactive if the FTA is positive

168. A RPR-card test yielded the following results:

	1:1	1:2	1:4	1:8	1:16
patient	R	R	R	Rm	NR

The patient's result should be reported as

   A. reactive, 1 : 4 dilution
   B. reactive, 1 : 8 dilution
   C. reactive, 1 : 16 dilution
   D. nonreactive

169. A ten-year-old male is seen by his pediatrician for a sore throat. A streptozyme screen is positive and the ASO titer is less than 60 Todd units. What is the next step?

   A. No further testing is necessary. The child does not have a group-A streptococcal infection
   B. Perform an anti-DNase B assay
   C. Perform an ELISA for ASO
   D. Repeat the ASO neutralization test. It should be positive if the streptozyme test is positive

170. When performing a slide agglutination test for C-reactive protein (CRP), the CLS notices that the undiluted sample shows no agglutination, but the 1 : 5 dilution shows agglutination. How should these results be interpreted?

A. The patient's serum contains a high level of anti-CRP
B. The patient's serum contains no CRP
C. The reaction exhibits a postzone effect
D. The sample was incorrectly diluted

171. In the indirect-immunofluorescence test to detect antibody to nuclear antigens on the HEp2 substrate, the patient's titer was 160 and the pattern was speckled. What should be done next?

A. Confirm the presence of the ANA using mouse liver or kidney
B. Perform a double-diffusion assay to determine if the Sm antibody is present
C. Perform the *Crithidea luciliae* assay
D. Perform a passive hemagglutination assay to determine if SS-DNA is present

172. Which assay is an example of direct immunofluorescence?

A. Detecting immunoglobulin in serum using fluorochrome-labeled anti-human globulin
B. Detecting immunoglobulin in a skin biopsy using horseradish peroxidase–labeled anti-human globulin
C. Detecting C3 in the glomerular basement membrane using a fluorochrome-labeled anti-human C3
D. Detecting syphilis-specific IgG in the absorbed fluorescent treponemal assay

173. The following results were obtained on a slide agglutination test for the detection of rheumatoid factor:

Undiluted Patient's serum + IgG-sensitized sheep RBCs = Agglutination
Patient's serum diluted 1 : 10 + IgG-sensitized sheep RBCs = Agglutination
Positive Control + IgG-sensitized sheep RBCs = Agglutination
Negative Control + IgG-sensitized sheep RBCs = No Agglutination

These results should be intrepreted as

A. normal
B. negative
C. positive
D. false positive

174. A ligand assay to detect HBs antigen (HBsAg) is performed by incubating the patient serum and alkaline phosphatase-labeled HBs antigen with a paddle coated with monoclonal antibody directed against the antigen. After washing, the paddle is incubated with p-nitrophenol phosphate; the absorbance is read at 405 nm. Which statement is correct?

A. The absorbance will be directly related to the concentration of HBsAg in patient serum and bound-enzyme activity
B. This is a homogeneous, competitive assay

C. The greater the concentration of HBsAg in the patient serum, the lower the measurable enzyme activity
D. This is a heterogeneous, sandwich-type (noncompetitive) assay

175. In a competitive-radioimmunoassay (RIA) procedure to detect thyroxine, the ratio of counts per minute (CPM) of the bound fraction is compared to the total count. The total count in a competitive RIA procedure is the CPM when

A. no tracer is added
B. no unlabeled ligand is present
C. maximum binding by the unlabeled ligand occurs
D. minimum binding by the unlabeled ligand occurs

176. While performing the classic anti-streptolysin–O neutralization test, the laboratorian noticed that the cell control showed hemolysis, the streptolysin-O reagent control showed hemolysis, the negative serum control showed hemolysis in all tubes, the positive serum control showed hemolysis at all dilutions, and the patient serum showed hemolysis at all dilutions. What is the best explanation for these results?

A. The complement reagent is too concentrated
B. Distilled water was used as the diluent
C. The incorrect concentration of cells was used
D. The streptolysin-O reagent was incorrectly reconstituted

177. In the hemagglutination-inhibition assay to measure rubella antibody, no agglutination was observed in any dilution from $1:8$ through $1:512$. Assuming that the serum was treated to remove nonspecific inhibitors and natural agglutinins and that the controls were acceptable, this result indicates

A. an absence of rubella antibody in the test serum
B. a high titer of rubella antibody in the test serum
C. the patient is currently infected with rubella
D. the patient is susceptible to rubella infection

178. Interpret these infectious-mononucleosis test results from a patient complaining of fever and joint pain.

Heterophile presumptive test $1:148$
Davidsohn differential test
   Guinea-pig kidney absorption $1:14$
   Beef erythrocyte absorption $1:14$

A. The patient has infectious mononucleosis
B. The patient has Forssman antibodies from a Salmonella infection
C. The patient has serum sickness
D. Rheumatoid factor is causing a false-positive reaction in the heterophile presumptive test

179. A red-top tube for a cold-agglutinin assay was drawn on a patient during the evening shift. The CLS found the requisition and the tube of unsepa-

rated blood in the refrigerator the next morning. What should be done next?

A. Spin down the tube and assay the serum
B. Place the tube at 37°C for an hour before spinning down the tube and removing the serum to assay
C. Perform an elution on the red cells from the sample and run the assay on the eluate
D. Spin down the tube and heat-inactivate the serum before running the assay

180. A hemagglutination test for rheumatoid factor yields the following results:

	1:20	1:40	1:80	1:160	1:320
patient	agg	agg	agg	agg	no agg

agg = agglutination; no agg = no agglutination

This finding is

A. not suggestive of rheumatoid arthritis
B. suggestive of rheumatoid arthritis
C. inconclusive; paired sera should be tested
D. indicative of rheumatic fever

181. In flow-cytometric analysis, forward-angle light scatter (FALS) indicates cell

A. concentration
B. granularity
C. size
D. surface markers

182. 0.1 mL of serum is added to a test tube containing 0.4 mL of saline. If 0.2 mL of this mixture were transferred to a test tube containing 0.2 mL of saline, the final dilution would be

A. 1:2
B. 1:5
C. 1:10
D. 1:20

183. According to organizational theorists, the functions of management include all of the following *except*

A. planning
B. motivating
C. organizing
D. purchasing

184. Which of the following guarantees hospital employees the right to engage in collective bargaining?

A. Wagner Act
B. Clinical Laboratory Improvement Act (CLIA)
C. National Labor Relations Act
D. Taft-Hartley Act

185. Needles should be recapped

A. before disposal
B. never
C. never, because they must be cut before disposal
D. never, unless a special recapping device is used

186. Darkfield microscopy is accomplished by

A. decreasing the intensity of the light source
B. lowering the condenser
C. closing the aperture on the condenser
D. using a light ring in the condenser to supply oblique light

187. The government licensing agency for use of radionuclides is

A. OSHA
B. NRC
C. HCFA
D. NCCLS

188. Which of the following is used to measure the rpm of a centrifuge?

A. Ohmmeter
B. Rheostat
C. Voltmeter
D. Tachometer

189. In the clinical laboratory, the patient specimen labeled with a bar code improves the efficiency and accuracy of all of the following *except*

A. specimen tracking
B. patient identification
C. inventory control
D. result reporting

190. By attending an approved continuing-education program of one-hour in length, an individual can receive credit for

A. 10.0 CEUs (continuing education units)
B. 1.0 CEUs
C. 0.5 CEUs
D. 0.01 CEUs

191. The percentage of normally distributed population that is expected to fall *outside* of 2 SDs is

A. 2.5%
B. 5%
C. 15%
D. 95%

192. The danger of explosion from highly flammable solvents may be reduced by all of the following *except*

   A. disposal of flammable solvents in the sewer with large quantities of water
   B. using a fume hood
   C. storing at temperatures below their flashpoint
   D. maintaining small quantities outside of a flammable storage cabinet

193. Calculate the concentration in millequivalents (mEq) for a solution containing 58.5 mg/dL of NaCl. (Atomic weights: Na = 23; Cl = 35.5)

   A. 1.0 mEq/L
   B. 5.0 mEq/L
   C. 10.0 mEq/L
   D. 20.0 mEq/L

194. Additional tests have been requested on a patient. The phlebotomist has collected only a purple-top EDTA tube. Which of the following tests can be performed on this tube without interference from the anticoagulant?

   A. Calcium
   B. Alkaline phosphatase
   C. Creatinine
   D. Creatine kinase

195. A continuing-education format using group interaction facilitates the learning experience by

   A. presenting authoritative viewpoints
   B. inviting a wide range of informed opinion
   C. presenting information in an organized way
   D. developing teamwork and sharing experiences

196. A serial dilution is set up by pipetting 0.1-mL serum into 0.9-mL saline in tube 1, and serially transferring 0.5 mL through tubes 2, 3, 4, and 5, each of which contains 0.5-mL saline. What is the dilution in tube number 5?

   A. 1 : 16
   B. 1 : 80
   C. 1 : 128
   D. 1 : 160

197. When shipping specimens to a referral laboratory the most important variable to control during transport is

A. temperature
B. light
C. air pressure
D. vibration

198. When using anhydrous calcium sulfate (Drierite) as a dessicant, cobalt chloride is added

A. as an indicator of the water-absorption capacity of the dessicant
B. to increase the water-absorption capacity of the calcium sulfate
C. as an inert salt to increase the volume of the total dessicant package
D. to reduce dust formed by the calcium sulfate and increase length of use

199. The site of collection for a blood-culture specimen should be disinfected by applying

A. 70% alcohol and waiting until the area is dry before puncture
B. 2% povidone-iodine and waiting until the area is dry before puncture
C. surgical soap liberally and waiting 5 min before puncture
D. 2% povidone-iodine, waiting 2 min, and following with a 70% alcohol wipe

200. A measurement, taken at an angle to the incident beam, of the amount of light scattered or reflected by small particles in a sample cuvette is the principle of

A. fluorometry
B. nephelometry
C. turbidimetry
D. mass spectrophotometry

Key to the CLS Review Test

1. A	19. C	37. B	55. C
2. C	20. D	38. B	56. D
3. D	21. A	39. D	57. B
4. A	22. B	40. A	58. C
5. B	23. A	41. C	59. A
6. B	24. A	42. B	60. B
7. D	25. B	43. C	61. C
8. C	26. D	44. A	62. B
9. B	27. B	45. D	63. D
10. C	28. C	46. C	64. A
11. C	29. C	47. D	65. C
12. A	30. A	48. B	66. D
13. B	31. C	49. C	67. C
14. C	32. B	50. C	68. B
15. C	33. B	51. A	69. C
16. B	34. B	52. C	70. B
17. A	35. A	53. C	71. D
18. B	36. B	54. A	72. A

73. B	105. B	137. C	169. B
74. C	106. B	138. D	170. C
75. A	107. A	139. A	171. B
76. A	108. C	140. B	172. C
77. B	109. D	141. D	173. C
78. C	110. C	142. A	174. C
79. C	111. D	143. D	175. B
80. B	112. D	144. A	176. B
81. B	113. B	145. D	177. B
82. A	114. D	146. B	178. C
83. D	115. C	147. C	179. B
84. C	116. A	148. B	180. B
85. D	117. B	149. B	181. C
86. A	118. C	150. C	182. C
87. C	119. D	151. A	183. D
88. D	120. D	152. D	184. C
89. A	121. C	153. D	185. D
90. A	122. A	154. B	186. D
91. A	123. D	155. A	187. B
92. B	124. D	156. A	188. D
93. C	125. C	157. C	189. B
94. C	126. D	158. D	190. B
95. C	127. B	159. D	191. B
96. B	128. D	160. A	192. A
97. D	129. A	161. B	193. C
98. A	130. D	162. C	194. C
99. C	131. B	163. C	195. D
100. B	132. A	164. D	196. D
101. A	133. A	165. A	197. A
102. C	134. D	166. A	198. A
103. A	135. A	167. B	199. B
104. B	136. C	168. B	200. B